+ early
- erasure p 13
- spelling error p 127

34/35

Medications and Mathematics for the Nurse

Medications and Mathematics for the Nurse

ESTHER G. SKELLEY, RN, MA

Catherine H. White, RN, MS — Consultant
Angela R. Emmi, BSNEd, MS — Series Editor

DELMAR PUBLISHERS
COPYRIGHT ©1976
BY LITTON EDUCATIONAL PUBLISHING, INC.

All rights reserved. Certain portions of this work copyright ©1959, 1967, and 1971 by Delmar Publishers, Inc. No part of this work covered by the copyright hereon may be reproduced or used in any form or by any means — graphic, electronic, or mechanical, including photocopying, recording, taping, or information storage and retrieval systems — without written permission of the publisher.

LIBRARY OF CONGRESS CATALOG CARD NUMBER: 76-5302

Printed in the United States of America
Published Simultaneously in Canada by
Delmar Publishers, A Division of
Van Nostrand Reinhold, Ltd.

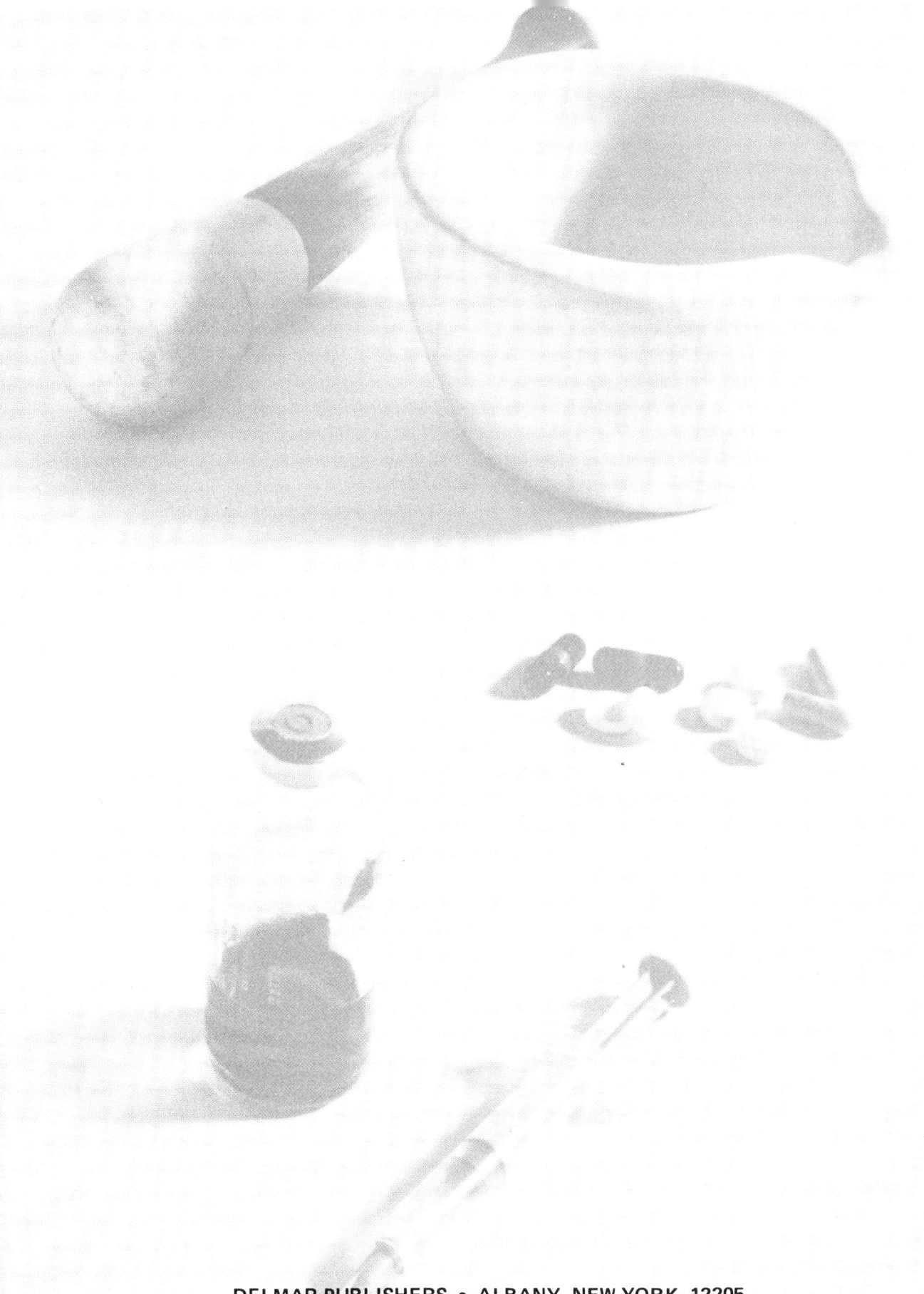

DELMAR PUBLISHERS • ALBANY, NEW YORK 12205
A DIVISION OF LITTON EDUCATIONAL PUBLISHING, INC.

Preface

This edition of *Medications and Mathematics for the Nurse* has been reorganized and its contents expanded to provide the student with a review of basic mathematics and updated drug information. More emphasis is placed on the role of the nurse and the specific effects of the drugs which are being administered. Additional photographs have been added to illustrate the techniques in the administration of medications by oral, inhalation or parenteral means. The unit on intramuscular injections includes several new descriptive illustrations. Also, more coverage has been given to disposable equipment, how to handle it and how to destroy it properly. Conversion to the metric system is shown and metric symbols predominate in the manner of presentation; in cases where both systems are in use, the metric reference is given first.

Medications and Mathematics for the Nurse is divided into five sections. Each section is made up of several units; these units contain stated objectives which are tested by end review questions. In addition, the Section has an achievement test which evaluates the student's understanding of the information covered in all of the units.

The first two sections deal with basic mathematics and the calculations of dosages. Practice problems are interspersed throughout the units; the answers to these problems are in the back of the book for the student's self-evaluation. The remaining sections deal with the administration of drugs and related substances. Emphasis is placed upon the nurse's responsibilities and upon safety precautions in pouring, giving, and charting the medications. Updated material includes the discussion of psychotropic drugs and radioactive substances along with information about the sources of drugs, standards, dosages, and how drugs act when given for various body disorders.

Educational aids have been added to the Appendix. They include: an expanded glossary of terms; Look-alike and Sound-alike drugs; Possible Pharmacological Drug Reactions; Metric dosages and Apothecary equivalents; and a Temperature Conversion chart.

The instructor's guide provides a bibliography and answers to the practice problems, unit review questions and the self-achievement tests.

Other Delmar texts in the nursing series are:

Emotional Adjustment to Illness

How to Calculate Drug Dosages

Giving Medications Correctly and Safely

Body Structures and Functions

Contents

SECTION 1 REVIEW OF BASIC MATHEMATICS

Unit 1 Introduction to Systems of Measurement   1
Unit 2 Numerals and Fractions   5
Unit 3 Decimal Fractions and Percents 12
Unit 4 Ratio and Proportion 19
Unit 5 Temperature Conversion 22
Achievement Review 1 25

SECTION 2 CALCULATIONS OF DOSES AND SOLUTIONS

Unit 6 Symbols and Measurement 28
Unit 7 Methods of Calculating Dosages 35
Unit 8 Problems in Solutions 41
Unit 9 Calculating Children's Dosages 45
Achievement Review 2 48

SECTION 3 ADMINISTRATION OF MEDICATIONS

Unit 10 Drug Sources, Standards, and Dosages 53
Unit 11 Responsibilities in the Administration of Medications 62
Unit 12 Forms of Drugs and How They Act 70
Unit 13 The Medication Order 77
Unit 14 Basic Procedures in Administering Medications 83
Unit 15 Administration of Oral Medications 89
Unit 16 Types of Syringes and Needles 97
Unit 17 Administration of Medications by Injection 105
Unit 18 Administration of Drugs by Inhalation and Local
         Application 119
Unit 19 Administration of Radioactive Substances 128
Achievement Review 3 132

SECTION 4 DRUGS AND RELATED SUBSTANCES

Unit 20 Drugs Used to Counteract Infections 137
Unit 21 Drugs Used in Malignant Diseases 149
Unit 22 Antihistamines and Motion Sickness Drugs 154
Unit 23 Vitamins and Minerals 159
Unit 24 Serums, Vaccines, and Toxoids 167

v

Contents

Unit 25 Psychotropic Drugs 171
Achievement Review 4 177

SECTION 5 EFFECTS OF MEDICATIONS ON BODY SYSTEMS

Unit 26 Medications Used for Circulatory System Disorders 181
Unit 27 Medications that Affect the Respiratory System 191
Unit 28 Medications Used for Gastrointestinal System Disorders..... 197
Unit 29 Medications Used for Urinary System Disorders 210
Unit 30 Medications Used in Treatment of Endocrine Conditions 218
Unit 31 Medications Used for Musculoskeletal System Disorders..... 228
Unit 32 Medications that Affect the Nervous System............... 234
Unit 33 Medications that Affect the Reproductive System 254
Achievement Review 5 261

APPENDIX
   Glossary 266
   Look-Alike and Sound-Alike Drugs.......................... 269
   Possible Pharmacological Drug Interactions................... 270
   Metric Doses and Apothecary Equivalents..................... 271
   Temperature Conversion Chart 272

Answers to Practice Problems 274
Acknowledgments... 277
Index... 278

The author and editorial staff at Delmar Publishers are interested in continually improving the quality of this instructional material. The reader is invited to submit constructive criticism and questions. Responses will be reviewed jointly by the author and source editor. Send comments to:

Director of Publications
Delmar Publishers
50 Wolf Road
Albany, New York 12205

A current catalog including prices of all Delmar educational publications is available upon request. Please write to:

Catalog Department
Delmar Publishers
50 Wolf Road
Albany, New York 12205

Or call Toll Free: (800) 354-9815

Section 1 Review of Basic Mathematics

Unit 1 Introduction to Systems of Measurement

OBJECTIVES

After studying this unit, the student should be able to:

- Explain why nurses should have knowledge of drug dosages and calculations.
- Determine areas in which improvement in basic arithmetic is needed.
- Name three systems of measurements.
- Identify terms used in each system.

Every nurse should have a sound basic knowledge of the systems used to weigh and measure drugs. This is true even though many hospitals have prepackaged unit dose medications. Such medications are packaged and labelled in prescribed dosages so that they are ready to be administered to the patient for whom they have been ordered. However, some hospitals have not adopted the unit dose plan and there will be situations where a dose must be prepared by the nurse from stock material on hand. Also, awareness of drug dosages alerts the nurse to the possibility of errors. Knowledge of calculation methods strengthens drug information about normal dosages and provides the nurse with security regarding the administration of medications.

Arithmetic is a branch of mathematics that deals with real numbers. In order to learn individual weaknesses in arithmetic, the following pretest is recommended. Those areas which need improvement may be strengthened through study of the remaining units in this section.

ARITHMETIC PRETEST

1. Write as Roman numerals.
   a. 15 XV
   b. 19 XIX
   c. 40 XL
   d. 60 LX
   e. 95 XCV
   f. 98 XCVIII
   g. 110 CX
   h. 124 CXXIV

Section 1 Review of Basic Mathematics

2. Write as Arabic numerals.
   a. XXIV __24__
   b. XLI __41__
   c. IX __9__
   d. XXVI __26__
   e. XCVII __97__
   f. IV __4__
   g. XIV __14__
   h. XIX __19__

3. Write in words.
   a. 1,005,221 __ONE MILLION FIVE THOUSAND TWO HUND. TWENTY ONE__
   b. 125,936 __ONE HUND. TWENTY FIVE THOUSAND NINE HUND. THIRTY SIX__
   c. 48,224 __FOURTY EIGHT THOUS. TWO HUNDRED TWENTY FOUR__
   d. 2,001.5 __TWO THOUSAND ONE AND FIVE TENTHS__
   e. 1,200,000 __ONE MILLION TWO HUNDRED__

4. Change to whole numbers or to mixed numbers.
   a. $\frac{24}{12}$ = __2__
   b. $\frac{9}{4}$ = __2 1/4__
   c. $\frac{100}{25}$ = __24__
   d. $\frac{16}{3}$ = __1 5/3__
   e. $\frac{500}{25}$ = __20__
   f. $\frac{67}{15}$ = __4 7/15__

5. Round off the following numbers to the next largest number.
   a. 498 to the nearest hundred __500__
   b. 2,597,500 to the nearest thousand __2,598__
   c. 1,997,855 to the nearest million __2,000,000__

6. Add the following decimals.
   a. .05, .010, .156 = __.216__
   b. 1.005, 20.1, 400.5 = __421.605__
   c. .004, 42.015, 1004.05 = __1046.069__

7. Add the following fractions.
   a. 1/5, 1/2, 1/4 = __19/20__
   b. 1/6, 3/8, 3/4 = __31/24__
   c. 2 3/4, 4 1/8, 5 1/2 = __11 11/8__

8. Subtract the following fractions and mixed numbers.
   a. 2/3 − 1/2 = __1/6__
   b. 4/5 − 1/3 = __7/15__
   c. 4 1/2 − 2 1/3 = __2 1/6__
   d. 10 1/4 − 6 3/8 = __3 7/8__

2

Unit 1 Introduction to Systems of Measurement

9. Subtract the following.
   a. 2 (5 + 3) − 4 (2 + 1) = __4__
   b. 4 (3 − 2) − 3 (4 − 3) = __1__
   c. 4 (3 − 1) − 2 (3 − 2) = __6__
   d. 5 (5 + 5) − 3 (5 + 3) = __26__

10. Subtract the following decimals.
    a. 12.05 − 10.50 = __1.55__
    b. 9.00 − 5.50 = __3.50__
    c. 125.50 − 100.60 = __24.90__
    d. 95.05 − 5.25 = __89.80__

11. Multiply the following.
    a. 525 x .51 = __267.75__
    b. 550.10 x .05 = __27.5050__
    c. 594.99 x .99 = __589.0401__
    d. 841.08 x .08 = __67.2864__

12. Divide the following.
    a. 3/5 ÷ 3/10 = __2__
    b. 4/8 ÷ 1/16 = __8__
    c. 14.25 ÷ 3.5 = __4.071__
    d. 150.25 ÷ .25 = __601__

13. Which is larger?
    a. 5/6 or 5/8 __5/6__
    b. 3/4 or 1/3 __3/4__
    c. .75 or .749 __.75__
    d. .25 or .255 __.255__

14. Write as decimals.
    a. Forty-five and five tenths __45.5__
    b. Thirty-five and three hundredths __35.03__
    c. Two and five ten thousandths __2.0005__
    d. One hundred sixty and three thousandths __160.003__

15. Change the following fractions to decimals.
    a. 7/10 = __.7__
    b. 5 1/4 = __5.25__
    c. 2 1/2 = __2.5__
    d. 1/4 = __.25__

16. Change the following to percents.
    a. 1/2 __50%__
    b. .007 __.7%__
    c. 3/4 __75%__
    d. .05 __5%__
    e. 1/4 __25%__
    f. .50 __50%__

17. What is
    a. 5% of 75 __3.75__
    b. .5% of 500 __2.5__
    c. 6% of 400 __24__
    d. .7% of 750 __5.25__
    e. 10% of 500 __50__
    f. 25% of 500 __125__

18. Write in Arabic numerals.
    a. Four thousand two hundred and eighty __4,208__
    b. Six hundred thousand __600,000__
    c. Six million __6,000,000__
    d. Forty thousand two hundred and eight __40,208__
    e. Two hundred thousand and twenty __200,020__
    f. Five hundred three and five tenths __503.5__

Section 1 Review of Basic Mathematics

SYSTEMS OF MEASUREMENT

In nursing, three systems of measurement are used: the metric system, the apothecaries' system and the familiar household measurement system. The metric system is used extensively outside of the United States and is increasing in use within this country. It is an international language of measurement and its symbols are identical in all languages. However, until the time arrives that the metric system has replaced the others, the nurse must know the three systems and learn to convert one system to another.

Terms used in the metric system are: meters, grams, and liters. Prefixes are added to form such measurements as centimeters, millimeters, micrograms, milligram, kilogram, and milliliters.

Terms used in the apothecaries' system are: quart, pint, ounce, dram, minim and grain. Terms used in the household system are measuring cup, tablespoon, teaspoon and drop; the nurse would be most likely to use these measures when providing health care to patients in the home and when measuring intake and output.

As prescriptions and medical orders are often written in Roman numerals and fractions, a short review will follow in the next unit.

Unit 2 Numerals and Fractions

OBJECTIVES

After studying this unit, the student should be able to:

- Change Arabic numerals to Roman numerals.
- Change Roman numerals to Arabic numerals.
- Identify the different kinds of common fractions.
- Solve problems using common fractions.
- Distinguish between relative values of common fractions.

ARABIC AND ROMAN NUMERALS

The earliest systems of numbers came from the Arabians, Egyptians and Babylonians. Toward the end of the sixteenth century, there emerged two systems, the Arabic and the Roman. Prescriptions and medical orders are often written with Roman numerals so it is essential that the nurse be familiar with them, figure 2-1.

Roman numerals over 100 are seldom used in medicine. Numbers 1 through 10 have been included in figure 2-1 because they are used extensively after each numeral: X, XX, XXX, etc. However, when writing the number 40 in Roman numerals, the number 10 (X) must precede the number 50 (L) and is written as XL. In other words, 10 "taken away" from 50 equals 40, or 50 minus 10 equals 40 (50 - 10 = 40).

The same principle applies when writing 90. The letter C is the Roman numeral for 100. Therefore, 90 is written XC as ten is taken away from 100; that is 100 minus 10 equals 90 (100 - 10 = 90).

Study figure 2-1 and complete the practice problems that follow it in order to check understanding of numerals and conversion from one system to another.

Arabic Numerals	Roman Numerals	Arabic Numerals	Roman Numerals
1	I	30	XXX
2	II	40	XL
3	III	50	L
4	IV	60	LX
5	V	70	LXX
6	VI	80	LXXX
7	VII	90	XC
8	VIII	100	C
9	IX	500	D
10	X	1000	M
20	XX		

Fig. 2-1 Arabic and Roman Numerals

Section 1 Review of Basic Mathematics

Practice Problems

1. Complete the following in Roman numerals:

   a. 2 = II
   b. 4 = IV
   c. 6 = VI
   d. 9 = IX
   e. 14 = XIV
   f. 16 = XVI
   g. 19 = XIX
   h. 24 = XXIV
   i. 40 = XL
   j. 49 = XLIX
   k. 60 = LX
   l. 75 = LXXV
   m. 85 = LXXXV
   n. 98 = XCVIII
   o. 110 = CX
   p. 1969 = MCMLXIX
   q. 11 = XI
   r. 14 = XIV
   s. 21 = XXI
   t. 69 = LXIX

2. Complete the following in Arabic numerals:

   a. IV = 4
   b. V = 5
   c. VI = 6
   d. IX = 9
   e. XIV = 14
   f. XIX = 19
   g. XXIV = 24
   h. XXVI = 26
   i. XXIX = 29
   j. XXXIV = 34
   k. XLIX = 49
   l. LIV = 54
   m. LIX = 59
   n. LXI = 61
   o. XCIV = 94
   p. CXIX = 119
   q. MCMLXX = 1970
   r. VIII = 8
   s. XVI = 16
   t. XXIII = 23

COMMON FRACTIONS

Medicine orders may be written in either the metric system or in the apothecaries system. If they are written in the apothecaries system, common fractions are used. Consequently, the nurse must know how to add, subtract, multiply and divide common fractions. She must also know how to convert common fractions into decimal fractions. Medicine glasses and other containers have markings of the metric system. Decimal fractions will be reviewed in Unit 3.

The Concept of Fractional Parts

A common fraction is a part of a whole number. In the fraction 2/5, the 2 above the line is the *numerator*, and the 5 below the line is the *demoninator*. The line separating the numerator from the denominator expresses the process of division: the numerator is divided by the denominator. For example, in 2/5, the 2 is divided by the 5.

Unit 2 Numerals and Fractions

Kinds of Common Fractions

Simple fractions are fractions which contain only one numerator and one denominator such as 1/2, 3/4, and 2/5.

Compound fractions are those in which an arithmetical process is necessary in either the numerator or denominator, as in

$$\frac{3 \times 5}{16} \quad \text{or} \quad \frac{9}{5-2}$$

Complex fractions may have simple fractions in either the numerator or the denominator, or both, as in

$$\frac{\frac{1}{3}}{4} \quad \text{or} \quad \frac{\frac{1}{3}}{\frac{3}{4}}$$

Proper fractions have a numerator which is smaller than the denominator, as in 3/4 or 2/3.

Improper fractions have a numerator which is larger than the denominator, as in 20/5 or 16/3.

A *mixed number* contains a whole number and a fraction, as in 5 3/4 or 4 1/2.

Equivalent fractions are those which have the same value, as in 1/3 = 2/6 or 3/5 = 6/10.

Reducing Fractions

It is always easier to work with common fractions reduced to their *lowest terms*. For example, it is easier to work with 3/4 than 75/100. Fractions may be reduced to their lowest terms by dividing both the numerator and denominator by the same number.

Examples: $\quad \frac{15}{60} \div \frac{15}{15} = \frac{1}{4} \quad$ or $\quad \frac{20}{100} \div \frac{10}{10} = \frac{2}{10} = \frac{1}{5}$

Practice Problems

3. Reduce the following fractions to their lowest terms.

   a. $\frac{4}{16}$ = _1/4_   d. $\frac{6}{24}$ = _1/4_

   b. $\frac{5}{15}$ = _1/3_   e. $\frac{25}{30}$ = _5/6_

   c. $\frac{24}{80}$ = _3/10_   f. $\frac{30}{50}$ = _3/5_

Changing Improper Fractions to Mixed Numbers

Improper fractions can be changed to mixed numbers by dividing the numerator by the denominator.

Example: $\quad \frac{9}{8} = 8\overline{)9}^{\,1\frac{1}{8}}$

Section 1 Review of Basic Mathematics

Practice Problems

4. Change the following improper fractions to mixed numbers.

   a. $\frac{7}{5}$ = __1 2/5__   d. $\frac{3}{2}$ = __1 1/2__

   b. $\frac{8}{7}$ = __1 1/7__   e. $\frac{16}{13}$ = __1 3/13__

   c. $\frac{12}{11}$ = __1 1/11__   f. $\frac{19}{15}$ = __1 4/15__

Changing Mixed Numbers to Improper Fractions

To change mixed numbers to improper fractions, multiply the whole number by the denominator and add the numerator to the product.

Examples: a. $3\frac{1}{3}$ = $\frac{(3 \times 3) + 1}{3}$ = $\frac{10}{3}$ = $3\frac{1}{3}$

b. $4\frac{3}{4}$ = $\frac{(4 \times 4) + 3}{4}$ = $\frac{19}{4}$ = $4\frac{3}{4}$

Practice Problems

5. Change the following mixed numbers to improper fractions. Check your work by changing the fractions back into mixed numbers.

   a. $3\frac{2}{3}$ = __11/3__   d. $5\frac{2}{5}$ = __27/5__

   b. $4\frac{1}{6}$ = __25/6__   e. $6\frac{1}{3}$ = __19/3__

   c. $2\frac{3}{4}$ = __11/4__   f. $7\frac{2}{5}$ = __37/5__

Addition of Common Fractions

When adding common fractions, the denominators must be the same figure. The following fractions can be added because their denominators are the same.

$$\frac{1}{3} + \frac{2}{3} = \frac{3}{3} \text{ or } 1$$

To add fractions which have *unlike* denominators, change the fractions to equivalent fractions by finding the lowest common denominator.

Example:

$\frac{2}{5} + \frac{3}{10} + \frac{1}{2} = ?$ $\frac{2}{5} = \frac{?}{10}$ $\frac{2}{5} = \frac{4}{10}$

$\begin{array}{c} \frac{2}{5} \\ \frac{3}{10} \\ \frac{1}{2} \\ \hline \end{array}$ $\begin{array}{c} \frac{4}{10} \\ \frac{3}{10} \\ \frac{5}{10} \\ \hline \frac{12}{10} = 1\frac{1}{5} \end{array}$

Ten is the lowest possible number that is divisible by each denominator. Therefore, change all the fractions to equivalent fractions with 10 as the denominator. Divide the lowest common denominator by the denominator of the fraction (10 divided by 5 equals 2). Multiply the quotient by the numerator of the fraction (2 times 2 equals 4). When all the fractions have been changed to the lowest common denominator, add as usual.

8

Unit 2 Numerals and Fractions

Addition of Mixed Numbers

Add the fractions first, and then the whole numbers. If improper fractions must be added, these must be changed to mixed numbers first. The whole number is then added with the other whole numbers.

Example: $2\frac{3}{4} + 2\frac{1}{2} + 3\frac{1}{8}$

$$\begin{array}{r|r} 2\frac{3}{4} & \frac{6}{8} \\ 2\frac{1}{2} & \frac{4}{8} \\ 3\frac{3}{8} & \frac{3}{8} \\ \hline 7 & \frac{13}{8} = 1\frac{5}{8} \\ + 1\frac{5}{8} & \\ \hline 8\frac{5}{8} & \end{array}$$

Practice Problems

6. Add the following fractions and mixed numbers. Reduce the answers to their lowest terms.

    a. $\frac{1}{4} + \frac{3}{4} = $ _1_

    b. $\frac{1}{3} + \frac{4}{9} + \frac{3}{18} = $ _17/18_

    c. $\frac{1}{2} + \frac{1}{3} + \frac{1}{6} = $ _1_

    d. $\frac{1}{5} + \frac{14}{25} + \frac{11}{50} = $ _49/50_

    e. $15\frac{3}{5} + \frac{4}{50} + 3\frac{3}{25} = $ _18 4/5_

    f. $3\frac{3}{10} + 5\frac{3}{15} + 4\frac{2}{5} = $ _12 9/10_

Subtraction of Common Fractions

In subtraction, first find the least common denominator. Subtract the smaller numerator from the larger one. Reduce the remainder to its lowest terms.

Examples: a. $\frac{3}{4} - \frac{1}{4} = \frac{2}{4}$ or $\frac{1}{2}$

b. $\begin{array}{r|r} 2\frac{1}{4} & \frac{4}{16} \\ -1\frac{3}{16} & \frac{3}{16} \\ \hline 1 & \frac{1}{16} \end{array}$ $(1\frac{1}{16})$

When the numerator of the fraction in the *minuend* (top number) is smaller than the numerator of the *subtrahend* (bottom number), it is necessary to borrow from the whole number in the minuend.

Example: $\begin{array}{r|r} 4\frac{1}{4} & 3\frac{5}{4} \\ -1\frac{3}{4} & 1\frac{3}{4} \\ \hline & 2\frac{2}{4} = 2\frac{1}{2} \end{array}$ Since the numerator of the fractional minuend is smaller than that of the subtrahend, borrow 1 from the whole number and add it to the fractional minuend.

$1 = \frac{4}{4}$ $\qquad$ $\frac{4}{4} + \frac{1}{4} = \frac{5}{4}$

Section 1 Review of Basic Mathematics

Then the fractions and whole numbers are subtracted as usual.

Practice Problems

7. Subtract the following fractions and mixed numbers. Reduce the answers to their lowest terms.

   a. $\frac{7}{8} - \frac{3}{6} = $ __3/8__

   b. $\frac{11}{12} - \frac{5}{6} = $ __1/12__

   c. $\frac{1}{3} - \frac{1}{4} = $ __1/12__

   d. $10\frac{3}{4} - 7\frac{1}{4} = $ __3 1/2__

   e. $16\frac{5}{6} - 14\frac{3}{8} = $ __2 11/24__

   f. $175\frac{7}{12} - 15\frac{1}{24} = $ __160 13/24__

Multiplication of Common Fractions

In order to multiply common fractions, the numerators are multiplied and then the denominators. Place the product of the numerators over the product of the denominators, and then reduce the resulting fraction to its lowest terms. Whenever possible, cancel fractions as this will shorten the operation.

Examples:

a. $\frac{1}{2} \times \frac{3}{4} = \frac{3}{8}$

b. $\frac{1}{3} \times \frac{3}{4} = \frac{1}{\cancel{3}_1} \times \frac{\cancel{3}^1}{4} = \frac{1}{4}$

c. $\frac{7}{8} \times \frac{2}{7} = \frac{\cancel{7}^1}{\cancel{8}_4} \times \frac{\cancel{2}^1}{\cancel{7}_1} = \frac{1}{4}$

Practice Problems

8. Multiply the following fractions and then reduce the products to their lowest terms.

   a. $\frac{2}{3} \times \frac{3}{4} = $ __1/2__

   b. $\frac{4}{5} \times \frac{1}{8} = $ __1/10__

   c. $\frac{4}{9} \times \frac{3}{8} = $ __1/6__

   d. $\frac{5}{7} \times 5\frac{1}{4} = $ __3 3/4__

   e. $\frac{3}{8} \times 1\frac{1}{4} = $ __15/32__

   f. $\frac{5}{12} \times 4\frac{3}{4} = $ __1 47/48__

Division of Common Fractions

In order to divide common fractions, the second fraction is inverted. Inverting a fraction means simply "turning it upside down". When 3/4 is inverted, it becomes 4/3. After inverting the second fraction, proceed as in multiplication.

Examples:

a. $\frac{9}{10} \div \frac{3}{5} = \frac{9}{10} \times \frac{5}{3} = \frac{\cancel{9}^3}{\cancel{10}_2} \times \frac{\cancel{5}^1}{\cancel{3}_1} = \frac{3}{2}$ or $1\frac{1}{2}$

b. $6 \div \frac{1}{4} = \frac{6}{1} \times \frac{4}{1} = 24$

c. $\frac{1}{4} \div 6 = \frac{1}{4} \div \frac{6}{1} = \frac{1}{4} \times \frac{1}{6} = \frac{1}{24}$

10

Unit 2 Numerals and Fractions

Practice Problems

9. Divide the following fractions and then reduce the answers to their lowest terms.

   a. $\frac{1}{5} \div \frac{1}{10}$ = **2**

   b. $\frac{1}{150} \div \frac{1}{100}$ = **109/150**

   c. $\frac{2}{5} \div \frac{10}{15}$ = **3/5**

   d. $3 \div \frac{5}{3}$ = **1 4/5**

   e. $\frac{2}{3} \div 5\frac{1}{2}$ = **4/33**

   f. $\frac{3}{4} \div \frac{8}{9}$ = **27/32**

RELATIVE VALUES OF COMMON FRACTIONS

A nurse must be able to recognize the relative values of a series of fractions; for example, when reading medication labels that express strength in fractional amounts she must know how they compare to other strengths. The following methods may be used to arrive at an answer.

- Change the fractions to a common denominator. The fraction with the largest numerator is the largest.

   Example: Which is the largest, 1/4, 1/15, or 1/3?

   $\frac{1}{4} = \frac{15}{60}$ $\frac{1}{15} = \frac{4}{60}$ $\frac{1}{3} = \frac{20}{60}$ Therefore, 1/3 is largest.

- Compare the numerators. If they are all the same, the fraction with the smallest denominator is the largest. In the example above, all the numerators are the same (1), and 1/3 has the smallest denominator. Therefore, 1/3 is the largest fraction.

- Change the fractions to decimals by dividing the denominator of each fraction into its numerator. The largest decimal fraction is the largest amount. (Refer to Unit 3 for review of Decimal Fractions).

Practice Problems

10. In each problem, underline the largest quantity and encircle the smallest quantity.

   a. $\frac{1}{3}$ $\frac{1}{8}$

   b. $\frac{1}{30}$ $\frac{1}{150}$ $\frac{1}{4}$

   c. $\frac{1}{5}$ $\frac{3}{20}$ $\frac{1}{100}$

   d. $\frac{1}{150}$ $\frac{1}{125}$ $\frac{1}{100}$

   e. $\frac{1}{3}$ $\frac{1}{2}$ $\frac{1}{5}$

   f. $\frac{1}{4}$ $\frac{3}{8}$ $\frac{3}{4}$

Unit 3 Decimal Fractions and Percents

OBJECTIVES

After studying this unit, the student should be able to:

- Read and write decimals correctly.

- Convert common fractions to decimal fractions and decimal fractions to common fractions.

- Add, subtract, multiply, and divide decimal fractions.

- Convert common fractions and decimal fractions to percents and percents to common fractions and decimal fractions.

- Find the percent of a given quantity.

When working with decimal fractions, it should be remembered that the location of the decimal point is important. Numbers which *precede* the decimal point are *whole numbers*; those which follow the decimal point are *decimal fractions*. The chart below should be studied for better understanding.

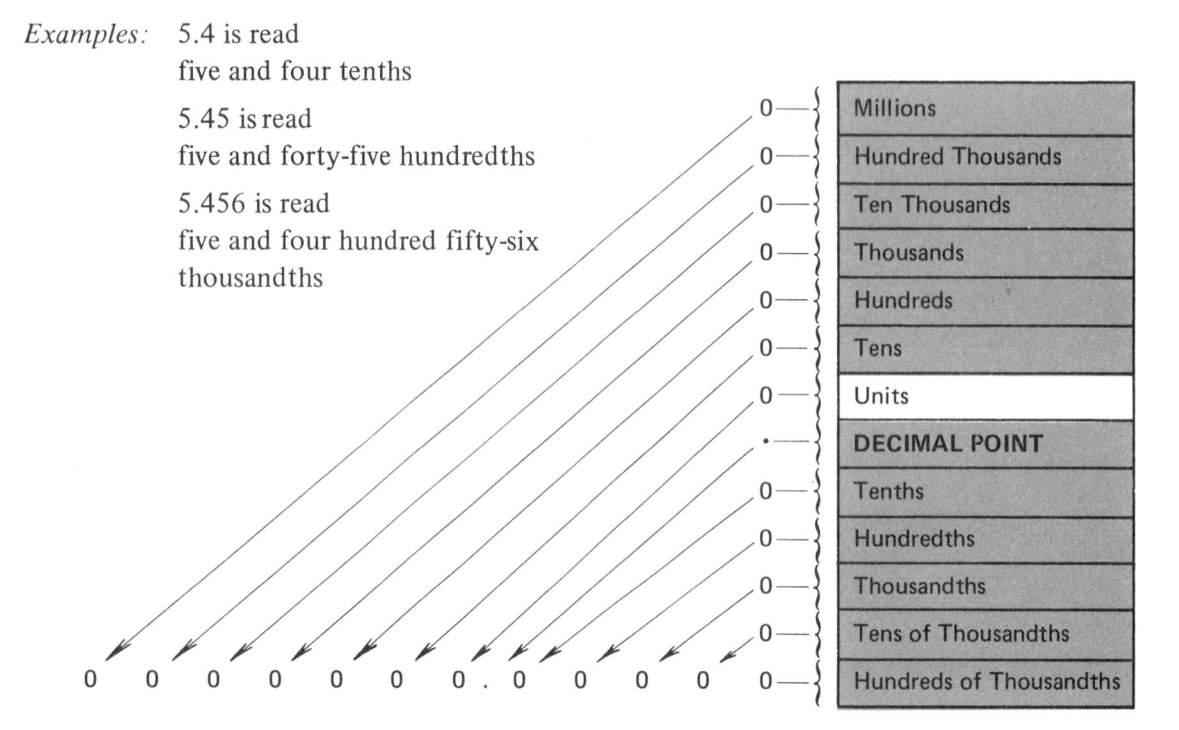

Examples: 5.4 is read
five and four tenths

5.45 is read
five and forty-five hundredths

5.456 is read
five and four hundred fifty-six thousandths

0 —	Millions
0 —	Hundred Thousands
0 —	Ten Thousands
0 —	Thousands
0 —	Hundreds
0 —	Tens
0 —	Units
• —	DECIMAL POINT
0 —	Tenths
0 —	Hundredths
0 —	Thousandths
0 —	Tens of Thousandths
0 —	Hundreds of Thousandths

0 0 0 0 0 0 0 . 0 0 0 0 0

Unit 3 Decimal Fractions and Percents

Practice Problems

1. Write the following numbers in words.
   a. 75.35 _SEVENTY FIVE AND THIRTY FIVE HUNDREDS_
   b. 1.005 _ONE AND FIVE THOUSANDTHS_
   c. .05 _FIVE HUNDREDTHS_
   d. 5.0 _FIVE_

CONVERSION OF COMMON FRACTIONS AND DECIMAL FRACTIONS

- To change a common fraction to a decimal, divide the denominator of the fraction into the numerator. Place the decimal point after the numerator and in the proper position of the quotient (answer).

   Example: Express 3/4 in decimal form.

   $$4 \overline{) 3.00} \quad .75$$
   $$\underline{2\ 8}$$
   $$20$$
   $$\underline{20}$$

- Decimal fractions are fractions that have denominators that are powers of ten; that is 10, 100, 1000, etc. The denominators may be omitted and a decimal point used to show it is a decimal fraction.

- To change a decimal or decimal fraction to a common fraction, write the decimal in the form of a fraction and reduce to lowest terms.

   Examples: a. Express .45 as a fraction.

   $$\frac{45}{100} = \frac{9}{20}$$

   b. Express .33 1/3 as a fraction.

   $$.33\frac{1}{3} = \frac{100}{\frac{3}{100}} = \frac{100}{300} = \frac{1}{3}$$

Practice Problems

2. Change to decimals.
   a. $\frac{3}{25}$ = _.12_   d. $\frac{6}{300}$ = _.02_
   b. $\frac{3}{5}$ = _.6_   e. $\frac{1}{75}$ = _.013_
   c. $\frac{5}{500}$ = _.01_   f. $\frac{4}{50}$ = _.08_

3. Change to common fractions.
   a. .25 _1/4_   e. $.66\frac{2}{3}$ = _1/6_
   b. .50 _1/2_   f. $.1\frac{1}{3}$ = _2/15_
   c. .75 _3/4_   g. $.11\frac{1}{9}$ = _1/9_
   d. .20 _1/5_

Section 1 Review of Basic Mathematics

ADDITION OF DECIMAL FRACTIONS

- When adding decimals, always place the decimal points one under the other.

    Example: Add 1.025, .12, and 20.02

    ```
      1.025
       .12
     20.02
     ─────
     21.165
    ```

    The answer is read: twenty-one and one hundred sixty-five thousandths.

Practice Problems

4. Add the following decimal fractions.
   a. 1.027, 21.50, 0.16 = *22.687*
   b. 305.25, 1.005, 0.05 = *306.305*
   c. 2,100.75, 21.50, 0.0021 = *2,122.2521*
   d. 750.20, .750, 1.255 = *752.205*

SUBTRACTION OF DECIMAL FRACTIONS

- When subtracting decimals, always place the decimal points one under the other. Then subtract in the usual manner.

Practice Problems

5. Subtract the following decimal fractions.
   a. 500. - 1.025 = *498.025*
   b. 275.005 - 70.001 = *205.004*
   c. 149.5 - 147.05 = *2.45*
   d. 350.21 - 349.20 = *1.01*
   e. 900.0 - 2.075 = *897.925*

MULTIPLICATION OF DECIMAL FRACTIONS

When multiplying decimal numbers, it is not necessary to line up the decimal points under each other.

- Multiply the decimal numbers as whole numbers; however, the number of places after the decimal points in the multiplicand and multiplier must be totaled. With this total of decimal places in mind, refer to the product (answer). Beginning with the last figure on the right, count in the number of places and place the decimal point.

    Example:
    ```
        250.5  multiplicand
         .75   multiplier
        ─────
        12525
        17535
        ─────
        187.875  (three places from the right)
    ```

The answer is read: one hundred eighty-seven and eight hundred seventy-five thousandths.

14

Unit 3 Decimal Fractions and Percents

Practice Problems

6. Multiply the following decimal fractions.
   a. 460.70 x 1.5 = _691.050_
   b. .650 x 1.25 = _.8125_
   c. 1.75 x .007 = _.01225_
   d. 35.05 x .5 = _17.525_
   e. 65.00 x 10 = _650.00_

DIVISION OF DECIMALS

When decimals are divided, the *divisor* becomes a whole number by moving the decimal point the required number of places to the right. The *dividend* decimal point must also be moved the same number of places to the right. The decimal point in the *quotient* must be placed directly above this point. Then divide as usual to the third place beyond the decimal point.

Example: Divide 5.50 by .25

```
                       22.0      (quotient)
       (divisor)   .25. ) 5.50.00   (dividend)
```

ROUNDING OFF NUMBERS

Sometimes, in working with decimals, an exact answer is not required. In such cases, the answer is rounded off to the nearest tenth, hundredth, or thousandth.

- If the last number of the answer after the decimal point is less than 5, it is dropped.
- If the last number of the answer is 5 or more than 5, it is treated as a whole and the number 1 is added to the preceding number.

Examples: Round off the following decimal fractions to the nearest tenth.

   1.83 = 1.8   5.225 = 5.2   83.26 = 83.3   12.55 = 12.6

Practice Problems

7. Divide the following decimal fractions. Round off the answers to the nearest hundredth.
   a. 382.93 ÷ 23.1 _16.58_   d. 38.6 ÷ 1.7 _.71_
   b. 48.5 ÷ 8.25 _5.88_   e. 648.72 ÷ 18.6 _34.88_
   c. 244 ÷ 3.1 _.71_

MULTIPLYING AND DIVIDING DECIMAL FRACTIONS BY MULTIPLES OF TEN

Since decimal fractions are based on multiples of 10 (tenths, hundredths, thousandths, etc.), it is easy to multiply and divide with these numbers.

- To *multiply* a decimal number by 10, the decimal point is moved one place to the *right*. To multiply a decimal number by 100, the decimal point is moved two places to the right. To multiply by 1000, the decimal point is moved three places to the right.

Section 1 Review of Basic Mathematics

- To *divide* by 10, the decimal point is moved one place to the *left*. To divide by 100, the decimal point is moved two places to the left. To divide by 1000, the decimal point is moved three places to the left. (It may be necessary to add zeros).

Examples:

.2 multiplied by 10 = 2.0

.3 multiplied by 100 = 30.0

.2 divided by 10 = .02

.3 divided by 100 = .003

When a number does not have a visible decimal point, it is understood that the point is at the end of the number, for example 22 is the same as 22.0.

Practice Problems

8. Multiply or divide as indicated.
   a. .525 x 10 = __5.250__
   b. 115 ÷ 100 = __1.15__
   c. 115 ÷ 1000 = __.115__
   d. 115 ÷ 10 = __11.5__
   e. .3 x 100 = __30.0__
   f. 8.325 x 1000 = __8325.000__
   g. 50.5 x 10 = __505.0__
   h. .505 ÷ 100 = __.00505__
   i. 5.05 ÷ 10 = __.505__

PERCENTAGE

The whole is expressed as 100%. Therefore, a certain percent indicates parts of 100. For example, 34% means 34/100 or .34 and 340% means 340/100 or 3.4 or 3 2/5. Since the strength of solutions is expressed in percentage, it is necessary for the nurse to be able to convert percents to decimal fractions and common fractions. This is done by considering the percent sign as a denominator of 100, and then dividing the number by this 100.

- To change a percent to a fraction, remove the percent sign and write the percent as the numerator of a fraction. Write 100 as the denominator of the fraction and reduce to lowest terms.

Example:

$$50\% = \frac{50}{100} = \frac{1}{2}$$

- If the percent is a mixed number or a fraction, the numerator of the complex fraction is divided by the denominator (100). The process may be simplified by merely multiplying the percent by 1/100.

Examples:

a. $5.5\% = 5\frac{1}{2}\% = \frac{5\frac{1}{2}}{100} = \frac{11}{2} \div 100 = \frac{11}{2} \times \frac{1}{100} = \frac{11}{200}$

b. $\frac{1}{4}\% = \frac{\frac{1}{4}}{100} = \frac{1}{4} \div 100 = \frac{1}{4} \times \frac{1}{100} = \frac{1}{400}$

Unit 3 Decimal Fractions and Percents

- To change a fraction to a percent, multiply by 100 and add the percent sign.

    Examples:

    a. $\dfrac{3}{4} = \dfrac{3}{\cancel{4}_1} \times \dfrac{\cancel{100}^{25}}{1} = 75\%$

    b. $\dfrac{29}{400} = \dfrac{29}{400} \times \dfrac{100}{1} = \dfrac{2900}{400} = 7\dfrac{1}{4}\%$

- To change a percent to a decimal, simply remove the percent sign and move the decimal point two places to the left. This is the same as dividing by 100. If the percent has a fraction, the fraction must be changed to decimal form before the decimal point may be moved.

    Examples:

    $50\% = .5 \qquad 5.5\% = .055 \qquad 1/4\% = .25\% = .0025$

- To change a decimal to a percent, move the decimal point two places to the right and add the percent sign. You are actually multiplying by 100.

    Examples:

    $.3 = 30\% \qquad .35 = 35\% \qquad .355 = 35.5\% \qquad .0355 = 3.55\%$

Practice Problems

9. Change the following common fractions to percents.

    a. $\dfrac{1}{4}$ = __25%__

    b. $\dfrac{1}{3}$ = __33⅓%__

    c. $\dfrac{2}{5}$ = __40%__

    d. $\dfrac{2}{3}$ = __66⅔%__

    e. $\dfrac{3}{25}$ = __12%__

10. Change the *largest* decimal in each series to a percent.

    a. .001   1.25   1.09   __1.25%__
    b. .7   .69   .349   __.70%__
    c. .08   .8   .185   __80%__
    d. .495   4.95   .049   __495%__
    e. .125   .005   .025   __12.5%__

11. Change each of the following percents to a fraction *and* a decimal.

    a. 2%   __1/50__   and __.02__
    b. 4 3/4%   __19/400__   and __.0475__
    c. 40%   __2/5__   and __.4__
    d. 19.3%   __193/1000__   and __.193__
    e. 64%   __16/25__   and __.64__

17

Section 1 Review of Basic Mathematics

DETERMINING QUANTITY IF A PERCENT IS GIVEN

- To find the percentage of a given number, convert the percent to a decimal or fraction; multiply the whole number by the decimal or fraction.

Example: How much is 5% of 48?

(Conversion to decimal)	(Conversion to fraction)
5% = .05	5% = $\frac{5}{100}$ or $\frac{1}{20}$
48 x .05 = 2.4	48 x $\frac{1}{20}$ = $\frac{48}{20}$ or $2\frac{2}{5}$
Note: 2.4 = $2\frac{2}{5}$	

Practice Problems

12. Solve each of the following problems and give the answer as a decimal and as a fraction.

Problem	Decimal	Fraction
a. How much is 20% of 36?	7.2	7 1/5
b. How much is 8% of 60?	4.8	4 4/5
c. How much is 1/2% of 750?	3.750	3 3/4
d. How much is 350% of 15?	52.5	52 1/2
e. How much is 2% of 10?	.2	1/5

Unit 4 Ratio and Proportion

OBJECTIVES

After studying this unit, the student should be able to:
- Convert common fractions, decimal fractions, and percents to ratios.
- Set up proportions and solve for unknown quantities.

In the preceding units, the processes by which fractional quantities can be expressed as common fractions, decimal fractions, and percents were reviewed. Ratios and proportion will be covered in this unit.

RATIOS

A ratio is another way of expressing the relationship between parts and a whole. It is a comparison between a pair of numbers.

- A common fraction may be expressed as a ratio of the numerator to the denominator. The numerator of the fraction is always placed in front of the denominator when it is being expressed as a ratio. (The colon which follows the numerator means "is to"; therefore, the fraction 1/8 would be shown as the ratio 1:8 and stated as "1 is to 8".)

Practice Problems

1. Write the following common fractions as ratios.

   a. $\frac{1}{100}$ = _1:100_   d. $\frac{7}{10}$ = _7:10_
   b. $\frac{3}{5}$ = _3:5_   e. $\frac{5}{2}$ = _5:2_
   c. $\frac{5}{6}$ = _5:6_   f. $\frac{5}{8}$ = _5:8_

- To change a percent to a ratio, it should be remembered that the percent sign (%) indicates parts of a hundred. Therefore, when the percent sign is dropped, 100 is used as the second term of the ratio.

Examples:

   20% = 20:100   5% = 5:100   25.5% = 25.5:100

Practice Problems

2. Write the following percents as ratios.

   a. 25% _25:100_   d. .3% _.3:100_
   b. 6%   _6:100_   e. 420% _420:100_
   c. 85% _85:100_   f. 8.3% _8.3:100_

19

Section 1 Review of Basic Mathematics

- When a decimal fraction is changed to a ratio, the placement of the decimal point indicates that the second term of the ratio will follow. This can be more easily understood by first changing the decimal to a common fraction.

    Examples:

    .3 = 3/10 = 3:10   .03 = 3/100 = 3:100   3.0 = 3/1 = 3:1

Practice Problems

3. Write the following decimals as fractions. Reduce the fractions to their lowest terms and then change them to ratios.

    a. 0.1 = *1/10* = *1:10*   d. 1.25 = *125/100* = *125:100*
    b. .35 = *35/100* = *35:100*   e. .75 = *75/100* = *75:100*
    c. .02 = *02/100* = *02:100*   f. .50 = *50/100* = *50:100*

PROPORTION

Most problems in medications are solved by the process of *proportion*. A proportion is an equation which shows the relationship between two equal ratios. The first and fourth items of the proportion are called the *extremes*. The second and third items are called the *means*.

The double colon between the two ratios means the word "as". The following example is read: "1 is to 8 as 4 is to 32".

Example:

             Extremes
             1:8 :: 4:32
             Means

- The product of the extremes equals the product of the means in a proportion. The preceding example is used to illustrate this point.

    1 x 32 = 8 x 4

When setting up a *proportion*, one must be sure that the first and third terms refer to the same things. In other words, the first term of each ratio must refer to the same items. The same follows through with the second and fourth terms in a proportion; or, the second terms of each ratio. They must refer to the same items.

- To find an unknown term in a proportion, substitute an X for the unknown and multiply the means and the extremes. If three of the four terms of a proportion are known, the fourth can be found as the X factor.

    Examples:

Using whole numbers	Using a fraction	Using a decimal
4:5 :: X:10	1/4:X :: 1:16	2.5:X :: 12:24
5X = 40	1X = 1/4 x 16/1	12X = 24 x 2.5
X = 40 ÷ 5	X = 4/1	12X = 60
X = 8	X = 4	X = 60 ÷ 12
		X = 5

Practice Problems

4. Find X in the following proportions.
   a. 50:X :: 25:1000   X = 2000
   b. 9:15 :: X:5   X = 3
   c. 1/10X:2000 :: 1:100   X = 10
   d. 1/400:X :: 2:1600   X = 2
   e. 25:X :: 5:10   X = 50
   f. 8:10 :: X:30   X = 24
   g. 4:8 :: X:16   X = 8
   h. 0.2:8 :: 25:X   X = 100
   i. 0.5:15 :: X:60   X = 2.0
   j. 0.7:X :: 70:500   X = 5.0
   k. 1/2X:1000 :: 1:500   X = 4
   l. 1/4:X :: 20:400   X = 5

Unit 5 Temperature Conversion

OBJECTIVES

After studying this unit, the student should be able to:
- Convert temperatures from the Fahrenheit scale to the Celsius scale.
- Convert temperatures from the Celsius scale to the Fahrenheit scale.

The Fahrenheit and Celsius scales differ, figure 5-1. Observation and comparison of the two scales will show the freezing point and boiling point of each. In the Fahrenheit scale the freezing point of water is 32 degrees and the boiling point of water is 212 degrees. In the Celsius scale, the freezing point is 0 degrees and the boiling point is 100 degrees.

Five degrees on the Celsius scale equals nine degrees on the Fahrenheit scale. Therefore, the fractions 5/9 and 9/5 are used to convert temperatures from one scale to the other. These fractions indicate a ratio between two scales.

The nurse will find it necessary to be familiar with the conversion formula in her care of patients and in understanding her environment. Originally, *centigrade* was used instead of Celsius. However, *Celsius* is the metric term. Thermometers, respirators and other scientific equipment which reflect the different scales, the current trend toward use of the metric system as an international unit of measurement — all require a knowledge of these measurements.

FAHRENHEIT TO CELSIUS

To convert from Fahrenheit to Celsius temperature:
- Subtract 32° from the Fahrenheit temperature.
- Multiply the result by 5/9.

$$C = F - 32 \times \frac{5}{9}$$

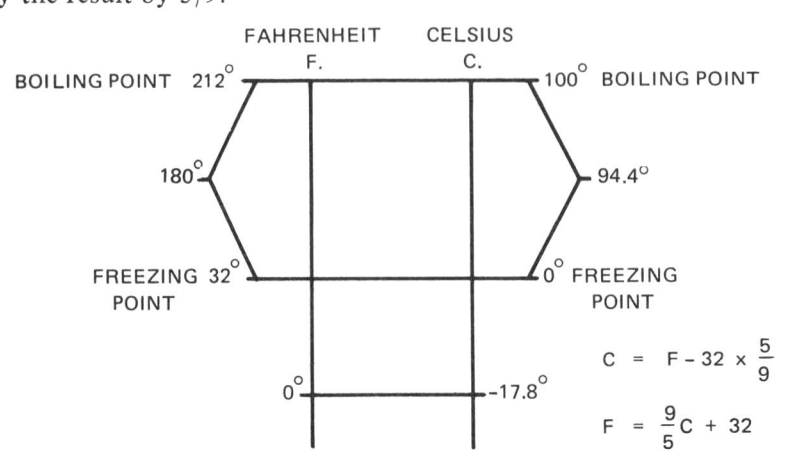

$$F = \frac{9}{5}C + 32$$

Fig. 5-1 Comparison of Fahrenheit and Celsius temperatures

Unit 5 Temperature Conversion

The formula for this conversion is written as follows:
    C = (F - 32) x 5/9

Example: Convert 105°F to Celsius.
    C = (F - 32) x 5/9
    C = (105 - 32) x 5/9
    105 - 32 = 73
    73 x 5/9 = 40.5
    C = 40.5°

Practice Problems

1. Convert the following Fahrenheit temperature to Celsius degrees. Give answers in decimal form, rounded off to the nearest tenth of a degree. Show the steps involved in the solution of the problems.
    a. 120°F = _C = 48.9_
    b. 100°F = _C = 37.8_
    c. 95°F = _C = 35_
    d. 90°F = _C = 32.2_
    e. 85°F = _C = 29.4_

CELSIUS TO FAHRENHEIT

To convert from Celsius to Fahrenheit temperature:
- Multiply the Celsius temperature by 9/5.
- Add 32°.

The formula for this conversion is written as follows:
    F = 9/5 C + 32

Example: Convert 25°C to Fahrenheit.
    F = 9/5 C + 32
    F = 9/5 x 25 + 32
    $\frac{9}{\cancel{5}_1} \times \cancel{25}^5 = 45$
    45 + 32 = 77
    F = 77°

Practice Problems

2. Convert the following Celsius temperatures to Fahrenheit. Give answers in decimal form, rounded off to the nearest tenth of a degree. Show the steps involved in the solution.
    a. 38°C = _F = 68°_
    b. 35°C = _F = 95_
    c. 75°C = _F = 167_
    d. 20°C = _F = 68_
    e. 45°C = _F = 113_

Section 1 Review of Basic Mathematics

NOTE: The following table is provided as an aid for study and comparison of temperatures. It will re-enforce what has been learned through the study and practice problems in this unit.

DEGREES FAHRENHEIT TO DEGREES CELSIUS AND VICE VERSA											
°F	°C	°F	°C	°F	°C	°F	°C	°F	°C	°F	°C
96	35.6	118	47.8	140	60	162	72.2	184	84.4	206.6	97
96.8	36	118.4	48	141	60.6	163	72.8	185	85	207	97.2
97	36.1	119	48.3	141.8	61	163.4	73	186	85.6	208	97.8
98	36.7	120	48.9	142	61.1	164	73.3	186.8	86	208.4	98
98.6	37	120.2	49	143	61.7	165	73.9	187	86.1	209	98.3
99	37.2	121	49.4	143.6	62	165.2	74	188	86.7	210	98.9
100	37.8	122	50	144	62.2	166	74.4	188.6	87	210.2	99
100.4	38	123	50.6	145	62.8	167	75	189	87.2	211	99.4
101	38.3	123.8	51	145.4	63	168	75.6	190	87.8	212	100
102	38.9	124	51.1	146	63.3	168.8	76	190.4	88	213	100.6
102.2	39	125	51.7	147	63.9	169	76.1	191	88.3	213.8	101
103	39.4	125.6	52	147.2	64	170	76.7	192	88.9	214	101.1
104	40	126	52.2	148	64.4	170.6	77	192.2	89	215	101.7
105	40.6	127	52.8	149	65	171	77.2	193	89.4	215.6	102
105.8	41	127.4	53	150	65.6	172	77.8	194	90	216	102.2
106	41.1	128	53.3	150.8	66	172.4	78	195	90.6	217	102.8
107	41.7	129	53.9	151	66.1	173	78.3	195.8	91	217.4	103
107.6	42	129.2	54	152	66.7	174	78.9	196	91.1	218	103.3
108	42.2	130	54.4	152.6	67	174.2	79	197	91.7	219	103.9
109	42.8	131	55	153	67.2	175	79.4	197.6	92	219.2	104
109.4	43	132	55.6	154	67.8	176	80	198	92.2	220	104.4
110	43.3	132.8	56	154.4	68	177	80.6	199	92.8	221	105
111	43.9	133	56.1	155	68.3	177.8	81	199.4	93	225	107.2
111.2	44	134	56.7	156	68.9	178	81.1	200	93.3	230	110
112	44.4	134.6	57	156.2	69	179	81.7	201	93.9	235	112.8
113	45	135	57.2	157	69.4	179.6	82	201.2	94	239	115
114	45.6	136	57.8	158	70	180	82.2	202	94.4	240	115.6
114.8	46	136.4	58	159	70.6	181	82.8	203	95	245	118.3
115	46.1	137	58.3	159.8	71	181.4	83	204	95.6	248	120
116	46.7	138	58.9	160	71.1	182	83.3	204.8	96	250	121.1
116.6	47	138.2	59	161	71.7	183	83.9	205	96.1	255	123.9
117	47.2	139	59.4	161.6	72	183.2	84	206	96.7	257	125

Achievement Review 1

Section 1 Review of Basic Mathematics

A. Complete the following problems.

1. Write as Roman numerals.
   a. 19 __XIX__
   b. 24 __XXIV__
   c. 49 __XLIX__
   d. 51 __LI__
   e. 98 __XCVIII__
   f. 102 __CII__

2. Write as Arabic numerals.
   a. IV __4__
   b. VI __6__
   c. IX __9__
   d. XIV __14__
   e. LX __60__
   f. LXXX __80__

3. Reduce to lowest terms.
   a. 25/75 __1/3__
   b. 6/10 __3/5__
   c. 18/20 __9/10__
   d. 20/24 __5/6__
   e. 14/28 __1/2__
   f. 100/1000 __1/10__

4. Change to mixed or whole numbers. If answers contain fractions, reduce to lowest terms.
   a. 40/19 __2 2/19__
   b. 56/24 __2 1/3__
   c. 12/4 __3__
   d. 15/3 __5__
   e. 60/20 __3__
   f. 60/25 __2 2/5__

5. Change to improper fractions.
   a. 1 4/5 __9/5__
   b. 5 5/7 __40/7__
   c. 12 1/3 __37/3__
   d. 14 5/6 __89/6__
   e. 25 1/4 __101/4__
   f. 11 2/5 __57/5__

B. Fraction Problems. Reduce answers to lowest terms.

6. Addition
   a. 1/3 + 3/4 = __13/12__
   b. 1/9 + 2/3 + 1/6 = __17/18__
   c. 2 1/4 + 3/16 + 5/8 = __3 1/16__
   d. 2 1/5 + 3/20 + 3/10 = __2 13/20__
   e. 1 1/3 + 2 4/9 + 3 3/18 = __6 17/18__

25

Section 1 Review of Basic Mathematics

7. Subtraction
   a. 2 5/8 - 1 1/4 = __1 3/8__
   b. 14 1/4 - 12 5/16 = __15/16__
   c. 55 1/6 - 28 1/12 = __27 1/6__
   d. 5/6 - 1/4 = __7/12__
   e. 4/6 - 5/8 = __1/24__

8. Multiplication
   a. 1/4 x 5/8 = __5/32__
   b. 3/6 x 12/36 = __1/6__
   c. 4/9 x 3/8 = __1/8__
   d. 1/8 x 16/32 = __1/16__
   e. 4/5 x 3/8 = __3/10__

9. Division
   a. 1/3 ÷ 6/9 = __1/2__
   b. 1/25 ÷ 4/50 = __1/2__
   c. 3 1/3 ÷ 2 3/6 = __1 1/3__
   d. 40 ÷ 10 1/2 = __3 17/21__

C. Decimal Problems

10. Addition
    a. 1.224 + 0.30 + 421.5 = __423.024__
    b. 140.25 + .0035 + 2.150 = __142.4035__
    c. 1,000,321. + 2.25 + 0.15 = __1,000,323.400__
    d. .0036 + 1.4 + 2,001.0 = __2,001.4036__

11. Subtraction
    a. 55.5 - 50.3 = __5.2__
    b. 5.95 - 0.36 = __5.59__
    c. 40.15 - 15.60 = __24.55__
    d. 100.02 - 98.95 = __1.07__

12. Multiplication
    a. 10.5 x .05 = __.525__
    b. 25.2 x 1.5 = __37.80__
    c. 1.15 x 2.55 = __2.9325__
    d. 100.25 x .5 = __50.125__

13. Division
    a. 250 ÷ 1.5 = __166.__
    b. 7.5 ÷ .05 = __150__
    c. 80. ÷ 6.4 = __8__
    d. 2.25 ÷ .2 = __11.25__

14. Identify the larger decimal by encircling it.
    a. (.50) or .050
    b. (.75) or .725
    c. .0385 or (.04)
    d. (1.45) or .145

D. Conversion Problems

15. Convert each to a fraction and a ratio.
    a. .02% __1/5,000__   __1:5,000__
    b. .3   __3/10__   __3:10__
    c. .08   __8/10__   __8:10__
    d. .5   __5/10__   __5:10__
    e. .15   __15/10__   __15:10__

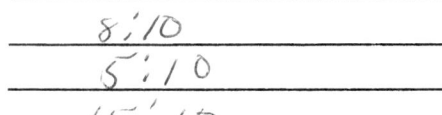

26

16. Change percent to: ratio, fraction, and decimal. (Reduce ratios and fractions to lowest terms.)
    a. 10% .10   1/10   1:10
    b. 20% .20   20/10   20:10
    c. 25% .25   25/10   25:10
    d. 50% .50   50/10   50:10
    e. 75% .75   75/10   75:10

17. Convert to Fahrenheit and Celsius degrees, as indicated.
    a. 230°F. 110   C
    b. 21°C   69.8   F.
    c. 5°C   41   F.
    d. 40°C   104   F.
    e. 100°F. 37.8   C
    f. 98.6°F. 37   C

E. Ratio-Proportion Problems

18. Find the unknown factor.
    a. x:4 :: 1:12   x = 1/3
    b. 500:x :: 5:25   x = 2500
    c. 1:250 :: x:500   x = 2
    d. 1/2:1000 :: x:500 x = 4
    e. 6:18 :: x:24   x = 6
    f. 5:15 :: x:60   x = 20
    g. 4:28 :: x:84   x = 12
    h. 9:36 :: x:72   x = 18
    i. 1/3:x :: 6:18   x = 1
    j. 7:x :: 14:28   x = 14
    k. 5:15 :: 10:x   x = 30
    l. 4:20 :: x:25   x = 5

Section 2 Calculations of Doses and Solutions

Unit 6 Symbols and Measurement

OBJECTIVES

After studying this unit, the student should be able to:

- Recognize and define metric terms of measurement.
- Differentiate between terms used in metric, apothecaries, and household measures.
- Convert measurements of weight and volume in metric, apothecaries, and household systems.
- Correctly identify and write all symbols and abbreviations described in this unit.

In order to begin working with problems in drugs and solutions, it is imperative that the basic arithmetic problems in the preceding section have been satisfactorily completed. The achievement review results will show where more study is needed. Only by study of the basic rules so that they are thoroughly understood, and application of these rules, can the nurse be able to solve the more complicated problems; those which involve calculation of dosages and preparation of solutions.

Once the nurse has learned the basic mathematics, understanding of the metric, apothecaries and household systems of measurement must be mastered.

THE METRIC SYSTEM

The international standard of measurement is the Metric System. Conversion to this system is taking place in medicine and nursing as well as in other areas. The metric measures pertain chiefly to length, weight, volume and temperature. (The conversion of temperature readings from Fahrenheit to Celsius degrees was covered in the preceding unit. The Celsius temperature, previously referred to as the centigrade temperature, is a metric measurement.)

The *meter* is the basic unit of *Length*. A meter is 39.37 inches long. A decimeter therefore, would be 3.94 inches long. A centimeter would be about 0.39 inches long; a millimeter would be about .04 inches long. Meters are not used in drugs and solutions but members of the health team often find reference to this unit in laboratory reports, charts and other data requiring linear measurements. Also, it is conceivable that references to tubing length may eventually be made a part of procedure instructions such as: "insert the rectal tube about one decimeter" (instead of 4 inches). However, these measures of length have not yet been widely used in metric outside of the laboratories. The student must be aware of this trend toward international use of the metric system.

The *gram* is the basic unit of *Weight* (or mass). A measure of weight tells how heavy an item is. A gram weighs about the same as one milliliter of water (1 ml) or about 15 grains.

The *liter* is the basic unit of *Volume*. This measure tells us how much space an item occupies. The liter is used for liquid measures. It is about the same as one quart or 1000 milliliters or the volume occupied by 2.2 pounds of distilled water at 4°C.

For practical purposes, a milliliter is considered equivalent to a cubic centimeter. Both terms belong to the terminology of the metric system; however, *milliliter* is the accurate and preferred term for the liquid measurements.

Briefly, the general terms which refer to the metric system are grams, liters, and meters (*and their prefixes*). It is important to keep this in mind when converting dosages to the metric system.

Prefixes, such as those shown below demonstrate the definite relationships to the measure.

  kilo = 1000.   (one thousand)
  milli = .001   (one-thousandth)
  centi = .01   (one-hundredth)
  deci = .1   (one-tenth)

Since the metric system is based on 10 and multiples of 10 (100, 1000, etc.) the measurements can be expressed in decimals, and decimals can be used in the calculations. Fractions should preferably be changed to their decimal equivalents when working with the metric system. (The unit on Decimals and Fractions should be reviewed at this time.) Metric units of measure are shown in figure 6-1. Weight is used for dry and Volume is used for liquid measurements.

To express one unit of measure in terms of the next *smaller* unit, *multiply* by 1000. Therefore, 2 grams equals 2000 milligrams and 0.5 grams equals 500 milligrams.

To express one unit of measure in terms of the next *larger* unit, *divide* by 1000. Therefore, 2 milligrams equals .002 grams and 50 milligrams equals 0.05 grams.

WEIGHT	VOLUME	LENGTH
1 kilogram (kg) = 1000 grams	1 kiloliter (kl) = 1000 liters	1 kilometer (km) = 1000 meters
1 gram (Gm) = 1000 milligrams	1 liter (L) = 1000 milliliter (ml)	
1 milligram (mg) = 1000 micrograms (mcg or µg)	or 1000 cubic centimeters (cc or cm^3)	1 meter (m) = 1000 millimeters (mm)

Figure 6-1 The Metric System

Practice Problems

1. a. How many milligrams are in 4.25 grams? In 42 1/2 grams? _4250 – 42500_
   b. How many milliliters are in 2 liters? In 1/5 liter? _2000 – 200_
   c. What part of a liter is 250 milliliters? 25 milliliters? _1/4 (.25) 1/40 (.025)_
   d. What part of a milligram is 80 micrograms? 800 micrograms? _8/100 (.08) 8/10 (.8)_

Section 2 Calculation of Doses and Solutions

2. Write the following measurements in the metric system.
   a. one thousand milliliters _1000 mL_
   b. one-quarter milligram _.25 mgm_
   c. five milligrams _5 mgm_
   d. six-tenths gram _.6 Gm_
   e. twelve and five-tenths grams _12.5 Gm_
   f. one-half milliliter _.5 ml_

THE APOTHECARIES' SYSTEM

Most hospitals have replaced the apothecaries' system with the metric; however, the latter is still used at times, figure 6-2. The student will recognize that some apothecaries' measurements are also used as household measures. However, it should be noted that this system shows 12 ounces making up one pound.

As there will be occasions when the apothecaries' system is still used, the symbols and abbreviations must be learned so that the prescribed dose for the patient is recognized and converted when necessary. Lack of knowledge about these symbols and abbreviations can result in danger for the patient. Sometimes, death may occur as the result of an accidental overdose; for example, giving a patient an ounce instead of a dram of a prescribed liquid medication. On the other hand, giving less than the prescribed dose may harm the patient by delaying his recovery. ACCURACY IN THE ADMINISTRATION OF MEDICATIONS CANNOT BE OVEREMPHASIZED. THE PATIENT'S LIFE MAY DEPEND ON IT.

Abbreviations and Symbols

Frequently used symbols and abbreviations in the apothecaries' system are:

m for minim   qt for quart

℈ or dr for dram   gal or C for gallon

℥ or oz for ounce   lb for pound

O or pt for pint

WEIGHT (Dry)	VOLUME (Wet)
60 grains = 1 dram (4 Gm) 480 grains = 1 ounce (30 Gm) 8 drams = 1 ounce (30 Gm) 12 ounces = 1 pound (360 Gm)	60 minims = 1 fluid dram (4 ml) 480 minims = 1 fluid ounce (30 ml) 8 fluid drams = 1 fluid ounce (30 ml) 16 fluid ounces = 1 pint (500 ml) 32 fluid ounces = 1 quart (1000 ml or 1 L) 4 quarts = 1 gallon (4000 ml or 4 L)

Figure 6-2 Apothecaries System (showing Metric approximates)

In this system, Roman numerals are used when writing numbers of less than 100. Arabic numbers are used for numbers over 100, for fractions, and for mixed numbers. The abbreviation $\overline{ss}$ is used, however, to indicate one-half. The following rules and examples will clarify the explanation:

- The unit of measure is written *before* the number; e.g. dram.
- The symbol for the unit of measure is used; otherwise, the abbreviation may precede the number; e.g. ℨ or dr.
- The number is written in small Roman numerals. ℨii̇̇
- A line is drawn over the numerals.
- When using the Roman numeral one, a dot is placed over the number (i̇).

Example: The unit of measure is dram.
The symbol for dram is ℨ
The abbreviation for dram is *dr*
Two drams may be written as ℨii̇̇

Example: The unit of measure is grain
There is no symbol for grain
The abbreviation for grain is *gr*
Twelve grains may be written as gr $\overline{xii}$

Practice Problems

3. Identify each of the following measurements.
   a. gr i̇i̇i̇   *3 grains*
   b. ℨ x̄v̇ı̇   *16 drams*
   c. m x̄i̇x̄   *19 minims*
   d. ℨ s̄s̄   *one half ounce*
   e. gr x̄x̄x̄   *30 grains*
   f. oz ı̇x̄   *9 ounces*

4. Use the appropriate symbols, abbreviations and Roman numerals in the following:
   a. 4 ounces   *ℨ ĪV̄*
   b. 8 grains   *gr. V̄IIĪ*
   c. 2 1/4 pints   *O Iİ 1/4*
   d. 15 minims   *m X̄V̄*
   e. 1/2 grain   *gr. s̄s̄*

5. Answer the following.
   a. How many ounces are in 2 apothecary pounds?   *24*
   b. How many grains are in ℨs̄s̄?   *30*
   c. How many ounces are in ℨx̄L̄?   *5*
   d. How many drams are in ℨx̄?   *80*
   e. How many minims are in 6 fluid drams?   *360*
   f. How many minims are in ℨs̄s̄?   *30*

Section 2 Calculations of Doses and Solutions

HOUSEHOLD MEASURES

The household measures are used primarily in the home. As this system gives only approximate measurements, it is seldom used in medicine. However, patients on intake and output surveillance need accurate reporting and members of the health team should know these measurements. Also, patients who must take medicine at home and others who need to administer liquids to them should be aware of these values, figure 6-3.

Drop (gtt.) =	approximate liquid measure depending on kind of liquid measured and the size of the opening from which it is dropped.
60 drops	1 teaspoon (tsp.)
1 dash	Less than 1/8 teaspoon
4 teaspoons	1 tablespoon (tbsp.)
2 tablespoons	1 ounce (oz)
4 ounces	1 juice glass
6 ounces	1 teacup
8 ounces	1 glass
16 tablespoons or 8 ounces	1 measuring cup (c.)
2 cups	1 pint (pt)
2 pints	1 quart (qt)
4 quarts	1 gallon (gal)

Figure 6-3 Common Household Measures

HOUSEHOLD		METRIC (Dry)		APOTHECARIES'
	=	0.060 gram or 60 milligrams	=	1 grain
1/8 teaspoon	=	0.5 gram (Gm)	=	7 1/2 grains
1/4 teaspoon	=	1.0 gram	=	15 grains
1 teaspoon	=	4 grams	=	60 grains or 1 dram
1 tablespoon	=	15 grams	=	4 drams
2 tablespoons	=	30 grams	=	1 ounce
2.2 pounds	=	1 kilogram		

Figure 6-4 Equivalent Dry Measures

HOUSEHOLD		METRIC (Liquid)		APOTHECARIES'
1 drop (gtt.)	=	0.060 milliliter	=	1 minim
15 drops	=	1 milliliter (1 cubic centimeter)	=	15 minims
1 teaspoon (tsp.)	=	4 milliliters	=	1 fluid dram
1 dessert spoon	=	8 milliliters	=	2 fluid drams
8 teaspoons or 2 tablespoons (tbsp.)	=	30 milliliters	=	1 fluid ounce
1 juice glass	=	120 milliliters	=	4 fluid ounces
2 measuring cups	=	500 milliliters	=	1 pint
4 measuring cups	=	1000 milliliters or 1 liter	=	1 quart or 2 pints

Figure 6-5 Equivalent Liquid Measures

Equivalent Weights and Measures

By mastering the weights and volumes given in figures 6-4 and 6-5, it will be possible to convert measurements from one system to another. This process is necessary to calculate dosages and prepare solutions.

When converting from one system to another, *multiply* to find the smaller measure.

Example: How many milliliters are in 3 drams?
    1 dr = 4 ml   4 x 3 = 12 ml

Example: How many milligrams are in 3 grains?
    1 gr = 60 mg   60 x 3 = 180 mg

When converting from one system to another, *divide* to find the larger measure.

Example: How many grams are in 30 grains?
    15 gr = 1 Gm   30 ÷ 15 = 2

Example: How many milliliters are in 6 minims?
    1 ml = 15 m.   6 ÷ 15 or 15)6.0 = 0.4   0.4 ml

Practice Problems

6. Convert the following household measures to milliliters. Remember to change fractions to decimals.
    a. 20 gtts. *1.2 ml*   b. 3 tsp. *12 ml*   c. 1 1/2 c. *375 ml*

7. Convert the following apothecaries' measures to milliliters.
    a. m. x̄ *.6 ml*   c. ℥ v *150 ml*
    b. ℥ iii *12 ml*   d. 0 ss *250 ml*

8. Convert the following metric measures to apothecaries' or household measures as indicated.
    a. 8 Gm = *2* tsp.   b. 10 Gm = *1/3* oz.   c. 75 mg = *1 1/4* gr

9. Indicate which of the following measurements may be considered equal by placing a checkmark in the space provided.
    a. 1 cc = 1 ml ✓   d. 1 ml = 1 Gm ✓
    b. 1 mcg = 1 m. _____   e. 1 kg = 1 L   ✓
    c. 1 L = 1 lb _____

PROBLEMS IN WEIGHT IN KILOGRAMS

Weight expressed in kilograms is frequently requested before basal metabolism tests or before anesthesia.

- To change pounds to kilograms, divide the weight in pounds by 2.2. There are 2.2 pounds in one kilogram.

Example: Weight in pounds is 132. What is the weight in kilograms?
    132 ÷ 2.2 = 60.0 kg

Section 2 Calculations of Doses and Solutions

Practice Problems — divide by 2.2
10. a. 184 lbs = __83.6__ kilograms
    b. 210 lbs = __95.5__ kilograms
    c. 85 lbs = __38.6__ kilograms
    d. 54 lbs = __24.5__ kilograms

- To change kilograms to pounds, multiply the kilogram weight by 2.2.

Example: 25 kilograms x 2.2 = 55 lbs

Practice Problems multiply by 2.2
11. a. 30 kilograms = __66__ lbs   c. 65 kilograms = __143__ lbs
    b. 45 kilograms = __99__ lbs   d. 75 kilograms = __165__ lbs

Unit 7 Methods of Calculating Dosages

OBJECTIVES

After studying this unit, the student should be able to:
- Calculate the amount of oral medication to be given from stock solutions.
- Calculate insulin dosage according to a syringe calibrated in units.
- Calculate dosage for an injection in terms of the strength of the drug on hand.

Medications are available in fixed forms, prescription bottles, and stock bottles. The nurse should be able to interpret the labels on these preparations in terms of the dosage prescribed for her patients.

FIXED FORMS

The fixed or prepackaged form means that each separate dose has been measured and labelled by the pharmacist or by the drug manufacturer. However, if the dosage *ordered* happens to be larger or smaller than the fixed form, the nurse must determine the proper multiple as ordered. For example, if the fixed form is phenobarbital 15 mg and a 45-mg dose is ordered, three 15-mg tablets are given. When the dosage ordered is smaller than the fixed form, the proportion must be determined; if a tablet is scored, it is simple to break it along the scored line and administer half the tablet. However, *if a tablet is not scored, do not attempt to break it to give a fraction of it.* Obtain the medication in a dosage form (smaller tablet, liquid preparation, etc.) which can be measured accurately.

PRESCRIPTION BOTTLES

The prescription bottle of liquid medicine is usually ordered in drams, ounces or minims. Patients in the home usually have liquid prescriptions ordered in household or utensil dosage such as teaspoons and tablespoons. Since household measures are approximate measures, the physician may request that the dosage be measured in a calibrated medicine dropper, minim glass, or medicine glass, figure 7-1. Disposable medicine glasses are available. The figure illustrates metric, apothecaries and household measures.

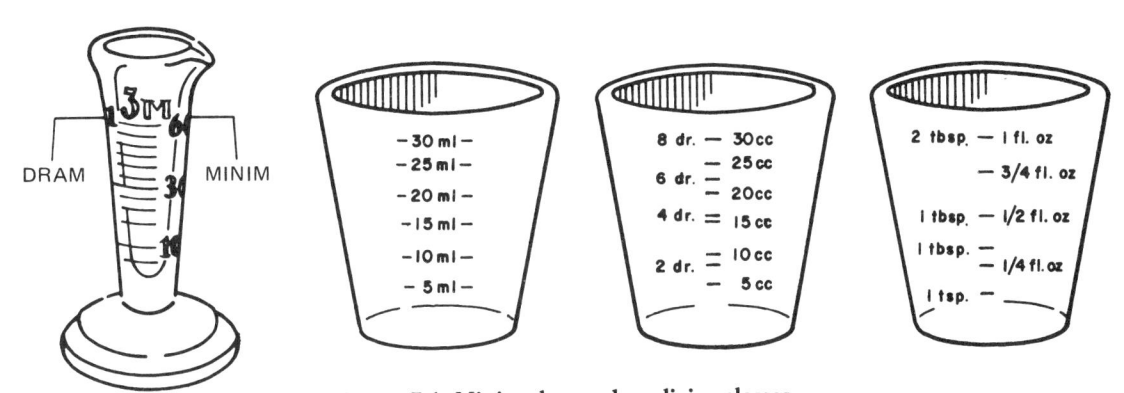

Figure 7-1 Minim glass and medicine glasses

Section 2 *Calculations of Doses and Solutions*

STOCK BOTTLES

Stock bottles contain large quantities of medicines; buying in large quantities reduces the cost of the medication. The label on the bottle gives the *strength* of the solution, or the amount of the drug per cubic centimeter, milliliter, dram, unit, or ounce. For example, the label on the bottle might indicate: 1 ml = gr 1/8. The proportion method is used to determine the correct amount of the solution. (Additional problems will be analyzed and discussed in the next unit.)

Example: Morphine sulfate gr 1/4 is ordered. The stock bottle contains many doses. The label on the bottle reads: 1 ml = gr 1/8. How much should be given?

Proportion method (reviewed in Unit 4): Prescribed drug is to the desired amount as the amount solute (drug) is to the stock solution.

1/4 gr:X :: 1/8 gr:1ml

1/8X = 1/4

X = 1/4 ÷ 1/8 or 1/4 x 8/1

X = 8/4 or 2 ml

Practice Problems

1. Calculate the amount of stock solution to be given in each of the following.
   a. Give atropine sulfate, gr 1/150.
      (The stock label reads 15 ml = 1/100 gr) __10 ml__
   b. Give terramycin suspension 0.75 Gm.
      (The stock label reads 5 ml = 250 mg) __15 ml__
   c. Give chloral hydrate gr x̄.
      (The stock label reads 5 ml = 0.3 Gm) __10 ml__
   d. Give elixir of phenobarbital gr s̄s̄.
      (The stock label reads 1 ml = 4 mg) __7.5 ml__
   e. Give ferrous sulfate 200 mg.
      (The stock label reads 1 ml = 40 mg) __5 ml__

CALCULATING INSULIN DOSAGES

Dosages of insulin are based upon (1) the degree of diabetes present, (2) the amount of physical activity of the patient, (3) the weight of the patient, (4) his metabolic rate. Unit 30 on endocrine disorders will discuss the need for and effects of insulin.

It is extremely important that the exact dosage of insulin be administered. The loss of one or two units of insulin in measuring or injecting it can cause a severe upset in the patient. An overdose may lead to insulin shock while an underdose may lead the patient toward diabetic coma.

Insulin is always measured in units (U). If U 40 solution is ordered, the nurse uses a U 40, red-scaled syringe and U 40 solution of insulin. If U 80 solution is ordered, a U 80, green-scaled syringe is used and, preferably, U 80 insulin. The use of different syringes is not encouraged because of the danger of error. Confusion between syringes and solutions

Unit 7 Methods of Calculating Dosages

have resulted in grave errors. *The nurse must be alert to measurements and use the syringe which is calibrated for the solution prescribed.* (Rarely, there may be times when the correct syringe is not available, so that the nurse must measure a U 80 solution in a U 40 syringe and vice versa). Also, some syringes have markings of U 40 on one side and U 80 on the other.

Insulin is also manufactured in U 100 vials. In any case U 80, U 40, and U 20 are all calibrated to the 1 milliliter or cubic centimeter scale. U 80 is most often used as the strongest solution and U 20 as the weakest. For example, U 40 has half the strength of U 80, and U 20 has half the strength of U 40. If an order states that the patient is to receive U 30 of a U 40 solution of insulin, the nurse should use a U 40 syringe, and administer 30 units according to the scale on the syringe.

- If the nurse *must* give U 20 from a bottle labelled U 40 and has to use a U 80 syringe, it would be calculated as follows.

    Method 1
    Desired dose: U 20 Insulin   *[handwritten: DESIRED : HAVE :: X : Syringe]*
    Syringe on hand: U 80
    Solution on hand: U 40 Insulin
    $\dfrac{U\ 20 \times U\ 80}{U\ 40} = \dfrac{1600}{40} =$ U 40 to be given in the U 80 syringe

    Method 2: Proportion
    U 20:U 40 :: X:U 80
    40X = 1600
    $X = \dfrac{1600}{40} =$ U 40 to be given in the U 80 syringe.

CAUTION: The use of different syringes is not encouraged because of the chance for error. Correctly calibrated syringes are available. The subject has been covered because, on occasion, the appropriate syringe may not be on hand at the time the insulin must be administered.

Practice Problems

2. Show complete calculations for administration of the doses as prescribed by the physician and encircle the final answer.

    a. Insulin U xxx from U 80 solution, using a U 80 syringe.
       [handwritten: U 30 : U 80 :: X : U 80   80X = 2400   X = 30]

    b. Insulin U x from U 40 solution, using a U 40 syringe.
       [handwritten: U 10 : U 40 :: X : U 40   40X = 40   X = 10]

    c. Insulin U xx from U 80 solution, using a U 80 syringe.
       [handwritten: U 20 : U 80 :: X : U 80   80X = 1600   X = 20]

    d. Insulin U xx from U 40 solution, using a U 80 syringe.
       [handwritten: U 20 : U 40 :: X : U 80   40X = 1600   X = 40]

Section 2 Calculations of Doses and Solutions

CALCULATING HYPODERMIC SOLUTIONS

Drugs for hypodermic use are prepared by the manufacturer in the form of tablets, ampules, and rubber-stoppered vials. Stock solutions usually come in various strengths. No more than 2 milliliter may be given in a subcutaneous injection; no more than 5 milliliters may be given in an intramuscular injection.

The tablet form is popular because of the ease of accountability. If the proper strength tablet is available, it may simply be dissolved in sterile water, drawn up in a sterile syringe and administered. Always use water for injection, USP. *Never use tap or distilled water.*

A problem may arise when the proper strength tablet is not available. The nurse has to calculate the dosage from the strength of the tablet on hand. When the tablets on hand are not the prescribed dosage, the formulas in the following example are used to compute the correct dosage.

Example: Morphine sulfate 10 mg s.c. is ordered.
The tablets on hand are 15 mg.

Formula A

$$\frac{\text{amount desired}}{\text{amount on hand}} = \text{part of tablet to be used}$$

$$\frac{10}{15} = \frac{2}{3} \text{ of a tablet to be used.}$$

Formula B

To calculate the same problem by proportion:
10 mg: 15 mg :: X tablet: 1 tablet
15X = 10
$$X = \frac{10}{15} \text{ or } \frac{2}{3} \text{ tablet}$$

Since the tablet cannot be divided into fractions accurately, it must be dissolved in an amount of sterile water which can be measured accurately. The correct fractional amount of solution is then given to the patient. Remember that this amount should be no more than 2 ml (30 minims) for a subcutaneous injection and no more than 5 ml for an intramuscular injection. The following procedure is used to determine the amount of water to be used as a solvent. (Unit 17 discusses administration in detail.)

- Invert the fraction which expresses the part of the tablet to be used.

- Select the amount of solution to be given to the patient by choosing a number which is evenly divisible by the denominator of the inverted fraction and which is no more than should be given by the method of injection used. For example, 2 ml (shown also as 30 minims marked on syringes).

- Multiply the inverted fraction by the number of tablets to be used and by the amount of solution to be given to the patient. The answer is the amount of *solution solvent to be used, not administered.*

| Inverted fraction | x | Number tablets | x | Number ml to be given to patient | = | Number ml to be prepared |

38

Unit 7 Methods of Calculating Dosages

Example: Find the amount of water necessary to dissolve 2/3 tablet for a *subcutaneous* injection.

1. Invert the fraction. 2/3 inverted is 3/2.
2. Select the amount to be given to the patient. The amount 1.2 ml is within the range for subcutaneous injection, and it is evenly divisible by 2, the denominator of the inverted fraction.
3. Multiply to find the number of milliliters to be prepared. Note that 1.2 is changed to 1 2/10 for the purpose of calculation.

$$\frac{3}{2} \times 1 \text{ tablet} \times 1\frac{2}{10} \text{ ml (same as 18 minims)}$$

$$\frac{3}{{}_1\cancel{2}} \times \frac{1}{1} \times \frac{\cancel{12}^6}{10} = \frac{18}{10} \text{ or } 1\frac{8}{10} = 1.8 \text{ ml or cc}$$

One tablet is to be *dissolved* in 1.8 ml and *1.2 ml of this solution is to be drawn up in the syringe and administered to the patient.* (2/3 of the tablet).

Examples:

1. How would you give a subcutaneous injection of morphine sulfate 5 mg from 15 mg tablets?

    a. $\dfrac{\text{Amount desired}}{\text{Amount on hand}}$ = Part of the tablet to be used

    $\dfrac{D}{H} = \dfrac{5}{15} = \dfrac{1}{3}$ tablet

    b. Invert fraction. 1/3 inverted is 3/1.
    Choose amount (which will be given to the patient) and is divisible by denominator.

    c. Multiply.
    $\dfrac{3}{1} \times 1$ tablet $\times$ 1 ml = 3 ml amount of solvent

    d. One tablet is to be dissolved in 3 ml water, and 1 ml will be drawn up in the syringe and administered to the patient.

2. How would you administer a subcutaneous injection of Pantopon gr 1/4 when you have gr 1/3 tablets on hand?

    a. $\dfrac{\text{Amount desired}}{\text{Amount on hand}}$ = Part of tablet to be used

    $\dfrac{\frac{1}{4}}{\frac{1}{3}} = \dfrac{1}{4} \div \dfrac{1}{3} = \dfrac{1}{4} \times \dfrac{3}{1} = \dfrac{3}{4}$ tablet to be used

    b. Invert fraction. 3/4 inverted is 4/3.
    Choose amount divisible by denominator.

    c. Multiply.

    $\dfrac{4}{3} \times 1 \text{ tablet} \times 1\dfrac{2}{10} \text{ ml}$ $\dfrac{4}{{}_1\cancel{3}} \times \dfrac{1}{1} \times \dfrac{\cancel{12}^4}{10} = \dfrac{16}{10} = 1\dfrac{6}{10}$

Section 2 Calculations of Doses and Solutions

    d. One tablet is to be dissolved in 1.6 ml water, and 1.2 ml will be drawn up in the syringe and administered to the patient.

3. How would you administer an *intramuscular* injection of 6 mg if the tablets on hand are 4 mg?

    a. $\dfrac{\text{Amount desired}}{\text{Amount on hand}}$ = Part of tablets to be used

$$\frac{D}{H} = \frac{6}{4} = 1\frac{1}{2} \text{ tablets}$$

    b. Change mixed number to improper fraction and invert fraction.
       1 1/2 = 3/2. 3/2 inverted is 2/3.

    c. Choose amount divisible by denominator (e.g. 3 ml) and multiply.

$$\frac{2}{3} \times 2 \text{ tablets} \times 3 \text{ ml}$$

$$\frac{2}{\cancel{3}_1} \times \frac{2}{1} \times \frac{\cancel{3}^1}{1} = 4 \text{ ml}$$

    d. Two tablets will be dissolved in 4 ml water and 3 ml of this solution is to be drawn up in the syringe and administered to the patient.
    *Note that the amount of solution to be given is larger than in the previous examples because the intramuscular method of injection is ordered.

Practice Problems

Calculate the following dosages for hypodermic injection. Give (a) the number of tablets to be dissolved, (b) the amount of sterile water to be used as solvent, and (c) the amount of solution to be given to the patient.

3. The dose ordered is .12 mg s.c. The tablets on hand are .6 mg.
    a. _____1 Tab_____   b. _____1/5 Tab_____   c. _____1 CC OF WATER_____

4. The dose ordered is 15 mg I.M. The tablets on hand are 25 mg.
    a. _____1 Tab_____   b. _____5 CC_____   c. _____3 CC OF WATER_____

5. The dose ordered is 10 mg I.M. The tablets on hand are .03 Gm. Convert to milligrams before calculating.
    a. _____   b. _____   c. _____

6. The dose ordered is gr 1/60 s.c. The tablets on hand are .6 mg. Convert to milligrams before calculating.
    a. _____   b. _____   c. _____

Unit 8 Problems in Solutions

OBJECTIVES
After studying this unit, the student should be able to:
- Calculate the amount of pure drug needed to make a certain solution.
- Calculate the amount of stock solution needed to make a dilute solution.
- Calculate the amounts of solvent and solute in a solution of a given percentage.

A solution is a liquid preparation which contains a dissolved substance. It consists of a *solvent*, the liquid in which a substance is dissolved, and a *solute*, the substance added to the solvent. Solutions are usually made from stronger stock solutions or from pure drugs. Pure drugs may be in solid or liquid form. A pure drug is always considered 100-percent pure unless stated otherwise on the label.

MAKING SOLUTIONS WITH PURE DRUGS

The strength of a solution may be expressed according to the percent, weight, or volume of the active ingredient (solute). Two methods may be used to calculate the amount of solute needed to make a solution of a given strength.

Formula A is a simple method:

$$\frac{\text{strength desired}}{\text{strength on hand}} \times \text{Quantity desired} = \text{Amount of solute}$$

Formula B is the proportion method:

Amount of drug : Amount of desired solution :: Strength of desired solution : Strength on hand

Either formula may be used to find out the amount of pure drug needed to make a solution of a given percentage. Remember that a pure drug is 100-percent pure and, therefore, 100 is substituted in the formulas for strength on hand. For the purposes of calculation, 1 gram may be considered equal to 1 milliliter.

Example: How many grams of sodium bicarbonate are needed to prepare 1000 milliliters of a 5% solution?

Formula A

$$\frac{\text{Percent desired}}{\text{Percent on hand}} \times \text{Quantity desired} \quad (\text{or } \frac{D}{H} \times Q)$$

$$\frac{5}{100} \times 1000 \text{ ml} = 50 \text{ Gm sodium bicarbonate}$$

Section 2 Calculations of Doses and Solutions

Formula B

Amount of drug is to amount of desired solution as percent of desired solution is to percent on hand.

X Gm:1000 ml :: 5:100

100X = 5000

$X = \frac{5000}{100}$

X = 50 Gm sodium bicarbonate

Practice Problems

1. Using both formulas, find the amounts requested in the following problems.

    a. How many grams of potassium permanganate are needed to prepare 250 milliliters of a 2% solution? 5 gms - A

    b. How many grams of sodium chloride are needed to prepare 250 milliliters of a 1% saline solution? 2.5 - A

    c. How many grams of sodium chloride are needed to prepare 1 pint of a 5% solution? 25 gms - A

2. a. How much of a 25% stock solution of formaldehyde is needed to prepare 1 liter of a 2% solution? 80cc

    b. How much of an 80% stock solution of magnesium sulfate is needed to prepare 250 milliliters of a 20% solution? 62.5cc

    c. How many milliliters of a 50% stock solution are needed to prepare 1 gallon of a 4% formaldehyde solution? 320 ml.

42

Unit 8 Problems in Solutions

MAKING DILUTE SOLUTIONS FROM STOCK SOLUTIONS

Solutions are frequently diluted from stronger stock solutions. Again either formula may be used; D/H x Q or proportion method remembering that ratios must refer to similar items (see formula B below).

Example: How many milliliters of a 10% saline solution are needed to prepare 500 milliliters of a 2% solution?

Formula A

$$\frac{2}{\cancel{10}_1} \times \frac{\cancel{500}^{50}}{1} = 100 \text{ milliliters of 10\% saline}$$

Formula B

(Amount is to amount as percent is to percent)

X:500 :: 2:10

10X = 1000

$X = \frac{1000}{10}$

X = 100 ml

ADDING THE SOLUTE

When making solutions, subtract the amount of the drug from the volume of the completed solution in order to find out how much water or other solute should be added. Also, keep in mind that when making a solution from a stock solution you do *not* have a 100-percent drug.

Example: Prepare 1 gallon of a 4% formaldehyde solution from a 50% stock solution. Calculation shows that 320 milliliters of stock solution will be used. Subtract the volume of the stock solution required from the volume of 1 gallon (4000 ml) to determine the amount of water to be added.

$$\begin{array}{r} 4000 \text{ ml} \\ -320 \\ \hline 3680 \text{ ml} \end{array}$$

Practice Problems

3. a. How much water must be added to make 1 quart (1000 ml) of a 2% solution if 20 Gm of sodium bicarbonate is in the solution at the time?

[Handwritten answer: 980 ml. Solution − Solvent = Solute. 1000 − 20 = 980 ml]

Section 2 *Calculations of Doses and Solutions*

3. b. If 100 Gm of sodium chloride is used to make 1000 ml of a 10% saline solution, how much water must be added?

$$\begin{array}{r} 1000 \\ \underline{100} \\ 900\,ml \end{array}$$

Solution
− solvent
Solute

c. How much water must be added to 100 ml of a 10% solution to make 1 pint (500 cc) of a 2% solution?

$$\begin{array}{r} 500 \\ \underline{-100} \\ 400\,ml \end{array}$$

Solution
− Solvent
Solute

44

Unit 9 Calculating Children's Dosages

OBJECTIVES

After studying this unit, the student should be able to:
- Calculate children's dosages by Young's rule, Fried's rule, and Clark's rule.
- Select the proper rule to use based on age and size of the child.

Children's dosages are calculated according to age and weight. They are naturally only a portion of an adult dosage. It is possible to calculate the child's dosage from the given adult dose. Three major rules are used for this calculation.

CAUTION: Whenever dosages involve using a capsule or a small fraction of a tablet, do not try to break the tablet or capsule. Refer such problems to the pharmacy so that a more accurate form of dosage may be obtained. Also, remember that barbiturates and narcotics are *rarely* ordered for children.

I. Young's Rule

$$\frac{\text{age of child}}{\text{age of child} + 12} \times \text{average adult dosage} = \text{child's dose}$$

Example: What dosage will be given to a 3-year old child when the adult dose is 50 mg?

$$\frac{3}{3 + 12} \times 50$$

$$\frac{3}{15} \times 50 = \frac{150}{15} = 10 \text{ mg}$$

$$\frac{\cancel{3}^1}{\cancel{15}_5} \times \cancel{50}^{10} = 10 \text{ mg is the child's dose}$$

(The child's dose in this case is 1/5 of the adult dose.)

II. Fried's Rule is used for calculation of infant dosage under two years of of age. It may be used for older children.

$$\frac{\text{age in months}}{150} \times \text{adult dose} = \text{infant's dose}$$

Example: What dosage will be given to a 15-month old infant when the adult dose is 50 mg?

$$\frac{15}{150} \times 50 \text{ mg}$$

$$\frac{1}{10} \times 50 = 5 \text{ mg is the child's dose}$$

(The child's dose in this case is 1/10 of the adult's dose.)

Section 2 Calculations of Doses and Solutions

    III.   Clark's Rule

$$\frac{\text{child's weight in pounds}}{150} \times \text{adult dose} = \text{child's dose}$$

Example: Do the same problem using the child's weight instead of age. The adult dose is 50 mg. What dosage will be given to a 24-pound child?

$$\frac{24}{150} \times 50 \text{ mg} = 8 \text{ mg child's dosage}$$

Practice Problems

Calculate the following, using the proper rule.

1. If the adult dose of tincture of digitalis is 1 ml, how much will be given to a 50-pound child?

2. The adult dose of Gantrisin® is 2 Gm for a maintenance dose. What will be the dosage of Gantrisin® for a 12-year old child?

3. The adult dosage of castor oil is ʒi . What amount of castor oil should be given to a 4-year old child?

4. The adult dose of potassium iodide is 15 drops. What dosage will be given to a 3-year old child?

5. The oral dosage of hykinone (vitamin K) is 2 mg. What dose will be given to a 12-year old child?

6. If the adult dosage of morphine sulfate is 10 mg, what will the dose be for a 3-year old child?

7. A 20-pound infant has been ordered a dose of cortisone acetate. If the adult dosage is 150 mg, what will the child's dose be?

8. If the adult dose of phenobarbital is 30 mg b.i.d., what is the dosage for a 25-pound infant?

Achievement Review 2

Section 2 Calculations of Doses and Solutions

1. Convert to milliliters.
   a. ℨiv = __16__
   b. ℨviii = __32__
   c. ℨxii = __48__
   d. ℨxvi = __64__

2. Convert to grams.
   a. gr 30 = __2__
   b. gr 45 = __3__
   c. gr 60 = __4__
   d. gr 75 = __5__

3. Convert to grams.
   a. ℨii = __60__
   b. ℨiv = __120__
   c. ℨvi = __180__
   d. ℨviii = __240__

4. Convert to milligrams.
   a. gr 1/4 = __15__
   b. gr 1/2 = __30__
   c. gr 5 = __300__
   d. gr 10 = __600__

5. Convert to minims.
   a. 1 ml = __15__
   b. 2 ml = __30__
   c. 4 ml = __60__
   d. 5 ml = __75__

6. Convert to drams.
   a. 4 ml = __1__
   b. 16 ml = __4__
   c. 12 ml = __3__
   d. 32 ml = __8__

7. Convert to ounces.
   a. 30 Gm = __1__
   b. 60 Gm = __2__
   c. 90 Gm = __3__
   d. 120 Gm = __4__

8. Convert to grains.
   a. 15 mg = __1/4__
   b. 30 mg = __1/2__
   c. 60 mg = __1__
   d. 120 mg = __2__

9. Express in kilograms.
   a. 260 lbs = __118.1__
   b. 145 lbs = __65.9__
   c. 96 lbs = __43.6__
   d. 38 lbs = __17.3__

Achievement Review

10. Show complete calculations in the following problems to determine what amount should be given to the patient.

   a. The ordered dose of potassium iodide is 2 Gm. The dosage on hand is labelled .5 Gm = 1 ml. The patient should be given

   b. The doctor orders caffeine sodium benzoate gr $\ddot{\overline{11}}$ by hypodermic. The ampule on hand is labelled 0.5 Gm = 2 ml.

   c. Cortisone acetate, 80 mg is ordered. The label reads 25 mg = 1 ml.

   d. Penicillin, U 50,000, I.M., is ordered. The label reads U 20,000 = 1 ml.

   e. The physician has ordered gr $\overline{x}$ of aspirin. If the stock bottle reads aspirin 0.3 Gm, how much is given?

Section 2 Calculations of Doses and Solutions

11. a. If the adult dosage of enteric coated Chlor-trimeton is 10 mg q4h, calculate the dosage for a 6-year old child.

    b. The adult dosage of dramamine is 50 mg q4h as needed. What will be the dosage for a 60-pound child?

    c. If the adult dosage of bonamine is 25 mg b.i.d., what will be the dosage for a 15-month child?

    d. If the adult dosage of paregoric is 10 ml, what dosage should be given to an 8-year old child?

12. a. Prepare to give morphine sulfate gr 1/6 s.c. from the stock vial which reads 1 ml = gr 1/8.

Achievement Review

b. The label on the insulin vial reads 1 ml contains U 40. Calculate the number of milliliters there will be in U 15.

c. Prepare to give 30 units of insulin from the vial which reads 1 ml contains 40 Units. What will you give?

d. Calculate the number of milliliters needed to give 250,000 units from a penicillin vial which is labelled 500,000 units per cc. Convert your answer to minims, also.

13. Complete the following for liquid measures.
    a. One liter is _____ milliliters or _____ quart(s).
    b. One ounce is _____ milliliters or _____ tablespoon(s).
    c. One fluid dram is _____ milliliters.
    d. Sixty milliliters is _____ fluid ounces.
    e. One full teacup is _____ milliliters or _____ ounce(s).
    f. One full eight-ounce glass is _____ milliliters.
    g. One pint is _____ milliliters.
    h. Sixty drops is _____ minims or _____ dram(s) or _____ milliliters.

14. Complete the following for weight measures.
    a. One kilogram is equal to _____ pounds.
    b. Thirty milligrams is _____ grain(s).
    c. Thirty grams is _____ grain(s) or _____ dram(s) or _____ ounce(s).
    d. One milligram is _____ gram.
    e. One gram is _____ milligrams.

Section 2 Calculations of Doses and Solutions

15. Match Columns A and B by placing the item from Column B in its correct area in Column A.

Column A	Column B
_____ a. 1 dram	1) 240 milliliters
_____ b. 1 grain	2) 1 kilogram
_____ c. 1 ounce	3) 30 milliliters
_____ d. 15 grains	4) 1 milligram
_____ e. 15 minims	5) 1000 milliliters
_____ f. 6 ounces	6) 1 kiloliter
_____ g. 2.2 pounds	7) 1 gram
_____ h. 1 quart	8) 60 milligrams
_____ i. 1/60 grain	9) 1 meter
_____ j. 8 ounces	10) 4 milliliters
	11) 1 milliliter
	12) 180 milliliters

16. a. Prepare 1 liter of 5% magnesium sulfate solution from stock crystals. How much water will be added to make the desired 1000 ml of solution? How many grams?

    b. Prepare 2000 ml of a 1:1000 solution of zepharin from a 10% stock solution. Indicate how much stock solution and how much water is needed.

Section 3 Administration of Medications

Unit 10 Drug Sources, Standards, and Dosages

OBJECTIVES

After studying this unit, the student should be able to:

- Give examples of drugs obtained from plant, animal, mineral, and synthetic sources.
- List common sources for drug listings and summarize the information given in them.
- Identify selected federal legislation regulating the manufacture, advertising, sale, and prescription of drugs.
- Define specific terms which describe dosages.

A drug is a substance or mixture of substances which has been found by clinical experience to be of definite value in the diagnosis and treatment of disease. Drugs cure diseases, or they may merely assist the body to overcome its own difficulties. Drugs are also valuable in helping to formulate diagnoses by outlining areas of internal organs to be x-rayed. Other drugs are used as preventive substances such as dilantin sodium which, if regularly taken, will prevent epileptic seizures in the average case. Vaccines of various types are also used to prevent certain diseases. Antibiotics, such as penicillin, are used to cure or help nature overcome an infection.

There were no standards for the preparation of drugs until comparatively recent times. The strength and pureness of a drug in the beginnings of drug preparation varied with the individual producer. Dosages prescribed were usually based on little or no scientific research. All this has changed with our modern approach to drugs.

SOURCES OF DRUGS

The beginnings of drug preparation date back many centuries. Principal sources for remedies were herbs, roots, bark, and other forms of plant life. These remedies, for the most part, were prepared in a powder form and then added to a liquid so that they could be administered orally. Poultices, and lotions were prepared from plant leaves and the fats or secretions from certain species of animals for the purposes of local application. Such sources are also used for obtaining our present-day drugs, but others have been added.

Section 3 Administration of Medications

Plants

Many plants contain properties which are of medicinal value. These properties may come from the plant root, stem, leaves, or fruit. Following are examples of plant drug sources.

The leaf of purple foxglove is a source for digitalis. Preparations from digitalis leaf are the most frequently ordered heart tonic or stimulant.

The seed of the castor bean plant is a source from which castor oil is extracted. It is commonly used as an irritant cathartic.

The whole plant of kelp, a brown algae, grows in salt water and is a rich source of iodine, figure 10-1. Iodine is essential in treating simple goiter.

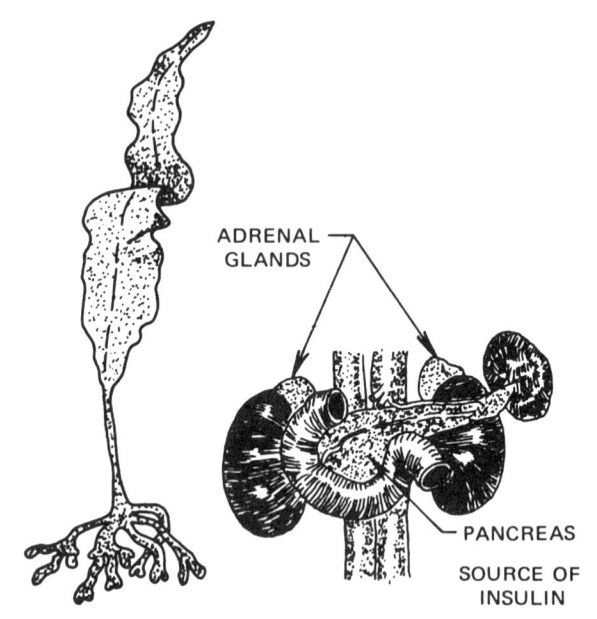

Fig. 10-1 Kelp   Fig. 10-2 Animal Drug Source

Animals

A number of essential extracts are obtained from animal tissues; the pancreas and adrenal glands are two examples, figure 10-2.

Insulin is obtained from the pancreas of cows and hogs. Its purpose is to aid in the utilization of blood sugar by the tissues. It also controls the level of the blood sugar. As a drug, it is used in the treatment of a condition known as diabetes mellitus. Although it does not cure diabetes, insulin is essential to the life of a diabetic when needed; in cases where the condition can be controlled by diet, the drug may not be necessary.

Adrenalin and cortisone are extracted from the adrenal gland. Adrenalin is a powerful heart stimulant. Cortisone is used in the treatment of rheumatoid arthritis, skin conditions, etc.

Minerals

Many naturally occurring mineral substances are used in medicine in a highly purified form. Sulphur, a nonmetallic element, and coal tar, a derivative of coal, are examples of mineral sources for drugs. After careful processing sulphur is used as a constituent of the sulfa drug family. The sulfa drugs, now prepared synthetically, have widespread use in the treatment of many types of infections.

Synthetic Drugs

Synthetic or chemically compounded (artificially prepared) medicine is another source for drugs. This source differs from the others in that artificial means are used to produce the drug as compared to the natural origin of other sources. In this process, a drug is obtained by combining a number of ingredients by scientific means. The result may be a drug which is the same as a natural drug, or it may be an entirely new substance.

For example, Chloromycetin is a drug now being chemically compounded; formerly it was produced only by natural means. An example of a drug which is obtained only by synthetic means is Sulfathiazole. Mineral sources are used in its preparation but, when chemically compounded, a new substance is produced. This new substance is not obtainable from any other source. The advantage of this synthetic method is that the medicines produced are usually less expensive and can be produced in a much greater volume.

DRUG LEGISLATION

The Federal Food, Drug, and Cosmetic Act

This law is enforced by the Food and Drug Administration of the Department of Health, Education, and Welfare. Its purpose is "to prohibit the movement in interstate commerce of adulterated and misbranded food, drugs, devices, and cosmetics." The act has been amended so that it now controls certification of insulin and antibiotics.

The Durham-Humphrey amendment of 1951 specifies which drugs must be dispensed by prescription and which may be sold over the counter.

The Kefauver-Harris amendment of 1962 requires that a new drug must be effective for the use intended and must be safe for use. It further requires that any adverse effects of new drugs be reported to the F.D.A. The 1962 amendment also requires that the generic name on drug labels must appear in type at least one-half as large as the trade name of the drug.

The Drug Abuse Control Amendments of 1965 (Harris Bill) strengthens interstate and intrastate control of the Federal Food, Drug, and Cosmetic Act over stimulants and depressants because of the danger of drug abuse.

In the early 1900's, it became necessary for federal legislation because of the increase in the use of chemicals in medicine. In order to protect the public, drug laws were enacted. Over the years, amendments were added to the early laws and new laws were made.

Social Security Amendments

There are many amendments pertaining to health care. Besides provisions for Medicare and Medicaid coverage, specific statements are included relating to persons who may dispense medications. For example,

> Item 1: Only (a) a licensed physician or a registered professional nurse or (b) under the direct supervision of a registered professional nurse, a licensed practical nurse, a student nurse in an approved school of nursing, or a psychiatric technician are permitted to administer medications and, in all instances, *in accordance with the Nurse Practice Act of each State.*
>
> Item 2: All medical orders are in writing and signed by the physician. Telephone orders are used sparingly, are given only to the registered professional nurse, and are signed or initialed by the physician as soon as possible.

Controlled Substance Act of 1970

This law controls the manufacture, importation, compounding, selling, dealing in and giving away of opium, cocaine, and their derivatives. It has replaced the Harrison Narcotic Act and includes harmful substances (e.g. LSD) in addition to narcotics. The nurse must

Section 3 Administration of Medications

keep an exact record of all narcotics and derivatives administered to patients. Missing narcotics must be reported to the nurse in charge immediately.

STANDARDIZATION OF DRUGS

The United States Pharmacopeia (U.S.P.) and The National Formulary (N.F.) require that drugs meet certain standards for purity and freedom from harmful contaminating substances, but they must also meet rigid standards as to the actual potency of the drug.

The active ingredient of a drug is determined by chemical analysis of assay. Some drugs cannot be satisfactorily analyzed chemically. The content, therefore, must be determined by testing it on animals. This method of testing is called bioassay. Insulin is standardized in this way. Drugs are also standardized by radioactive tagging. These drugs give off rays which have penetrating powers and must be tagged and identified.

Reasons for Standardization

Drugs are standardized in order that physicians ordering the drug can be guaranteed of its potency and purity. The United States Pharmacopeia and The National Formulary require that all drugs listed have been tested by the drug houses which manufacture the drugs. This requirement protects the doctor and his patient from substandard or substituted chemicals and assures that the potency of the drugs will be maintained at a constant level.

The 1962 amendment to the Federal Food, Drug, and Cosmetic Act, also known as the Kefauver-Harris Amendment, now requires that a new drug not only be safe for use, but also that it be effective for the purpose intended. Any adverse effects of a drug must be reported to the Federal Drug Administration. Thus we see the protective values of this legislation.

The Controlled Substances Act of 1970 has replaced the Harrison Narcotic Law and includes control of other substances as well as narcotics.

The Standardization Procedure

After drugs are assayed or bioassayed, the following steps are taken for standardization of the particular drug.

1. Animal testing.
2. Human testing under controlled conditions (investigational use only).
3. Application is made to the Food and Drug Administration with the test results.
4. The Food and Drug Administration releases the drug for general human consumption.

Upon release by the F.D.A., the drugs are listed in New Drugs until they have been proven of sufficient value to be included in the U.S.P. or N.F.

Listing of Official Drugs

The Federal Food, Drug, and Cosmetic Act specifies that a drug is official when it is listed in these publications:

1. The United States Pharmacopeia (U.S.P.) issued by the United States Pharmacopeial Convention. Drugs are admitted on the basis of therapeutic merit or

necessity. All drugs given in the U.S.P. must be of the purity and strength specified by the national committee. The following information is given for each drug: source, chemical and physical properties, means of identification and assay, method of storage, dosages, compounding instructions, and action. The U.S.P. is revised every five years.

2. The National Formulary (N.F.) is issued by the American Pharmaceutical Association. These drugs are not listed in the U.S.P. and are chosen on the basis of demand. When a drug is dropped from the U.S.P., it is maintained in the N.F. until it is no longer in sufficient demand to require listing. The N.F. is also revised every five years.

Other Reference Sources

1. The Physicians' Desk Reference, intended for the use of the physician, is published annually with the cooperation of drug manufacturers whose products are described.

2. New Drugs is published annually by the Council on Pharmacy of the American Medical Association. All of the drugs listed have reached a certain frequency of use; there is no implied endorsement of their effectiveness. The manual also lists the newer drugs that are being used but which have not been proven of sufficient value to be included in the U.S.P. or the N.F.

3. A hospital formulary may be compiled by the pharmacy committee through the pharmacy department of a hospital. It provides for drug simplification, especially with respect to drugs which tend to duplicate one another's effect or which offer chemical or pharmacologic variations of questionable merit.

DRUG DOSAGES

The dosage is the amount of drug prescribed for administration. It is solely determined by the doctor. Factors which will determine the amount of dosage are:

- The patient's weight, sex and age
- The disease
- How it is to be administered (oral, intravenous, intramuscular, topical, etc.)
- The patient's tolerance of the drug; that is, how well a drug can be taken without injurious effects.

Terms used to describe dosages are important for the nurse to know.

- An average dose is the amount of a medication which has proven most effective with a minimum of toxic effects.
- The initial dose is the first dose.
- The maintenance dose is given after the initial dose has reached the desired effect.
- The maximum dose is the largest amount of a medication which can safely be given to a patient.
- The lethal dose is the amount of dosage which could kill a patient.

Section 3 Administration of Medications

SUGGESTED ACTIVITIES

- With the permission of the nurse in charge, examine the medicine cabinet on the hospital unit where assigned. Observe, take notes and prepare a report on the following.
    a. Dosage forms of drugs contained in the medicine cabinet.
    b. The order in which the drugs are arranged.

- Refer to an encyclopedia or biology book and, using the form provided below, prepare a report listing the following.
    a. Three plants from which drugs are derived. Explain the use of each drug.
    b. Three animals from which hormones or other medicinal products are obtained. Explain the use of these products as therapeutic agents.
    c. Three minerals from which medicinal products are obtained. Explain the medical use of each product.

Sources	Its Medical Use
Plants	
1.	
2.	
3.	
Animals	
1.	
2.	
3.	
Minerals	
1.	
2.	
3.	

- Examine a recent edition of the following publications.

    Compare the contents.

    U.S. Pharmacopoeia

    National Formulary

    New Drugs

    Physician's Desk Reference

- Using the form illustrated, look up penicillin, streptomycin, and neomycin. Record the drug information as presented in each publication. Explain any differences in the information presented.

Drug	Information		
	U.S.P.	N.F.	P.D.R.
Penicillin			
Streptomycin			
Neomycin			
Explanation of Differences			

REVIEW

A. Briefly answer the following questions.

1. If a nurse wished to find some important and commonly used drug, what would be her best source?

2. If a drug were new on the market and its value had not been completely established, where would she find it?

3. What is a maintenance dose and when is it given?

4. How does a maximum dose differ from a lethal dose?

5. Based on information learned from the previous section, what two systems are used for measuring dosage and how do they differ?

Section 3 Administration of Medications

6. Give the purpose of the following drug legislation and explain the beneficial results of each.

    a. The Food, Drug and Cosmetic Act

    b. The Controlled Substance Act of 1970

7. List the four categories of drug sources and complete the chart.

Drug Source	Drug Obtained	Its Purpose or Function	Forms in which Available

8. Define the following terms.

    average dose —

    contaminating —

    extract —

    generic name —

    initial dose —

    lethal dose —

    maintenance dose —

    maximum dose —

    standardize —

    synthetic —

    trade name —

    tolerance —

EXTENDED STUDY

Learn the meaning and proper use of the following terms before proceeding to the next unit.

autoclave	oral
blood level	potent
contraindication	prescription
dosage	reaction
ethical	sedative
Harrison Act	sterile technique
hypnotic	symptom
injection	topical
intramuscular	Uniform Narcotics Law
narcotic	

Unit 11 Responsibilities in the Administration of Medications

OBJECTIVES

After studying this unit, the student should be able to:

- State the common policies regarding the administration of medications by the practical nurse.
- List common adverse drug reactions.
- State the proper methods of disposal of unused medications.
- Explain proper aftercare of equipment.

The nurse who is allowed to give medications is indeed a valuable aid to the physician, patient, and the nurse in charge. The performance of this important task entails certain responsibilities.

The administration of medications is one of the greatest responsibilities assigned to the practical nurse. Hospitals differ in their administrative procedures. Some hospitals do not permit anyone except a professional nurse to administer medications. This is particularly true in hospitals which are staffed by registered nurses and/or provide experience for student nurses enrolled in a school of nursing or an academic program for registered nursing. Other hospitals permit the practical nurse to administer the routine medications including sedatives at bedtime. (A *sedative* is a medication which is given to quiet a patient). Still others, especially the smaller institutions, frequently find it necessary to have the practical nurse distribute all the medications, including the intramuscular injections. (*Intramuscular injections* are medications given by needle into an area within the muscle substance).

Because of the wide range in hospital practices it is safer to teach the practical nurse student correctly while still under close supervision than to have the nurse pick up this knowledge on the job where adequate time may not be given to teaching this important part of nursing care. When the practical nurse cares for the chronically ill patient in the home, she is required to give medications to these patients. The administration of medicines can be dangerous if the nurse has not been taught and given opportunity to practice under the supervision of a qualified person.

THE MEDICATION

One may ask: From whom or from what source is the medication obtained? In the hospital or nursing home, the order for a medication is written by the doctor on the patient's order sheet. This sheet may be a part of the patient's chart or in the doctor's order book. An example of a medication order is shown in figure 11-1.

The pharmacist fills the *prescription* (the doctor's order for medication). In the hospital, the hospital pharmacy would perform this function. Outside, a patient who

ORDER SHEET				
	FITZPATRICK, DENNIS		8A	DR. JAMES
Patient's Name:	Last	First	(Room or Ward)	(Physician)
Date Ordered	Medication and Directions		Ordered by	Date Discontinued
2/18/76	Phenobarbital 60 mg. at h.s.		Dr. James	

Fig. 11-1 Sample Order Sheet

receives the prescription (in the doctor's office, or at home or as a refill of a medication he took while hospitalized) would need to have it filled by a *registered pharmacist* employed by a community pharmacy.

No medications are permitted to be given to patients without a written order from the doctor. The nurse must learn to read and interpret the doctor's order, the dosage, and method of administration of the drug. If a nurse does not understand the order, there should be no hesitancy to contact the professional nurse in charge, the physician, or the hospital pharmacist to obtain more detailed advice.

> Errors in medications can cause fatal results. Therefore, the greatest care must be exercised.

If a nurse is on a home case, the community pharmacist is contacted to compound the prescription written by the doctor. In a hospital, the routine procedure of that hospital will be followed; the head nurse or medication nurse usually takes care of procuring medications.

Dosage Amount

Every nurse should know the average dose of drugs and how to pour these medications. Accuracy is extremely important. If two drams of a medicine is ordered, two drams must be given; a graduated measuring glass or cup should be used for accurate measuring, figure 11-2. One should never feel that a teaspoonful of medicine may be given when a dram is ordered, or drops given when minims are ordered. The viscosity (thickness) of medications differ. If the physician orders 30 minims of medicine, a minim glass is used, figure 11-3. If he orders 30 drops (as in a home, or in

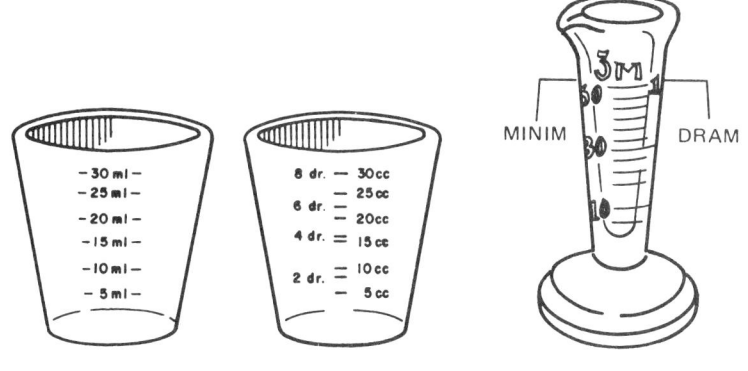

Fig. 11-2 Medicine Glasses: Metric and Apothecaries' Measures

Fig. 11-3 Minim Glass

Section 3 Administration of Medications

the hospital), a dropper is used. Substitutions should not be made unless absolutely necessary and approved by the attending physician.

How the Medication is Given

A nurse who follows the physician's written order will know whether the medicine is to be given by mouth (p.o.), by sterile injection (s.c., I.M., I.V.), by rectum (p.r.) or by local application (topical). Sterile technique must *always* be employed in giving medications by injection and scrupulously clean technique in giving oral medications. The nurse must learn how to maintain sterile technique when she is taught how to handle syringes and needles.

When Medication is to be Given

In writing a prescription the doctor specifies the interval at which medicines are to be administered. The reason for specifying definite intervals for giving medicines is to help nature maintain a certain *blood level* of the drug. In this way the desired results of the drug will be obtained. *The nurse has an ethical obligation to give medicines at the times directed by the doctor in his written prescription.* The nurse must stay with the patient until he has taken the medication. A medication should *never* be left with a patient.

Orders written either q.i.d. or 4 x D, and q.4 h. are sometimes confusing to the new nurse.

        q.i.d. or 4 x D means 4 times a day.

        q.4 h. means every 4 hours during the 24 hours.

All nurses must learn the meaning of these symbols and many others that are used before attempting to administer any medications. An extensive coverage of these symbols will be found in unit 13.

By Whose Authority

A nurse may work directly under the physician's supervision, as on a home case, or under the supervision of a professional nurse in the hospital or nursing home. In any situation, directions must be accurately followed and *any* unexpected symptoms which may occur as a result of administering medications to the patient must be reported promptly.

Contraindications for Using Drugs

No nurse should attempt to administer drugs without adequate training to do so through a study of the kinds of drugs, the dosages, and their expected reactions. On the basis of this study it will be possible to determine the favorable and unfavorable reactions of drugs which should be reported. This is an important aspect of administering medications.

It is not the responsibility of the practical nurse to determine when a drug should not be given (contraindications), but it is an asset to know the qualifying conditions or circumstances for its use. If a dosage should result in an unfavorable reaction, it should not be repeated until the doctor or nurse in charge has been contacted.

Some examples of common adverse drug reactions are: skin rash, pallor, flushed complexion, swelling of the joints, low blood pressure, irregular pulse, abnormal temperature,

Patient:	LANE, DONALD	Room 401
		Doctor: B. Langdon
Date	Time	Medication	Comments — Observations
7/5/75	8 a.m.	Digoxin 0.5 mg - p.o.	Pulse 70, regular. Drug retained.

Fig. 11-4 Recording of Drug on Patient's Chart

vomiting, loss of appetite, nausea, sharp pain, fainting, and the like. These and other recognized unfavorable symptoms should be learned by the practical nurse if she is to effectively participate in the administration of medications.

REACTIONS TO MEDICATIONS

Reactions to medications must be recorded and reported. The nurse who administers a drug to a patient must record this on the patient's chart immediately after giving it, figure 11-4. To record the patient's reaction to the drug, the nurse must know what signs to look for in order to be able to chart these for the doctor. For example, if a patient were given *tincture of digitalis* and the nurse observed that the pulse became irregular and/or the patient's face became flushed, the exact observation and time must be recorded on the chart. This must also be reported verbally to the nurse in charge. In this way the nurse may be able to avoid serious complications for the patient. After recording and reporting the reaction, the nurse should return to the patient's bedside to reassure him. If the patient's condition appears to be serious, the practical nurse should ring for the professional nurse and not leave the patient alone, even for a moment.

> Many of the drugs in current use are extremely potent in their effects. Being potent, it is possible that they can cause undesirable, as well as desirable, effects. These undesirable effects can range from mild to severe. Whatever the degree of reaction, a written report must be made of any adverse drug reaction that occurs.

Section 3 Administration of Medications

> 7. *Professional Use of Narcotic Drugs.* (1) Physicians and Dentists. A physician or a dentist, in good faith and in the course of his professional practice only, may prescribe, administer, and dispense narcotic drugs, or he may cause the same to be administered by a nurse or interne under his direction and supervision.
>
> (3) Return of Unused Drugs. Any person who has obtained from a physician, dentist, or veterinarian any narcotic drug for administration to a patient during the absence of such physician, dentist, or veterinarian shall return to such physician, dentist, or veterinarian any unused portion of such drug, when it is no longer required by the patient.

Fig. 11-5 Quotation from the Uniform Narcotics Law

MEDICATIONS NOT COMPLETELY USED

Upon discharge from the hospital, patients may leave some unused medications. It is customary to return these to the nurse in charge who will send them back to the pharmacy. Any narcotics remaining after the patient's discharge must be returned to the pharmacy or to the doctor if the nurse is caring for a case in the home; there are federal and state laws which govern the control of narcotics. These laws are the Controlled Substance Act of 1970 and the Uniform Narcotics Law. A quotation from the Uniform Narcotics Law explains this in more detail, figure 11-5. A careful and complete record of narcotics ordered, dispensed, and returned must be kept by hospitals and private physicians.

AFTERCARE OF EQUIPMENT

Plastic and disposable equipment has replaced many items which formerly were reusuable. However, some hospitals and other health-related facilities still use syringes, needles, medicine glasses and other articles which must be cleaned, packaged and autoclaved. Although there may be a central service department where unsterile equipment may be packaged and autoclaved, the nurse who uses these articles has the obligation to rinse them immediately after use and place them in the basket which is to be sent to central supply. Medicine glasses and other oral equipment are usually taken care of in the hospital unit. In small hospitals and in the home, nurses or assigned personnel must thoroughly, clean and sterilize the equipment usually by boiling. The use of disposable medicine cups, syringes, and needles has greatly simplified the work of the nurse and central service department. The nurse must not forget that to dispose of needles and plastic syringes means that they must be destroyed, not simply thrown away. This is especially true of needles; they should be broken off at the hub before being discarded. This can be done by using the sheath and bending the needle back and forth until it is broken off, figure 11-6. A small carton with an opening in the lid may be used to collect the discarded syringes, and destroyed. Some service trays are equipped with a bag for the disposable syringes and a container for the discarded needles.

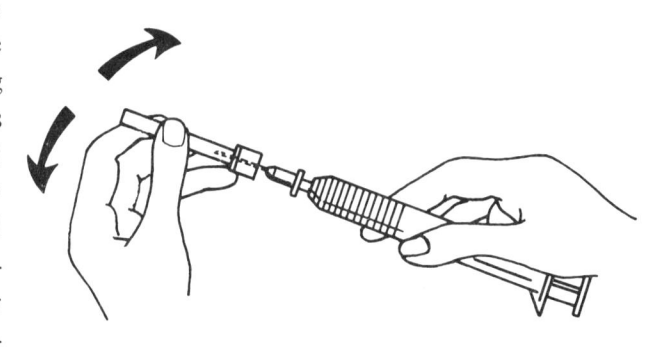

Fig. 11-6 Breaking off the Needle of a Disposable Unit

ETHICS APPLIED TO ADMINISTRATION OF MEDICATIONS

Ethical concepts are concerned with the administration of medications. Anyone who has access to a medicine cabinet may be tempted to take a medicine, as simple as an aspirin. The nurse must recognize the fact that the medicine in the hospital cabinet belongs to the institution or to a patient; therefore, no nurse or other employee may take it. Also, since drugs and narcotics may become habit-forming, the nurse must bear in mind the harm which may come to her when she takes medications without the advice of her doctor.

If the wrong medication is given to a patient, the supervisor or physician in charge must be notified immediately.

COPING WITH THE UNUSUAL

The nurse must be alert to the patient who brings his medicines to the hospital. A suitcase may be full of old drugs. This situation must be reported to the nurse in charge, who will discuss the matter with the patient's doctor. He will frequently have these drugs removed and write new orders for the medications his patient is to receive which will be supplied through the hospital pharmacy.

Again, if the wrong medication is given to a patient, the supervisor or physician in charge must be notified immediately.

SUGGESTED ACTIVITIES

- With prior arrangements made by the instructor, tour a hospital, clinic, and another health-related facility to find which medications and injections are administered by the practical nurse. Compare findings and discuss the role of the PN and the RN in these situations.

REVIEW

A. Answer the following questions in the space provided.

1. During visiting hours you observe a visitor giving your patient a bottle of medicine not ordered by her present doctor. What would you do in this situation?

2. Explain the aftercare of the following equipment used in giving medications: medicine glasses, tray, pitcher, glass syringes and stainless steel needles; and disposable needles and syringes.

Section 3 Administration of Medications

3. Returning from lunch at 1:00 P.M., the nurse observes a 12 o'clock medication untouched, on the patient's bedside table. Explain what is entirely wrong in this situation.

4. List five common unfavorable reactions which might occur following administration of a drug.

5. Why is time an important element in administering a medication?

6. If the wrong medication was given, what should be done?

7. a. What procedure should be followed to report and record the administration of a drug?

   b. Prepare an example of what would be shown on a patient's chart if he had been given Penicillin, 50,000 units by intramuscular injection at 10:00 A.M. and developed large red areas and itching on both ankles at 10:30 A.M. (include headings and today's date on the chart.)

8. What procedure should be followed with the patient who brings his own drugs to the hospital?

EXTENDED STUDY

Learn the meaning and proper use of the following terms which will be discussed in the next unit.

addiction	dissolve
aerosol	enteric coated
antiseptic	homogeneous
astringent	local action
atomizer	remote action
cohesive	side effects
compounded	stimulant
depressant	suspended

Unit 12 Forms of Drugs and How They Act

OBJECTIVES

After studying this unit, the student should be able to:

- List the forms in which drugs are prepared and give examples of these preparations.
- State methods of storing drugs and preserving them from deterioration.
- Define types of action and side effects.

The method for administering a drug is dependent upon its form, its properties, and the effects desired. If it is to be given orally, the drug may be in the form of a liquid, tablet, or powder. For injection purposes, it must be prepared in a liquid form. For topical use, it may come in liquid, powder or semisolid form.

FORMS OF DRUGS

Drugs are compounded in three basic types of preparations: liquid, solid, and semisolid. Variations in the form of a drug are largely determined by how easily the drug agents can be dissolved. It will be found that some are soluble in water, others in alcohol, and others may require a mixture of several solvents.

Liquid Preparations

Liquid preparations are those containing a drug which has been dissolved or suspended. The drug may be further classified as an aqueous or alcoholic preparation depending on the solvent used. The liquid preparations prescribed for internal use, except for the emulsions, are rapidly absorbed through the stomach or intestinal walls.

Emulsions. *Emulsions* are mixtures of oil and water, usually with a milky appearance. They separate into layers only after standing for long periods of time. Emulsions should be shaken before administering. An example of an emulsion is cod liver oil.

Solutions. One or more drugs can be dissolved in an appropriate solvent to make a solution. The solution will appear to be clear and homogeneous. An example of a solution is normal saline.

Mixtures and Suspensions. Drugs which are mixed with a liquid but are not dissolved are called mixtures or suspensions. The drugs are in the form of fine particles suspended in the liquid. These preparations must be shaken before being administered to the patient. Examples are milk of magnesia, and rhubarb and soda mixture.

Syrups. Drugs dissolved in a solution of sugar and water and flavoring are called syrups. An example is syrup of ipecac.

Elixirs. Drugs dissolved in a solution of alcohol and water which has been sweetened and flavored are elixirs. The bitter or salty taste of the drug is disguised when prepared as an elixir. Because of this, it is frequently used for children's medications. Examples are elixir of phenobarbital and elixir of terpin hydrate.

Tinctures. Tinctures are drugs dissolved in alcohol or alcohol and water. For the most part, they are made to represent 10% of the drug agent. Examples are tincture of digitalis and tincture of iodine. Tincture of iodine is one of the exceptions to the 10% rule for tinctures; it may be a 7% or 2% tincture.

Spirits. Alcoholic solutions of volatile (easily vaporized) drugs are called spirits. A spirit is also called an essence. Examples are spirits of peppermint and aromatic spirits of ammonia.

Fluidextracts. Drugs which have been processed to a concentrated strength using alcohol as the solvent are called fluid extracts. Examples include fluidextract of ergot, fluidextract of ipecac and cascara sagrada fluidextract.

Lotions. Aqueous preparations of suspended ingredients used externally (without massage) to treat skin conditions are lotions. They soothe and moisten the skin and can inhibit the growth of bacteria. An example is Bacitracin.

Liniments. These are drugs which are used externally and are applied with massage to produce a feeling of heat or warmth to the area. An example of a liniment is methyl salicylate.

Sprays. As their name implies, sprays are drugs prepared to such a consistency that they may be administered by an atomizer, figure 12-1. They are principally used to treat nose and throat conditions. The drug functions as an astringent (produces a shrinking or contracting effect) or as an antiseptic (inhibits growth or microorganisms). Oil is usually used as the solvent. Examples are ephedrine and Neo-synephrine® sprays.

Aerosols. Aerosols may be sprayed on the skin without touching it. This has a great advantage when the skin is irritated or burned. There are three types of aerosol preparations: surface, steam and foam aerosols.

- A *surface aerosol* may be prepared in liquid or powder form. They may contain an antiseptic, a burn remedy, or a desensitizing substance.

- A *steam spray aerosol* is applied in a spray under pressure. They may contain body lotions or rubbing solutions.

- A *foam aerosol* must be shaken before spraying in order to emulsify the substances to be sprayed. They may contain foam medications, ointments, creams, or lotions.

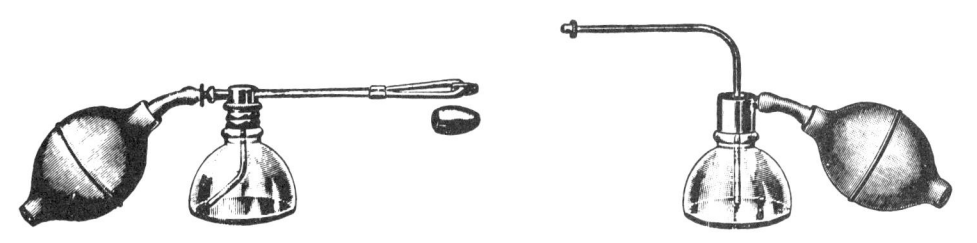

Fig. 12-1 Liquid Atomizer and Powder Blower

Section 3 *Administration of Medications*

Solid and Semisolid Preparations

Solid and semisolid preparations are drugs such as tablets and capsules. They have both external and internal uses, depending upon the drug agent and the drug form. Examples of drug forms for external use are suppositories, ointments, plasters, and medicated pads. Capsules and tablets are prepared for internal use.

Capsules. A capsule is a small two-part container; the container is made up of a gelatin substance into which the medication is placed.

Spansules are capsules enclosing delayed-action medications. They are used more extensively because of their convenience in maintaining the desired effect over a longer period of time.

Pills. These are small round medicinal preparations which are swallowed whole.

Tablets. These are small discs of varying thicknesses and sizes; they contain medicine and a cohesive substance. Tablets are formed by being compressed in a mold. The color of a tablet is usually added and is not due to the drug present.

Tablets may be coated to hide their bitter taste; also they will not be affected by the gastric juices. These are called *enteric coated* and will not dissolve and begin action until they reach the intestines. An example of an enteric coated tablet is Repetabs.

A tablet is often crushed and dissolved in a palatable liquid if it is to be administered to a child, or to an adult who has difficulty in swallowing. It is also administered in this manner to those who cannot be depended on to swallow a tablet such as in the case of some mentally or physically handicapped persons.

Scored tablets are those marked with indentations into halves and quarters so that they may be easily broken for proper dosage. A method used for breaking a scored tablet is to place it on a clean surface and separate it into sections by using a clean file.

Hypodermic tablets are a combination of a medication and milk sugar that dissolves completely and rapidly for hypodermic injection. An example of a hypodermic tablet is morphine sulfate 15 mg.

Troches or *lozenges* are hard circular or oblong discs made of a medication in a candy-like base. They dissolve on the tongue and are commonly used for the treatment of sore throats. Drinking of liquids is avoided after troches or lozenges are taken because their effect would be destroyed by the resulting dilution and washing away of the drug agent.

Suppositories. Suppositories are drugs which are usually shaped like a cylinder or cone for insertion into the rectum, vagina or urethra. A suppository consists of a drug agent or agents combined with a base of soap, glycerinated gelatin or cocoa butter oil. These bases are selected because they are readily fusible (will melt) when subjected to body heat. Medications may be administered in this form when oral medication is not possible. Suppositories are actually classified as drugs for *external use*. A rectal suppository is frequently used to alleviate pain from hemorrhoids, while vaginal suppositories are used to relieve minor vaginal irritations or infections.

Ointments. Ointments are semisolid preparations made for use on the skin surface. They are compounded either with an oily base or a water-soluble base to keep the drug agent in longer contact with the skin. Zinc Oxide ointment is frequently used.

HOW DRUGS ACT

Drugs may be used to cure disease or to restore a disturbed or diseased physical state to a normal or an improved state. In the latter case, drugs assist the body to overcome its own difficulties by causing a change in the activity of cells but not in their basic function. Most drugs may be classified into three general groups:

1. Those which act directly upon one or more tissues of the body.
2. Those which act upon microorganisms which invade the body (chemotherapy and antibiotics).
3. Those which replace body chemicals and secretions (hormones).

Classified Actions of Drugs

Certain drugs are prescribed because of the selective actions which result when they are administered. The terms applied to these actions are descriptive of the action which takes place.

Selective Action. This is the term applied to drugs which act upon certain tissues or specific organs of the body. They are principally the stimulants and depressants.

Stimulants are drugs which increase cell activity. An example is caffeine which stimulates the cerebrum.

Depressants are drugs which decrease the cell activity. An example is morphine, which depresses the respiratory center in the brain.

A change in the dosage of a drug will alter the degree of stimulation or depression of the cells and tissues.

Local Action. *Local action* is the term applied to external drugs which act upon the area to which they are admininstered. An example is the application of methyl salicylate to sore muscles or painful joints. The medication is rubbed into the skin overlying the area of pain.

Remote Action. The term applied to a drug which affects a part of the body distant from its site of administration is called *remote action.* An example is an apomorphine injection in the arm; this stimulates the vomiting center in the brain.

Specific Action. This is the term applied to a drug which has a particular effect upon a definite pathogenic organism. An example is the action of quinine upon the malarial parasite.

Some drugs should not be given at the same time as they may interact and cause unfavorable and harmful effects, see *Possible Pharmacological Drug Interactions* in the Appendix.

In fulfilling the desired actions there are also adverse drug reactions which can occur.

Side Effects. *Side effect* is the term applied to results which are not desired, and which may limit the usefulness of the drug. An example is the toxic side effects of digitalis: vomiting, diarrhea, and irregular heartbeat. Adverse drug reactions and untoward effects are also known as side effects.

Addiction. This is the term applied to a condition in which there is a dependence and craving for a narcotic or other habit-forming drug. Examples of habit-forming drugs are morphine, Demerol®, and phenobarbital.

LOSS OF DRUG POTENCY

Factors which determine the life of a drug are: date of manufacture, the type of the container, the method of storage and the unique properties of the drug.

Date of Manufacture or Preparation

Drugs such as antibiotics are stamped with an expiration date. Beyond this date it is unsafe to use them because of gradual deterioration or change in potency.

Type of Container

Screw cap or plastic-stoppered glass bottles are the most common type of containers used for medicines. Glass is a good container because it does not react chemically with most of the drugs. It also has an advantage because the amount of drug contained can be readily seen. Bottles should always be capped when not in use to prevent the deterioration of the medicine. Many drugs will undergo chemical changes when exposed to the air for any length of time. For example, alcoholic preparations will evaporate rapidly and make a drug more potent than it was when ordered.

Method of Storage

Certain medications must be kept refrigerated. Insulin, antibiotics, vitamins in oil, and hormone products will deteriorate if kept at room temperature. They must be returned to the refrigerator immediately following their use.

Unique Properties of the Drug

Some medicines require dark bottles; otherwise they will deteriorate when exposed to light. Others require an absorbent material which removes moisture in the air within the container; otherwise the moisture would be absorbed by the drug, thereby causing it to deteriorate.

Precautions in the Selection of a Drug for a Medicine Order

Any drug which shows any change in consistency, odor, or color should be discarded.

Any drug about which there is the slightest doubt should be discarded or, if in a hospital, returned to the pharmacy and reordered.

SUGGESTED ACTIVITIES

- Write to a pharmaceutical house and obtain a catalog listing drugs. Refer to the catalog and take notes on the following observations.

  a. Identify forms of drugs which are available.

  b. List any information given concerning the drug which applies to a better understanding of the drug (for example; side effects, interactions with other drugs, etc.).

Unit 12 Forms of Drugs and How They Act

- Make the following observations in the hospital or health-related facility which provides clinical practice, and prepare a report on your findings.
    a. The types of containers used for drugs.
    b. The methods used for storing drugs.
    c. Special precautions taken in the use of drugs to control deterioration.
- Refer to the medicine order book. Select five drugs which have been ordered and determine the type of action which should result when each drug is administered. List side effects, if any, which might occur.

REVIEW

A. Answer the questions in the space provided.

1. Why are drugs prepared in various forms?

2. What responses might be expected from:
    a. A stimulant?

    b. A depressant?

3. In the table below give an example of each form of drug and its use.

Forms	Drug	Its Use
Emulsion		
Mixture		
Solution		
Syrup		
Elixir		
Spirit		
Tincture		
Fluidextract		
Lotion		
Spray		
Liniment		

Section 3 Administration of Medications

4. On the following chart, list the forms of drugs prescribed for internal use. Give an example of each and tell how each is administered.

Forms	Drug	How Administered

EXTENDED STUDY

Learn the meaning and proper use of the following terms.

- complication
- diagnose
- doctor's narcotic registration number
- Kardex
- medicine card
- medicine order
- patient's chart
- prescription
- inscription
- superscription

Unit 13 The Medication Order

OBJECTIVES

After studying this unit, the student should be able to:

- State the methods by which orders for medications are given.
- Interpret a prescription.
- Read and write the abbreviations commonly used in doctors' orders and prescriptions.

It is the responsibility of the doctor to diagnose the cause of illness and to prescribe a medication. The medication prescribed is generally referred to as a medication or medicine order and may be given by a number of methods. Since it is usually the duty of the nurse to carry out the order, it is extremely important that the methods and their interpretations are known.

HOW MEDICATION ORDERS ARE GIVEN

The medication order is the drug order written by the doctor for a specific patient. It designates the drug to be used, the dosage, the form of the drug, the time or number of times it is to be administered, and the method by which it is to be given. Many times it includes directions for checking with the physician such as when any contraindications develop while using the drug, or when certain blood responses must be maintained.

Patient's Order Sheet and Kardex

For this method of giving a medicine order, the doctor writes the order directly on the patient's order sheet which is a part of the *patient's chart*. The chart is a comprehensive record prepared for each patient and includes all pertinent information about the patient and his illness. After the medicine order has been written by the doctor, the chart is then usually placed on the desk of the head nurse, who will copy the order onto the Kardex. From the Kardex, the nurse prepares the medicine cards. In some hospitals, the recording of doctors' orders is delegated to a ward secretary. However, *it is the responsibility of the nurse* in charge of the medications and treatments to verify all entries and assume responsibility for the safety of the patient.

The *Kardex* is a rotating file; each patient has a separate order card in the Kardex. The Kardex file may be arranged alphabetically according to the patient's name, or it may be arranged according to room number, figure 13-1, page 78. When the Kardex system is used, an order book (discussed in the following paragraph) is usually not in use.

Section 3 Administration of Medications

Date	Treatments	Hour
3/1/76	Steam inhalation - vaporizer in room	Continuously

Religion Roman Catholic	Diagnosis Bronchitis			
Name Simpson, Iris D.	Rm. No. 109	Age 33	Operation Date —	Dr. or Service L. St. Onge M.D.

Fig. 13-1 Kardex

Date	Patient's Name	Room	Medication	Written by (Doctor)	Checked by (Nurse)
9/16/75	McCall, Ella	1009	Acetylsalicylic Acid gr. X q.4.h.	Dr. R. Smith	M. Clark 9:15
9/16/75	Lawrence, Paul	1021	tr. Digitalis MX (m) p.c. breakfast q.d.	Dr. B. Long	M. Clark 9:25
9/16/75	Davidson, Lee	1037	elix. Terpin hydrate ʒi q.4.h. p.r.n.	Dr. J. Mertz	M. CLARK 9:46

Fig. 13-2 Doctors' order book

Order Book

The drug order book is the book in which the physicians write the orders for each of the patients on the hospital unit, figure 13-2. The nurse in charge is responsible for checking the order book, securing the medications ordered from the pharmacy, and writing the medicine cards so that medications may be given at the intervals specified in the order. These duties are sometimes done by the nurse responsible for medications and treatments.

In each case the head nurse checks the individual order, writes the medicine card, and checks that the drug is in the medicine cabinet.

Prescription

A prescription is a separate written order which is not part of the patient's chart; it may be used in the following situations.

- In the hospital
- Upon discharge from the hospital
- On an office visit
- On a home visit

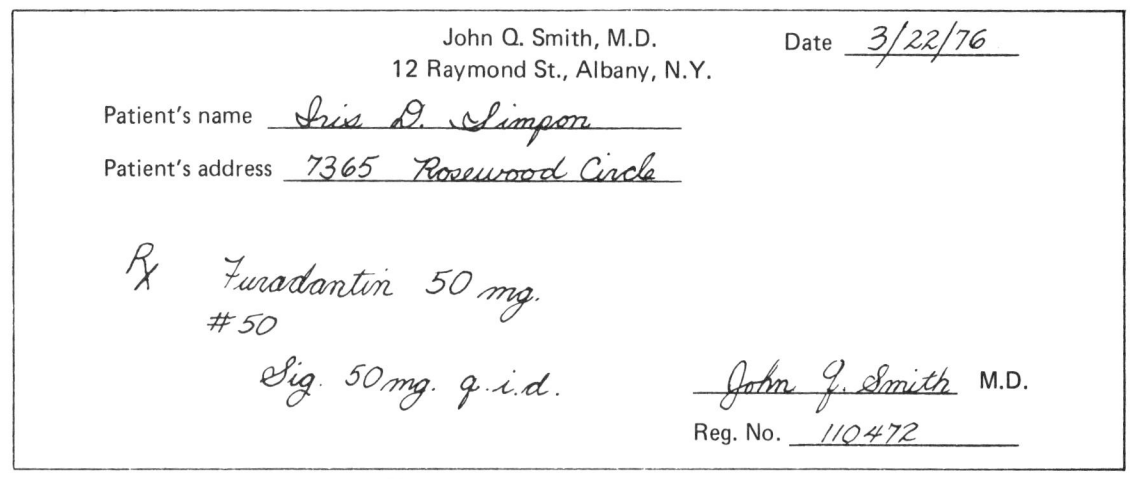

```
                    John Q. Smith, M.D.          Date  3/22/76
                    12 Raymond St., Albany, N.Y.
   Patient's name    Iris D. Simpson
   Patient's address  7365 Rosewood Circle


   ℞    Furadantin 50 mg.
        #50
             Sig. 50 mg. q.i.d.              John J. Smith   M.D.
                                           Reg. No. 110472
```

Fig. 13-3 Sample of a Prescription

The purpose of the prescription is to control the sale and use of drugs which can be safely or effectively used only under the supervision of a physician.

A prescription is made up of several parts: the superscription, inscription, subscription, signature and registration number.

The superscription includes the patient's name, the date, and the symbol R_x, meaning "take thou" or "I prescribe."

The inscription includes the names and amounts of the drugs to be compounded in the medication. The most important drug or base is listed first.

The subscription includes the directions to the pharmacist for compounding the prescription.

The signature includes the directions to the patient for taking the medicine. In most states, the doctor's registration number must also be recorded.

Verbal Orders

It is extremely unwise for a nurse to accept a verbal order for a medication except in a dire emergency, such as when a doctor is unable to reach the patient within a short time. A written order should thereafter be obtained *as soon as it is possible.* It should be noted, however, that the policies of hospitals differ in this matter, and some specifically state that verbal orders are not to be accepted under any circumstances.

If the nurse is required to telephone a doctor concerning a recent development or complication in the condition of the patient, the symptoms should be written down to be sure the nurse does not forget to tell the doctor everything that is important. Following the report the nurse should write down the suggestions and orders which the doctor may give. These must be read back to be sure that they have been correctly understood.

If a complicated order for medications is to be given, it is wise to have the doctor contact the pharmacist directly. In this way the nurse will be assured of the order's accuracy and will be relieved of the responsibility of accepting it.

THE MEDICATION ORDER AND THE MEDICINE CARD

The medication order is referred to for preparing the medicine card (also called a medicine ticket). The card, in turn, is used for reference in pouring medications.

Section 3 Administration of Medications

In most instances, cards are made out in various colors, each having a particular meaning. Hospital practices will vary, but usually a white card designates an oral medication, a red card, an intramuscular injection and a blue card, an emergency medication. It is approximately two by two inches in size. When prepared, it should be clearly printed and should contain specific information, figure 13-4.

- Room and bed number
- Patient's full name
- The name of the medication
- The route for administration (mouth, rectal, subcutaneously, etc.)
- The dosage of the medication
- The hours to be administered
- The date the medication was ordered

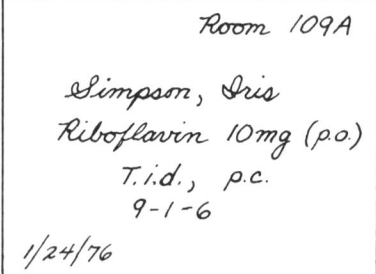

Fig. 13-4 Medicine Card

Abbreviation	Meaning	Abbreviation	Meaning
āā	(equal parts) of each	p.o.	by mouth
a.c.	before meals	per	through or by
ad lib	if desired, freely	p.r.	by rectum
b.i.d.	two times a day	p.r.n.	when required
c̄	with	q.d.	every day
cc.	cubic centimeter	q.h.	every hour
comp.	compound	q.2.h.	every two hours
CBC	complete blood count	q.3.h.	every three hours
dil.	dilute	q.i.d.	four times a day
dr	dram	q.n.	every night
elix.	elixir	q.s.	in sufficient quantity
ext.	extract	Ⓡ	trade name
Gm	gram	R$_x$	take
gr	grain	R.B.C.	red blood count
gtt(s).	drop(s)	s̄	without
h.	hour	s.c.	subcutaneous (injection)
h.s.	bedtime	Sig. or S.	write on label
I.M.	intramuscular	Sol.	solution
I.V.	intravenous	s.o.s.	if necessary
L.	liter	sp.	spirits
M	mix	s̄s̄.	one half
m(s)	minim(s)	s.s.	soap suds
ml	milliliters	stat.	immediately
mixt.	mixture	syr.	syrup
mg	milligram(s)	t.i.d.	three times a day
O.	pint	tr. or tinct.	tincture
oz	ounce	ung.	ointment
p.c.	after meals	W.B.C.	white blood count

Fig. 13-5 Common Medical Abbreviations

The card remains with the medication until it has been administered. When a medication is discontinued or changed, the card is destroyed by the nurse in charge.

ABBREVIATIONS

Abbreviations are the "shorthand" of the medical and nursing professions; they are a clear and concise means for writing orders. Without going into a detailed description, the doctor states what is to be done and how and when it should be done. This medical shorthand is an international language used by professional people concerned with the care of patients. In the study of the unit on arithmetic of solutions and dosage, you learned some abbreviations. All of the abbreviations in figure 13-5 should be learned if you are to properly fulfill your role in administering medications.

SUGGESTED ACTIVITIES

- Prepare a report on the methods used for obtaining and executing medicine orders in the hospital or other health facility where you are having your clinical experience.
- Make a study of a patient in whom you are particularly interested and prepare an example of the following.
   a. Items which must be recorded by the nurse on the patient's chart.
   b. The Kardex
   c. Completed medicine cards (use the colors as observed by the hospital or other health facility)

REVIEW

A. Answer the following questions.

1. Interpret the following medication order:

   Give Prednisolone 2.5 mg tablet T.I.D. pc.

2. Describe the procedure that should be followed when accepting a doctor's verbal order.

3. What is the purpose of a prescription?

Section 3 *Administration of Medications*

4. Tell how the patient's chart differs from the Kardex.

5. Describe the Kardex and tell how it differs from the medicine card.

B. Match the two columns by placing the letter of the word or statement from Column II in the most suitable space in Column I.

Column I	Column II
____ 1. a.c.	a. dram
____ 2. s.o.s.	b. three times a day
____ 3. I.V.	c. every day
____ 4. b.i.d.	d. if necessary
____ 5. elix.	e. white blood count
____ 6. aa	f. when required
____ 7. R$_x$	g. before meals
____ 8. q.s.	h. intravenous
____ 9. p.o.	i. to, up to
____10. oz – ℥	j. equal parts of each
____11. gtts.	k. two times a day
____12. dr – ʒ	l. with
____13. p.r.n.	m. elixir
____14. q.i.d.	n. ounce
____15. ss	o. four times a day
____16. t.i.d.	p. every four hours
____17. q.d.	q. drop(s)
____18. q.4 h.	r. take
____19. W.B.C.	s. extract
____20. c̄	t. by mouth
	u. one-half
	v. mixture
	w. sufficient quantity

EXTENDED STUDY

Learn the meaning and proper use of the following terms.

    precipitate   meniscus   surface tension

Unit 14 Basic Procedures in Administering Medications

OBJECTIVES

After studying this unit, the student should be able to:

- List routes for giving medications.
- Describe the basic rules and procedures for administering medications.

Medicine is administered by several routes. These routes, named in order of frequency of use, are: oral, injection (subcutaneous, intramuscular and intravenous), inhalation, local application to skin and mucous membrane, and rectal insertion.

Certain basic rules and procedures must be followed when giving a medication regardless of its form or the route by which it is to be given.

RULES FOR GIVING MEDICATIONS

When working with medications, the so-called six correct steps of accuracy should always be kept in mind. These are the important responsibilities of the nurse when pouring and administering medications.

---

1. Correct dose is measured.
2. Correct medicine is poured.
3. Correct patient is given the medicine.
4. Medicine is given at the correct time.
5. Medicine is administered by the correct channel or method.
6. Correct charting of the medication and any related information is done.

Six Correct Steps of Accuracy

In following the six steps of accuracy, *avoid distractions.* Do not talk with anyone while pouring or adminstering medications. The distraction may cause serious consequences. *Read the label on the medicine bottle carefully three times:*

- When the bottle is taken from the shelf of the medicine cupboard.
- When the drug is taken from the container.
- When the bottle is replaced on the shelf of the medicine cupboard.

OTHER RULES AND CONSIDERATIONS

- Read each medicine card carefully. If not clear, refer back to the patient's chart and Kardex. Check with the nurse in charge, who will clarify the matter and make any corrections.

Section 3 Administration of Medications

- Avoid handling medications with the fingers. In administering pills or capsules, use the container cap to drop the tablet into the medicine glass.

- Never return poured, unused medications to stock bottles or containers.

- Never take medicine from an unmarked or soiled container. Contact the pharmacy. It is the responsibility of the pharmacist to change the label.

- Do not give medicines you have not poured yourself unless the properly identified medication is received from the hospital pharmacy in ready-to-use form.

- Give medicines only upon written orders from the doctor, or when directed by the head nurse. However, it should be noted that the head nurse does not originate the medicine order; only a doctor can do this.

- Using the medicine card for reference, give all medications by mouth unless otherwise ordered. Refer to the medicine order whenever there is any doubt, or check with the head nurse, figure 14-1.

- Do not give an oral medication to a patient who is unable to swallow or is unconscious.

- Do not have any patient carry or administer medications to other patients.

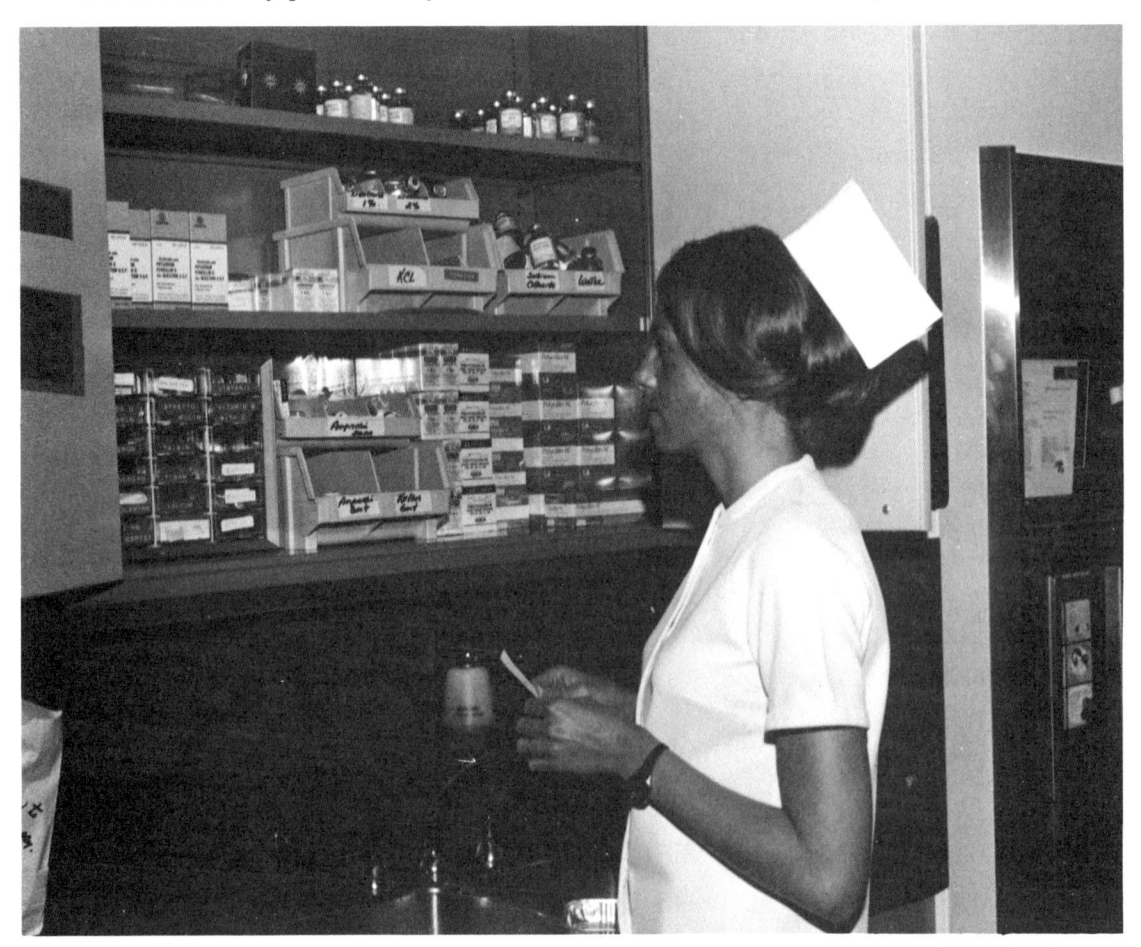

Fig. 14-1 Using the patient's medicine card for reference, the nurse carefully selects the medication.

Unit 14 Basic Procedures in Administering Medications

- To check that you are measuring the *correct dosage,* read the label on the bottle to see if the dosage is the same as the doctor ordered, figure 14-2. If not, calculate the correct dosage. *Be sure to have the nurse or doctor check your calculation before giving the medicine.*
- To be sure that the *correct medicine* is selected, *the label should be read three times* as previously described. Compare the label with the medicine ticket before pouring the medication, figure 14-3. If there is even the slightest difference between the label and the medicine ticket as to the identification of the medicine, check with the head nurse before pouring.

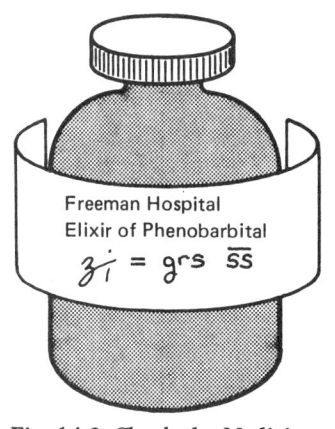

Fig. 14-2 Check the Medicine Label for the Correct Dosage

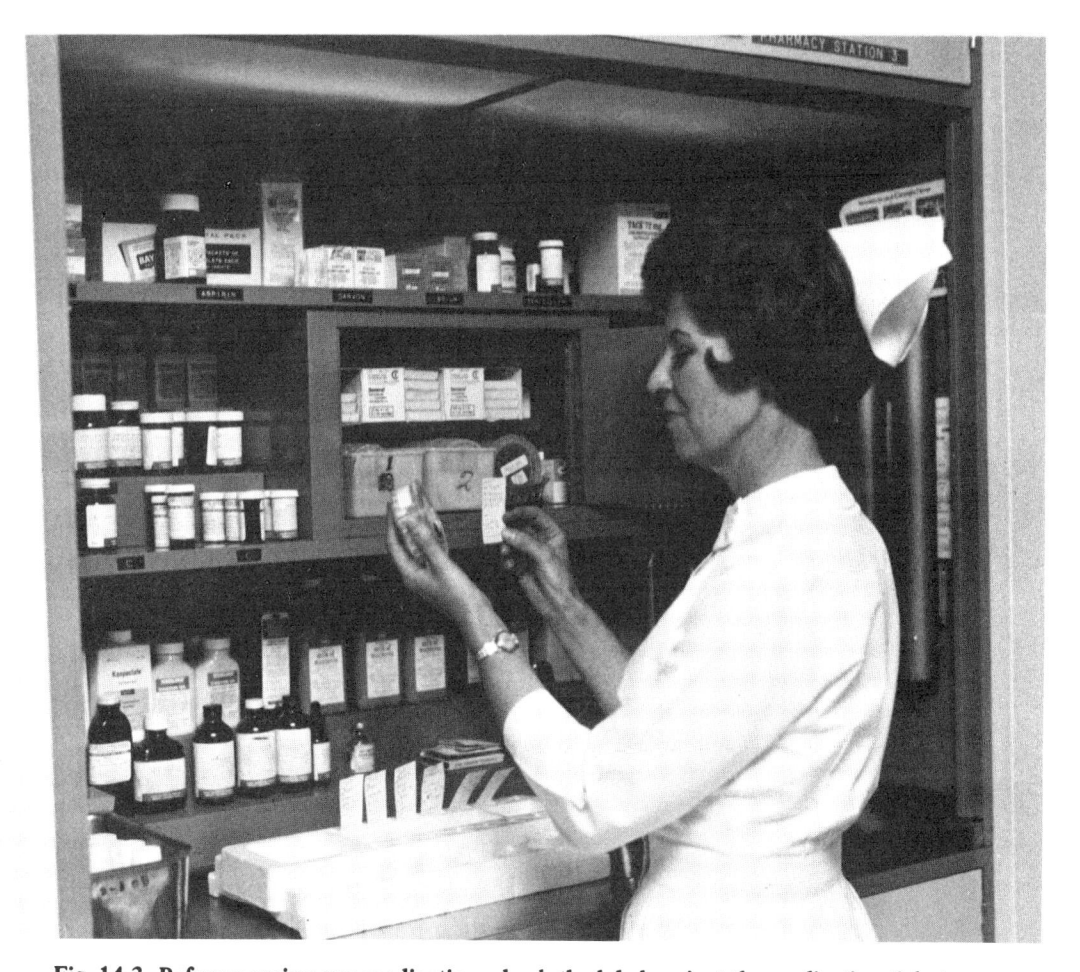

Fig. 14-3 Before pouring any medication, check the label against the medication ticket.

85

Section 3 Administration of Medications

- If the dosage of medication is larger than what you learned to be the maximum dose, check the order with the head nurse before administering it.
- Always shake a bottle in which there is a *precipitate* (a substance separated from a solution in the form of fine particles) before pouring it. An alternate rotating wrist movement will insure a more thorough mixture.
- When pouring liquid medications, hold the bottle with the label upward to avoid soiling it, figure 14-4. Cleanse the lip of the bottle before replacing it on the shelf.
- Measure the correct quantity, using proper utensils.
- When pouring liquid medications, hold the graduate or medicine glass at your eye level, indicating with the thumb of the left hand the level which the medication should reach. The correct level is the lowest part of the fluid surface, figure 14-5. Note that the medicine forms a concave surface (meniscus) as illustrated. The concave surface is caused by the fact that liquids tend to cling to the sides of their containers while surface tension contracts the center of the surface to keep it flat.

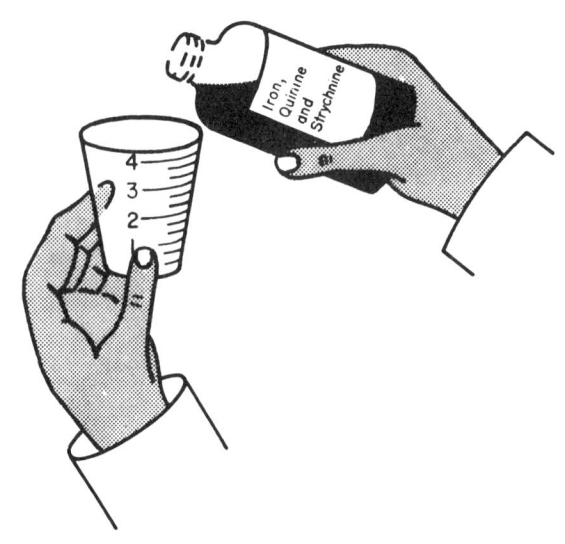

Fig. 14-4 The Bottle is Held with the Label Upward. Medication is Poured at Eye Level

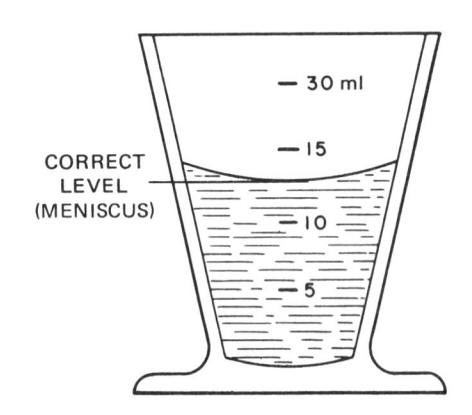

Fig. 14-5 Surface Appearance of Poured Medication

- Always replace the bottle cap after pouring the medicine. While pouring, the cap should be held or placed in such a position that the clean end (that portion which may come in contact with contents of the bottle) will not be contaminated.
- It is advisable not to mix liquid medications unless directed to do so. A chemical change may result, thus forming a precipitate.
- To be sure that the *patient is the correct one,* check the name on the medicine ticket with the name on the patient's wristband. Ask the patient his name. Should two patients of the same name have medications ordered, be sure that the first name of each appears on the medicine ticket.
- To be sure that the *time is correct*, check the medicine ticket or card. This is important because the doctor may want a certain blood level of the drug; this can be maintained only if his order is followed correctly.

Unit 14 Basic Procedures in Administering Medications

- To be sure that the *right method* or route of administration of the drug is used, again check the medicine card.
- Be sure the medicine and all pertinent information is charted.

SUGGESTED ACTIVITIES

- Practice the procedure for reading the label of a medicine bottle when selecting it from the medicine cupboard.
- Divide the class in several groups. One student may role play a nurse preparing a medication. The other students observe the procedure which was followed. The students then list the precautions that were taken and/or omitted.
- Make a report on the rules which must be followed in preparing and administering medications at the hospital where clinical experience is being obtained.

REVIEW

A. 1. Name the six steps to follow to insure accurate administration of medication and tell how each step is checked.

2. Explain why the level of a poured medication appears to be concave.

3. Under what circumstances may medications be administered by a patient?

4. Explain how the nurse should dispose of leftover medications.

5. If two liquid medications are mixed together and a precipitate results, should it be administered? _____ Give reason for your answer.

6. Explain what should be done to a mixture before pouring it.

7. Name four instruments or devices used for measuring medications.

8. If a nurse doubts the dosage shown on the medicine card, what should be done?

Section 3 Administration of Medications

9. Give a list of precautions which should be taken when pouring any medications.

10. Briefly explain why the practical nurse should have a registered nurse or physician check any dosage calculations before administering the medication to the patient.

11. Explain three reasons why it is unsafe to administer medications which have been measured by another nurse.

12. State three reasons why medications going to one patient may not be mixed together.

13. What reasons would you give nursing students to explain why they must not talk to anyone or have other distractions while pouring or measuring medications.

EXTENDED STUDY

Learn the meaning and proper use of the following terms.

absorption   buccal   sublingual

Unit 15 Administration of Oral Medications

OBJECTIVES

After studying this unit, the student should be able to:

- Demonstrate the procedure for preparing liquid and solid oral medications.
- Demonstrate the procedure for administering liquid and solid oral medications.
- State modifications in giving oral medications to children.

Some of the principles covered in the preceding chapter are repeated in this and the following units as the principles are basic to the administration of drugs by mouth, injection, inhalation and topical application. In addition, repetition is reinforcement of learning — a most important consideration in teaching and learning about medications.

Every morning before any medication is given all medicine cards should be checked against the Kardex for lost cards, omissions, stop dates, discontinued medications, etc. If the medication has been automatically stopped, or about to be stopped, as narcotics, hypnotics, and antibiotics are in some hospitals, a note should be left to remind the physician to renew the order if he wishes to do so.

The method by which a medicine is to be administered is determined by the condition of the patient, the disease or illness, the rate of absorption desired, and the form of drug available. The most common method of administering a medication is by mouth; this is sometimes referred to as *administration of oral medications*.

Drugs administered by mouth may be in solid or liquid form. Drugs taken in solid form are pills, tablets, lozenges, capsules and powders; they are usually taken with a drink of water. Some drugs are not swallowed but are placed in the mouth. A *sublingual* tablet is placed under the tongue. An example of a sublingual tablet is nitroglycerin used for angina (symptom of a heart condition). A *buccal* tablet is placed between the cheek and the gum and allowed to dissolve. A lozenge is another form of drug which is not swallowed; it is kept in the mouth and its effect is obtained by allowing the lozenge to dissolve slowly in the mouth.

Liquid preparations are the solutions, elixirs, syrups, etc. This form of medication is absorbed more rapidly than the solid forms. The color of liquid drugs sometimes appears unattractive and its taste may not be agreeable to the patient. However, in many instances these disadvantages are overcome by the use of artificial coloring and flavoring. A drug which has an agreeable taste and appearance will often have a favorable psychological effect upon the patient. In addition to the physical benefit a medication offers a patient, the psychological effect is also important.

Section 3 Administration of Medications

MEDICATIONS IN LIQUID FORM

It is important that the dosage of medicine be measured accurately, otherwise it may not fulfill its purpose when administered. Serious consequences can occur from an overdose or an underdose due to inaccurate measure.

Measuring Devices

The most common measuring devices for oral liquid preparations are the minim glass, the graduated medicine dropper, the medicine glass and the graduated cylinder.

The *minim glass* is a small measuring device graduated on one side in milliliters or cubic centimeters (metric unit of liquid measure) and on the opposite side in minims (apothecary unit of liquid measure). It is ideal for measuring small quantities of medicines in liquid or powder form. Its capacity usually does not exceed 60 minims (4 milliliters or cubic centimeters, 1 dram).

The *medicine glass*, like the minim glass, is graduated in both the metric and apothecary systems of measure. It differs in that it has a greater capacity; 30 milliliters or cubic centimeters (8 drams, one ounce); it may be used to administer the medication just as an ordinary drinking glass.

The *graduated cylinder* is available in either or both systems of measure. Its shape facilitates the reading of the measured dosage more accurately and clearly. It is sometimes called a graduate.

Graduated medicine droppers are obtained marked in milliliters. Their capacity usually does not exceed 2 ml. They are, therefore, used for measuring relatively small dosages, figure 15-1. A drop from this type of medicine dropper is closely equivalent to a minim. This is not true for the ordinary medicine dropper.

In the absence of other measuring devices, the syringe (with or without the needle) is a measuring device which can be used for measuring dosages for oral medications. It is graduated in milliliters and cubic centimeters.

Preparing Liquid Medications

The procedure for preparing any type of medication begins with careful attention to personal cleanliness. The hands and the equipment to be used should be scrupulously clean.

1. Assemble items which will be needed on the counter at which the medications are to be prepared — measuring utensils, medicine cards, medicine glasses, pitcher of water to dilute medications, and tray on which to carry the pitcher and poured medications. (If you are unfamiliar with the floor layout, it also may be necessary to obtain a floor plan to show the location of rooms.)

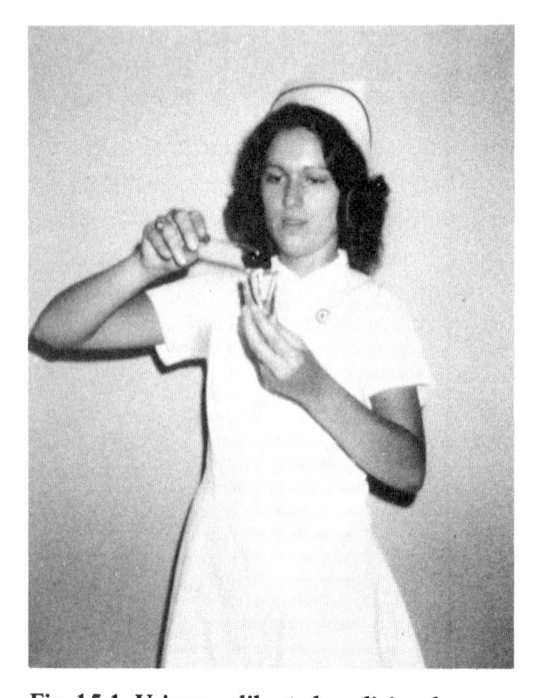

Fig. 15-1 Using a calibrated medicine dropper

2. Place each medicine card next to a medicine glass.
3. Check the drug listed on the medicine card with the label on the medicine bottle. The label should be read three times —
   - When taken from shelf
   - When poured from container
   - When returned to shelf
4. Calculate, if necessary, the correct dosage ordered. Be sure calculations are checked by the nurse in charge.

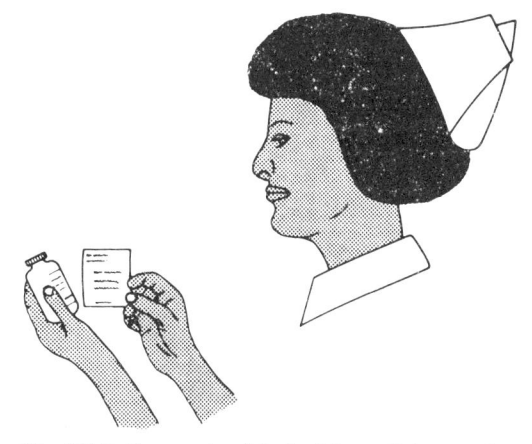

Fig. 15-2 Comparing label with medicine card

5. Check to see that the cap of the bottle is on securely. Shake the bottle to mix its contents thoroughly. This is particularly necessary when pouring drugs which are classified as mixtures. It is advisable to keep the thumb over the cap of the bottle when shaking it, to avoid its working lose.
6. Remove the cap and place it so that the *top* side is on the table. Never open more than one medicine bottle at a time. As each is used, replace the cap. This will help to avoid pouring the wrong medication and will assure that the cap is replaced on the right bottle.
7. Pour the medication, holding the medicine glass at eye level. Hold the thumbnail on the level to which the medication is to be poured. The label side of the bottle should be held toward the palm of the hand to avoid soiling the label as the medication is poured. Pour the medication to the level of the line marked by the thumbnail, figure 15-4.
8. Place the measured medicine in the medicine tray slot. Check the medicine card with the label on the bottle. Place the medicine card with the poured medication. (The card remains with the medication until the medication has been administered.)

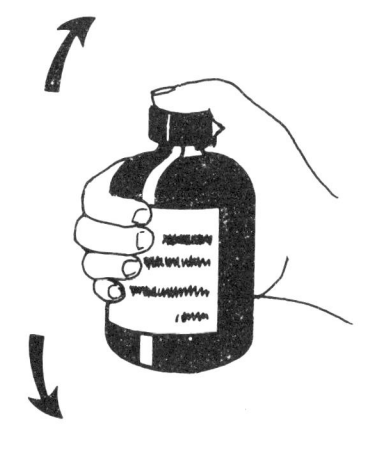

Fig. 15-3 Shaking medicine bottle

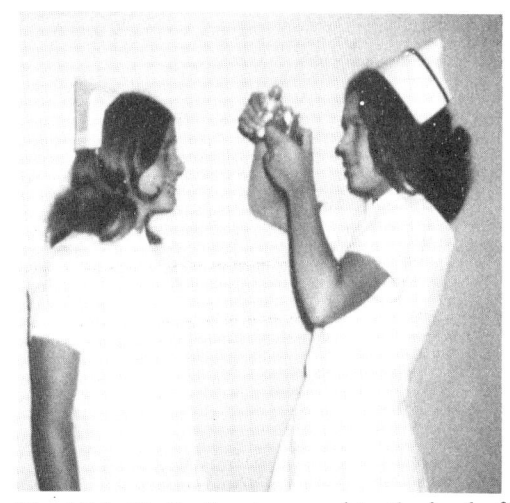

Fig. 15-4 Medication is poured to the level of the thumbnail.

Section 3 Administration of Medications

9. Wipe the lip of the bottle with a moist piece of clean paper towel or gauze before recapping it.
10. Reread the label on the bottle before replacing the bottle on the shelf.
11. Continue to pour the remaining medications due at this hour.
12. When finished pouring the medicines, clean up the area, lock the medicine cabinet, and return the key to the nurse in charge.

Giving Liquid Medications

Liquid prepackaged unit doses of medications are ordered from the pharmacy as are all other medications. They may be poured from the sealed container during the pouring of other liquid medications, or the containers may be placed with the medicine card on the tray and poured at the patient's bedside. Plastic ounce receptacles are used for these liquid medications.

After the medications have been poured and are ready to be given to the patient, the following procedure is recommended.

1. Carry the large or individual medicine tray to the bedside and place it securely on the bedside table. A wheeled medicine cart is now used in many places.
2. Check the name on the patient's wristband with the name on the medicine card. If there is any doubt in your mind, ask the patient his name.
3. Be pleasant. Hand the patient the medication and some water with a smile of interest and encouragement.
4. Remain with the patient until he has swallowed the medication.
5. Help any patient who is unable to manage the medicine glass or who is incapacitated in any way.
6. After the distribution of medications, discard disposable medicine glasses. If non-disposable medicine glasses have been used, rinse them under cold running water, wash them thoroughly in warm soapy water and rinse. Send glasses to the central service department or boil (or disinfect) as instructed.
7. Clean and replace equipment which has been used.
8. Chart the medications administered and record any reactions observed.
9. Return medicine cards to their proper location.

MEDICATIONS IN SOLID FORMS

Tablets and capsules are available in varying dosages and are ordered as such. When this is not possible, several may be administered to make up the required dosage. If a tablet size exceeds the dosage required, it may be broken into sections (scored or indented types are usually used for this purpose) to obtain the correct amount of dosage.

One or more capsules are administered to fulfill the correct dosage. Less than a capsule dosage is not given because of the difficulty in obtaining accurate measure.

A powder can be dissolved and given as a liquid preparation or poured from its paper into a spoon (water is sometimes added to float the powder). It is placed well on the back of the patient's tongue and followed by a drink of water.

Unit 15 Administration of Oral Medication

Preparing Solid (dry) Medications

Equipment to be used must be scrupulously clean. Wash the hands thoroughly before preparing to handle any medications.

1. Assemble the items which will be needed: measuring utensils, medicine cards, medicine glasses, pitcher of water, tray on which to carry the pitcher and poured medications, and a spoon or small paper cup for the pouring of tablets.

2. Arrange medicine glasses with medicine cards. If drug calculations were necessary, have them checked by the nurse in charge.

3. Check the label on the bottle with the medicine card three times.

4. Place the number of tablets in the lid or cap of the bottle and then into the medicine glass or paper container. Break scored tablets on clean area. A teaspoon may be used to pour tablets in place of the cap; this helps in the selection of the correct number of tablets, figure 15-5.

5. Place medications on the tray for administration at the bedside.

6. Clean up the counter area and lock the medicine cabinet.

Giving the Solid (dry) Medications

When unit doses are to be administered, they are obtained from the plastic dispenser cabinet (figure 15-6) and placed with the medicine card in the proper area on the plastic tray. These trays hold as many as 30 medication spaces. The tray is usually wheeled on a conveyor to the patient's bedside. The nurse opens the package for the patient to take the enclosed capsule or tablet. Following the dispensing of medications, the materials may be discarded. If nondisposable glasses and spoons are used, they must be sterilized for future use.

The procedure for giving tablets and capsules follows the same pattern used in giving liquid medications. However, a spoon or small paper cup will help in the administration of solid medications. The medication is placed well on the back of the patient's tongue and is then followed by a drink of water.

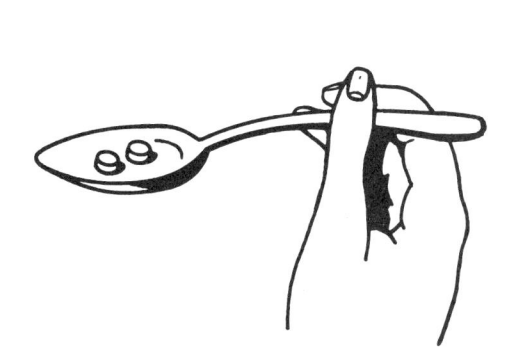

Fig. 15-5 Teaspoon for pouring tablets

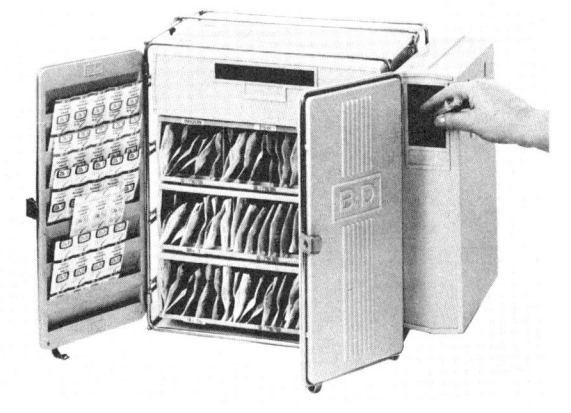

Fig. 15-6 Dispenser cabinet for unit doses provided by the manufacturer

Section 3 Administration of Medications

Elderly people frequently need help in placing tablets in their mouths and sometimes in swallowing. Time and patience are important in the administration of drugs to the elderly, figure 15-7.

Medicine trays or carts are never taken into an isolation area. Also, if patient is disoriented or mentally ill the medicine tray or cart is left at a distance from the patient so that a sudden movement on his part will not disarrange it.

In homes for the elderly the medicine cart must be kept under observation at all times. It is well to have a reliable aide go with the medication nurse (to watch the cart) while she gives the medication, *which sometimes takes time and necessitates the nurse turning her back on the medication cart.*

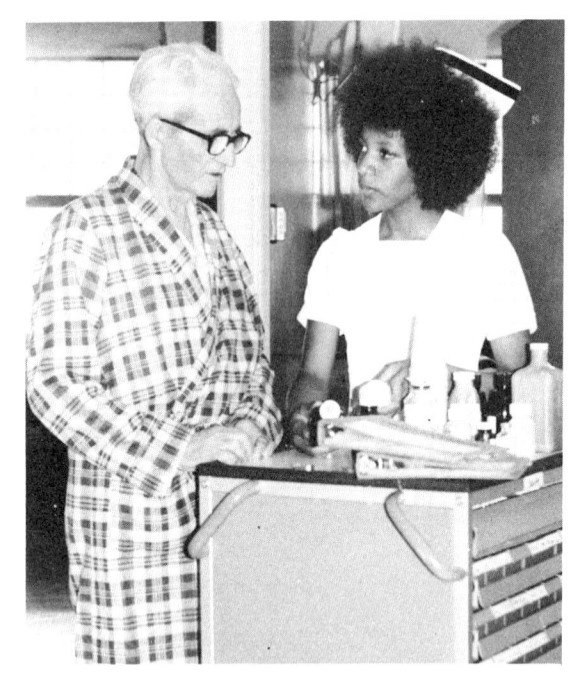

Fig. 15-7 A Nurse and patient discuss his medication.

PREPARING AND ADMINISTERING DRUGS TO CHILDREN

Drugs may be given to children in honey, applesauce etc. if their diet permits. Children, especially infants, are sometimes unable to swallow tablets of any size. A tablet should be crushed and its contents poured into a spoon. The crushed tablet should then be allowed to dissolve by adding just enough water to make a swallow. It is placed well on the back of the child's tongue and followed with a drink of water.

The method used to crush the tablet will depend on the equipment available. Use of a mortar and pestle is the most desirable method, but in the event these are not available, two spoons may be used as illustrated. However, great care must be used so that none of the tablet is lost in this process, figure 15-8 and 15-9.

Another method is to place the tablet in a medicine glass or pill dish and to crush it with a spoon or other suitable instrument.

Unpleasant medicinal tastes may be disguised by using aromatic flavors such as wintergreen, peppermint, spearmint, etc. They should not be added unless directed by the doctor and only in specified quantities. Excess amounts can cause serious harmful effects.

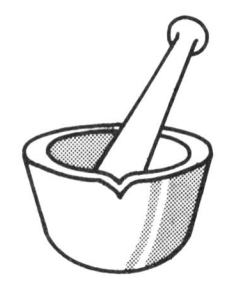

Fig. 15-8 Mortar and pestle

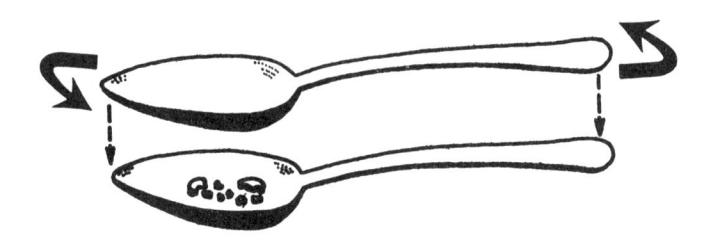

Fig. 15-9 Crushing tablets with spoons

PRECAUTIONS IN ADMINISTERING MEDICATIONS

The nurse who is given the responsibility of administering medications should take precautions. Some important points to remember are:

- Be alert to possible side reactions and toxic reactions. The absence of a reaction following an initial dose does not mean that no reactions will follow subsequent doses. Cumulative action must be considered and the patient observed for any signs.

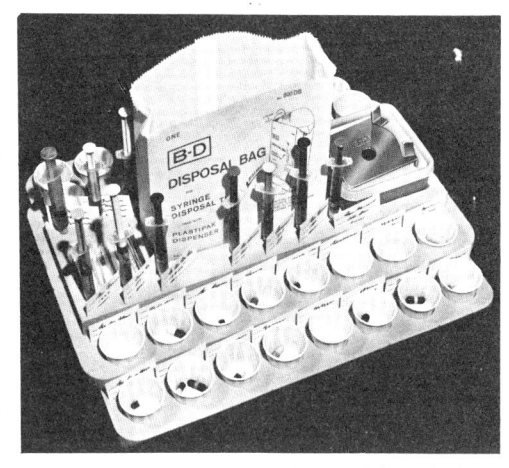

Fig. 15-10 This tray may be used for administering both oral medications and injections.

- Care must be taken that the right drug is given to the right person. Cards must be attached to medicine glasses and cups so that they cannot become loose and/or get mixed with other cards and medications, figure 15-10.
- If the patient asks about medications, suggest that he discuss it with his doctor. However, report any questions or signs of anxiety about the medications to the nurse in charge.

CHARTING OF MEDICATIONS

After the medications have been given they should be charted promptly. The information to be charted will include:

- The medication
- The amount given
- The exact time given
- The route of administration (by mouth, hypo, etc.)

Note any unusual reactions or symptoms following administration of the medication. Report this to the nurse in charge immediately and then chart it.

If the patient refuses to take a medication, report to the nurse in charge or the physician, if you are on a home case. Explain the reason for refusal. Chart the reason or reasons.

A drug which is given to a patient for pain or sleeplessness should be followed up to see if the desired results have been achieved. Chart the results.

SUGGESTED ACTIVITIES

- Refer to the Kardex and record the number of medications to be given orally. What is the percentage compared to all other methods of administering medications? Report your findings to the class.
- Practice measuring liquid medicine with:
  a. Graduated medicine dropper
  b. Medicine glass
  c. Minim glass

Section 3 Administration of Medications

- Practice the procedure for administering a liquid medicine orally. Remember to follow the six steps of accuracy.
- Practice the procedure for administering a pill or powder orally. Remember to follow the six steps of accuracy.

REVIEW

1. Name the two systems of measurement. Identify the terms used in each system (to measure liquid and dry forms of medication).

2. Explain the procedure for administering a liquid medication orally.

3. Explain the procedure for administering a tablet orally.

4. List the important items which are to be charted following the administration of medication.

5. Give the precautions to be taken when administering oral medications.

6. Name four devices used for measuring oral medications.

EXTENDED STUDY

Examine and practice handling various types of hypodermic syringes and needles.

Unit 16 Types of Syringes and Needles

OBJECTIVES

After studying this unit, the student should be able to:
- Describe the types of syringes and needles used for giving injections.
- Clean and sterilize nondisposable syringes and needles.

The nurse may be called upon to administer several types of injections. In giving injections it will be necessary for her to know about the syringes and needles which are used and how they are cared for.

SYRINGES

The components of a syringe consist of a barrel and plunger. These must fit together tightly if they are to be effective. Some manufacturers give assembly numbers to syringes and plungers so that they will be properly matched when assembled. Other manufacturers produce syringes which have interchangeable barrels and plungers. They are made so that any needle fits snugly and they may or may not be provided with a locking device for the needle. The syringes range in size from 1/4 ml or cc to 100 ml or cc. The size used will depend upon the amount and type of drug to be administered. Nondisposable syringes are usually made of Pyrex glass.

The barrels of most syringes are calibrated in the metric scale. There are also syringes which have special graduations, such as those used for insulin injections. Tuberculin syringes are calibrated in both the metric and apothecaries' scales.

Syringes are classified as either standard or special. A *standard* syringe is used for most types of injections; a *special* syringe is used for a particular type of injection. Examples of special syringes are the tuberculin and insulin syringes. Tuberculin syringes are used to administer intradermal skin tests. They can be used to measure minute quantities of testing materials such as 0.01 ml. The insulin syringe is used for administering insulin to a diabetic and is calibrated in units as well as milliliters or cubic centimeters.

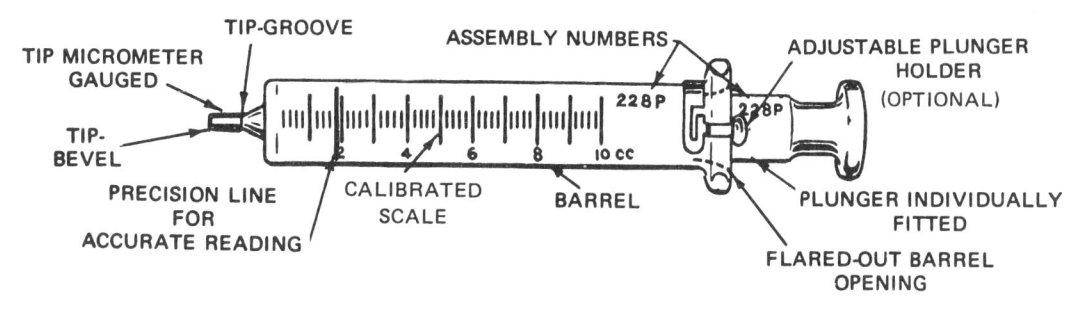

Fig. 16-1 Hypodermic syringe components

Section 3 Administration of Medications

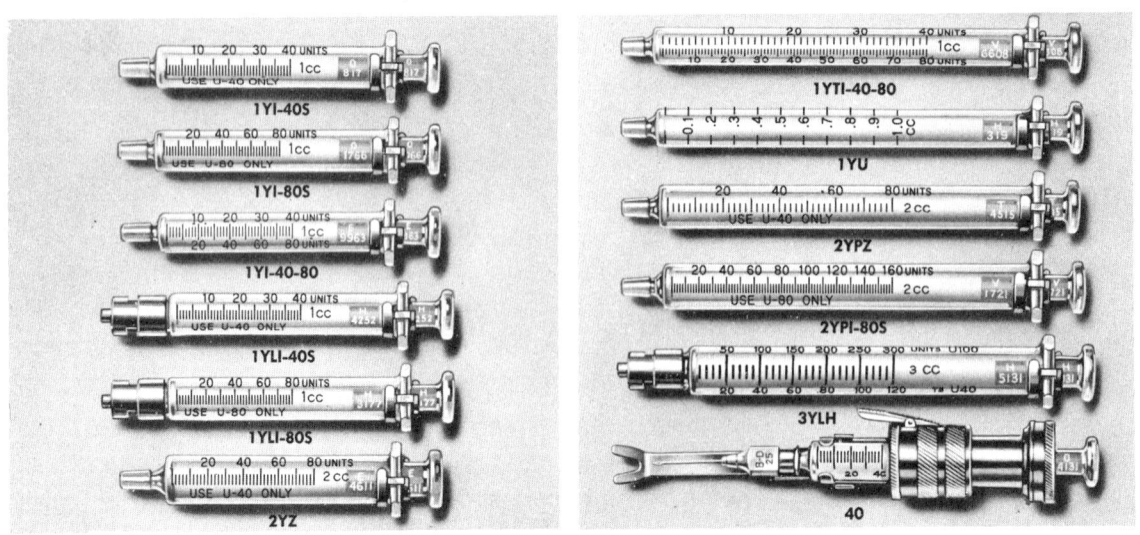

Fig. 16-2 Types of hypodermic syringes

Hospitals are now using sterile, prepackaged, disposable needles and syringes. These are timesaving for the nurse and safer for the patient. However, reusable equipment is still used to a limited degree; therefore, it is necessary to know how to clean and sterilize reusable equipment properly.

Care of Nondisposable Syringes

Syringes should be cleaned immediately after use by flushing with cold water or a neutral cleaning solution until all traces of the medication disappear. The needle and syringe parts are then separated and allowed to soak in a neutral cleaning solution for 5 to 20 minutes. If an oily medication or solution has been used, they should be left to soak for 1 to 1 1/2 hours. Any soil which has not been removed after soaking should be brushed or wiped away. The use of an abrasive cleaner should be avoided on glass parts because of the danger of scratching surfaces and removing graduate marks. After soaking and brushing, the syringe should be assembled and flushed with a cleaning solution, then rinsed under running tap water and, finally, flushed with distilled water or alcohol. The syringe is then ready for sterilization by the central service department. The use in hospitals of ultrasonic cleaning devices has greatly enhanced the efficiency and speed by which reusable needles and syringes can be cleaned.

It is seldom necessary to boil syringes because of the availability of disposable syringes. However, if a glass syringe *is* used, the syringe may be sterilized in an autoclave by steam under pressure, by ethylene oxide gas, by radiation, or by boiling it in water. By this latter method, distilled water is considered the best medium. Do not boil syringes in water containing an alkali because this will mar the glass surface. The syringes should be carefully placed in the sterilizer and boiled for 20 minutes. Unnecessary boiling shortens the life of the syringe. If spore-bearing bacilli are suspected, boiling is not recommended; autoclaving is used instead. Lack of proper sterilization has probably been a cause of the easy transmission of hepatitis.

Disposable Syringe Units

Disposable syringes with separate needles and disposable syringe-needle units are available. They are enclosed in peel-apart packages. Some have clear vinyl overwraps

Unit 16 Types of Syringes and Needles

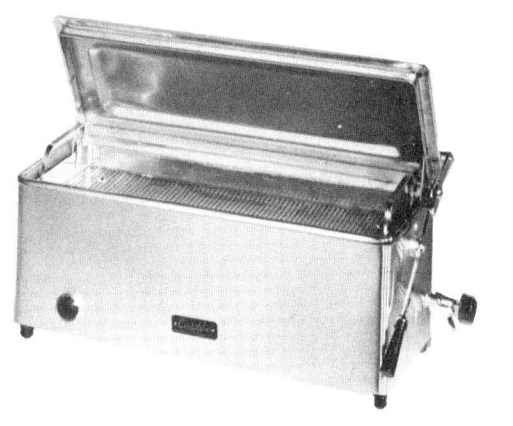

Fig. 16-3 Boiling water sterilizer

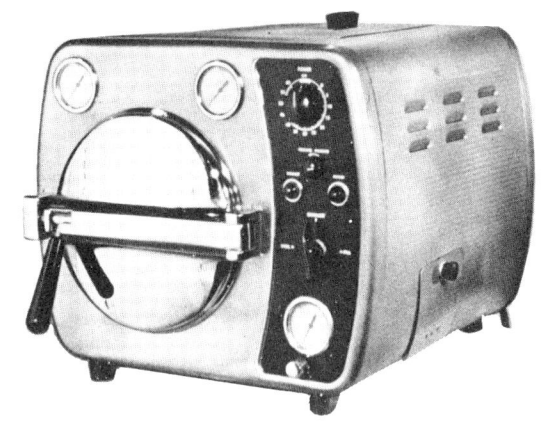

Fig. 16-4 Small autoclave

A

B

C

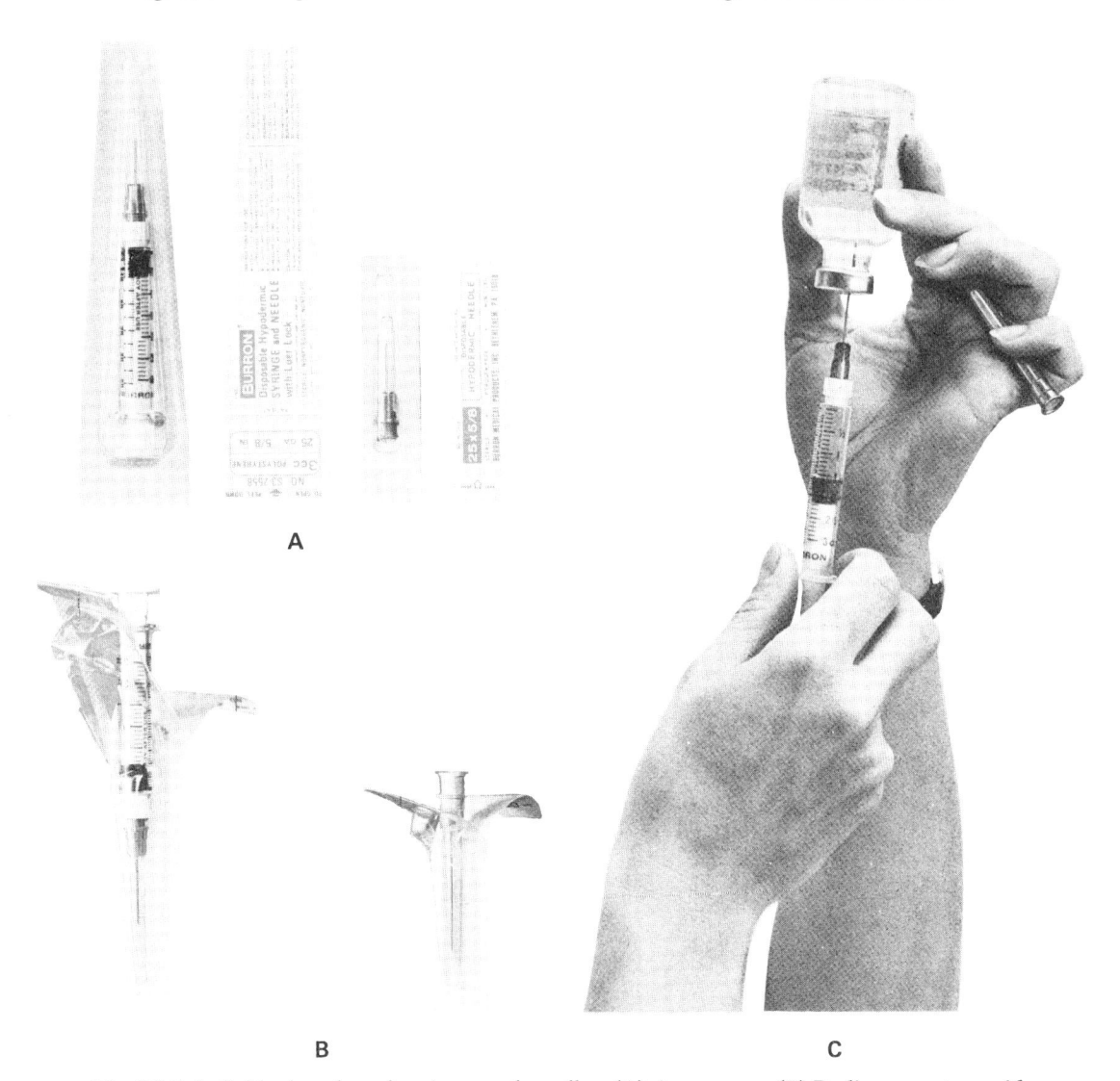

Fig. 16-5 Individual packaged syringes and needles; (A) Appearance (B) Peeling open to avoid contamination and (C) Using the disposable unit. (Courtesy of Burron Medical Products, Inc.)

Section 3 Administration of Medications

for protection and instant identification. Within the package is a sterile syringe (with or without a needle) whose tip is protected by a shield.

If the package contains a syringe-needle unit, the needle cannula is already affixed directly into the syringe barrel. To use the disposable syringe – needle unit, twist the caps off to break the vacuum; then remove the caps by pulling straight off, figure 16-6.

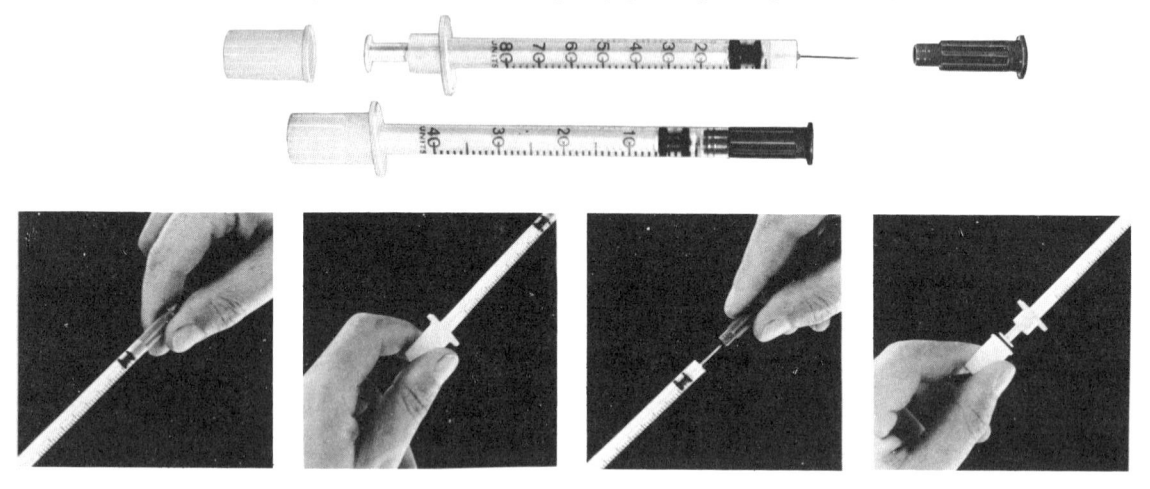

Fig. 16-6 Disposable insulin syringe-needle unit
(Courtesy Becton-Dickenson)

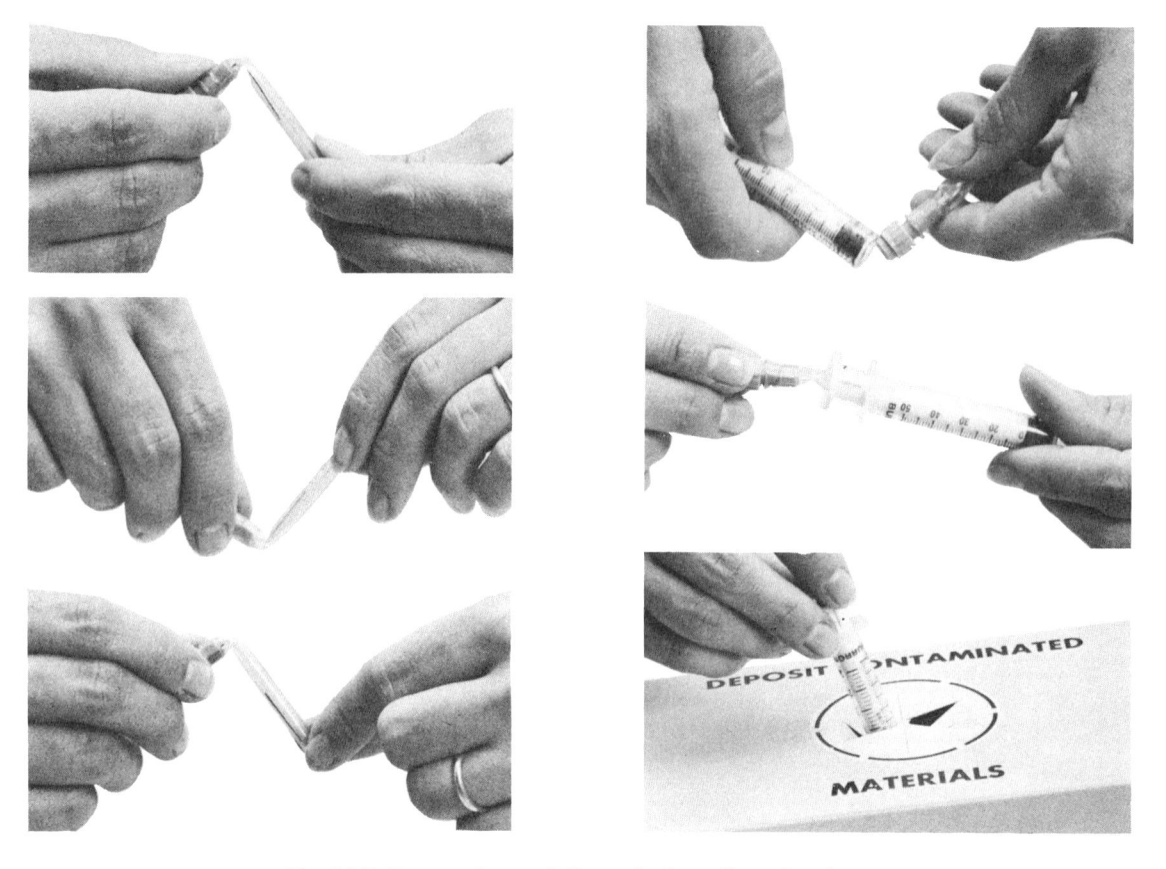

Fig. 16-7 Destruction and disposal of needle and syringe

After using a disposable unit, the nurse must be sure to destroy the needle and the syringe — not just throw them away. To destroy the needle, replace the needle guard and bend both the needle and guard downward, then upward and down again. The needle is then broken and encapsulated in the guard. The syringe may be destroyed by holding the barrel in one hand, the luer lock with the other and snapping outward. The syringe will break at the base of the syringe barrel. Then dispose of both items in a clearly marked materials box.

Some medications which are to be given hypodermically come in a prefilled, premeasured cartridge unit. Single dose antibiotics, narcotics, barbiturates and cardiovascular agents are often administered in this kind of cartridge-needle unit. The unit fits into a separate metal plunger, figure 16-8.

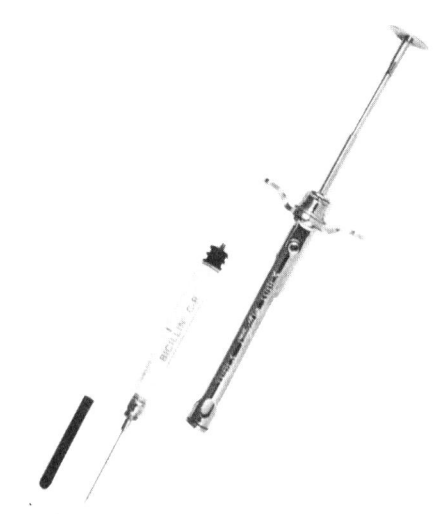

Fig. 16-8 A prefilled, premeasured sterile Cartridge Unit and Syringe

HYPODERMIC NEEDLES

Needles for syringes are either disposable or made of high-quality stainless steel. Lengths range from 1/2" to 3" and are measured from where the needle *joins* the hub to the tip of the point (hub not included). Special needles that have a stop are measured from the stop to the tip of the point. Diameters on needles are indicated by gauge numbers ranging from 13 to 27. The bigger the gauge number, the smaller the diameter of the needle. Gauge numbers are often stamped on the flat of the hub for ready reference. In choosing the size

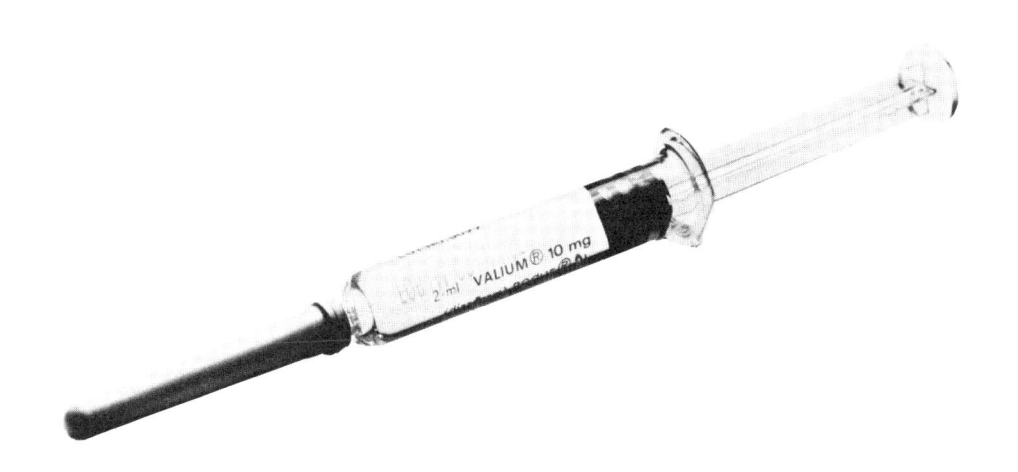

Fig. 16-9 Premeasured, prefilled dose of medication in disposable syringe
(Courtesy of Roche Labs)

Section 3 Administration of Medications

of a hypodermic needle for an injection, the nurse should be governed by four factors: safety, rate of flow, comfort of patient and depth of penetration. Sizes and their particular applications are shown in figure 16-10.

Attention should be given to the sharpness of a needle prior to its use. If a needle is dropped, the point is sometimes damaged. If a needle appears dull do not use it, as the injection will be a difficult and painful one.

The *nondisposable* needle should be cleaned immediately following its use by flushing it with cold water. If the cannula is clogged, needle wire is inserted in the bore from the hub end and carefully forced through to remove the congested matter. The inside of the hub is cleaned with a tightly wound cotton applicator. Stains may be removed by use of a

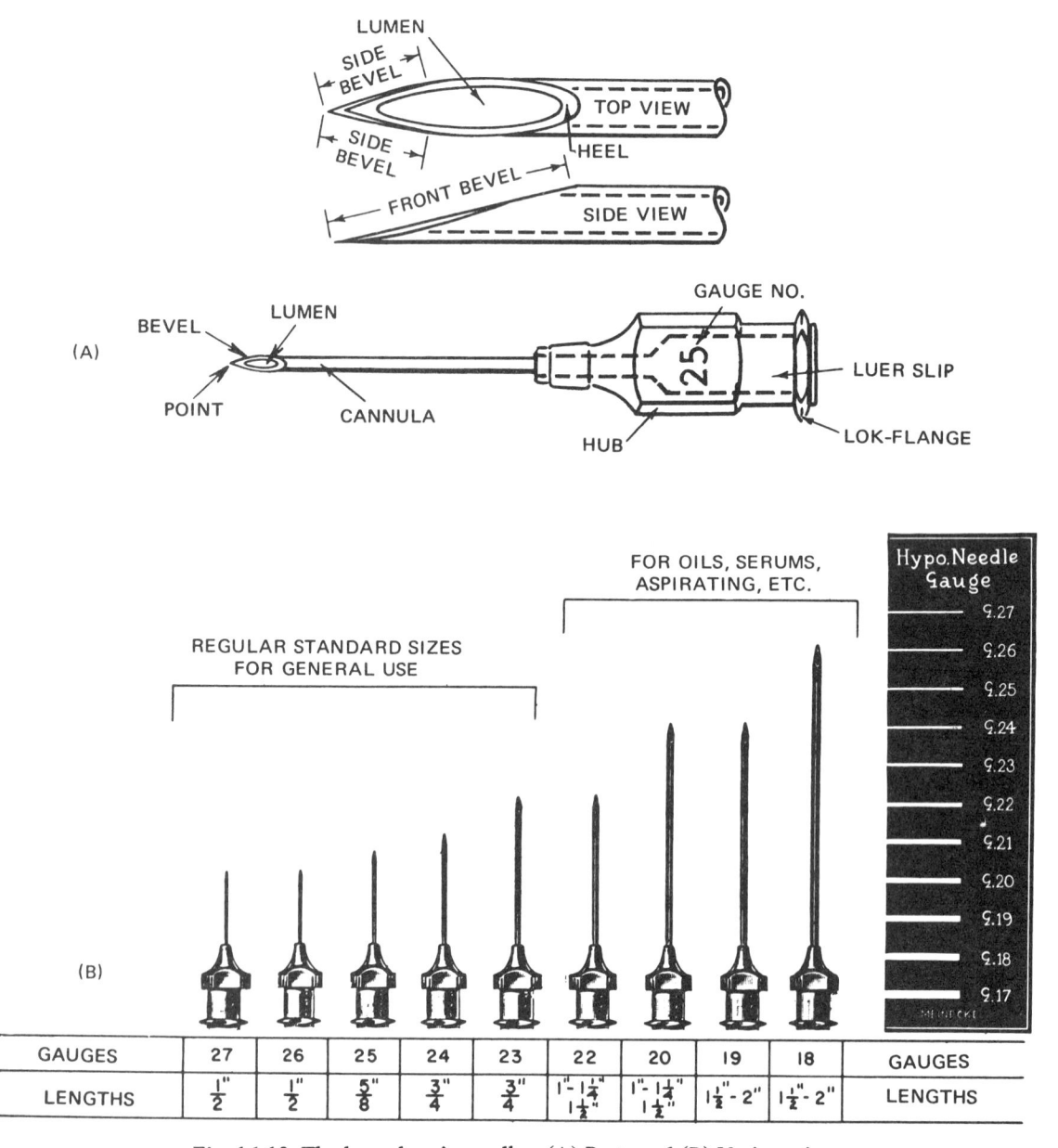

GAUGES	27	26	25	24	23	22	20	19	18	GAUGES
LENGTHS	$\frac{1}{2}"$	$\frac{1}{2}"$	$\frac{5}{8}"$	$\frac{3}{4}"$	$\frac{3}{4}"$	$1"-1\frac{1}{4}"$ $1\frac{1}{2}"$	$1"-1\frac{1}{4}"$ $1\frac{1}{2}"$	$1\frac{1}{2}"-2"$	$1\frac{1}{2}"-2"$	LENGTHS

Fig. 16-10 The hypodermic needle: (A) Parts and (B) Various sizes

household abrasive cleaner. If the needle should be stuck, soak the syringe and needle in cleaning solution for 5 minutes. Then, with the aid of pliers or forceps, loosen the needle by rotating the syringe counterclockwise, figure 16-11. Cleanse the syringe and needle as previously suggested.

Following these operations, the needle should be rinsed and washed thoroughly with a neutral cleaning solution. The final step is to flush the needle with alcohol or air, or with a quick-drying commercial needle drier. The needle is now ready for sterilization. It may be sterilized by boiling from 15 to 20 minutes. Stainless steel needles can withstand a temperature of 100° Celsius which is 212° Fahrenheit. If spore-bearing bacilli are suspected, boiling is not recommended. Spore-bearing bacilli are destroyed more effectively by steam under pressure (autoclave) or dry heat (hot air). A moist temperature of 120°C kills all vegetative bacteria and most spores within 15 to 20 minutes; and a dry temperature of 160°C kills all spores within 1 hour.

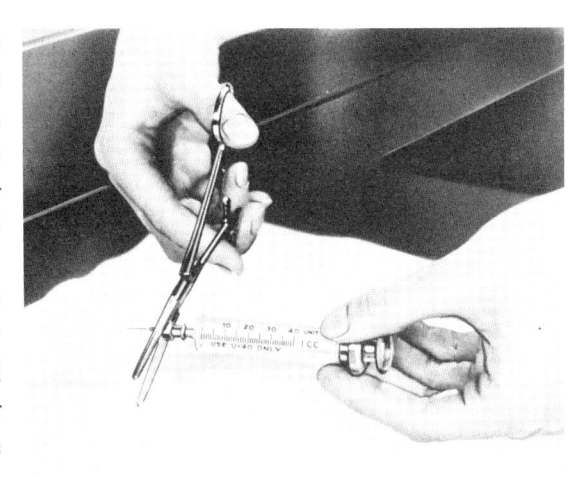

Fig. 16-11 Removing stuck needle

Disposable needles should have the needle points broken off at the hub before disposing of them. There is no reboiling with disposable needles.

SUGGESTED ACTIVITIES

- Observe how hypodermic needles are stored and cared for at the hospital with which you are affiliated and report your findings to the class.
- Sometimes we break syringes carelessly, not realizing the expense of replacement of such equipment. Go to a large drugstore and price the various types of syringes comparable to the ones used on your hospital service. Present your findings to the class.
- Obtain illustrations of different types of syringes and hypodermic needles from appropriate catalogs. Prepare a folder or booklet with these illustrations: include under each, its type and use.

REVIEW

1. On the illustration, identify the parts of the syringe.

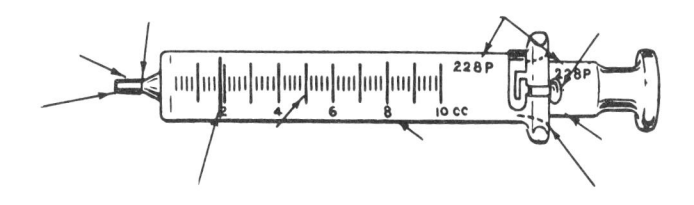

Section 3 Administration of Medications

2. What system(s) of measurement are shown on syringes?

3. Name a syringe used for measuring very small quantities.

4. How is the diameter of a needle designated?

5. Name 4 factors that govern what needle size should be used.

6. How is a needle measured for length?

7. State three reasons for the trend toward use of prepackaged, sterile, disposable needles and syringes.

8. Explain how to discard a disposable syringe and needle.

EXTENDED STUDY

Learn the meaning of proper use of the following terms.

subcutaneous	intradermal
intramuscular	25-gauge needle
intravenous	dispersion

Unit 17 Administration of Medications by Injection

OBJECTIVES

After studying this unit, the student should be able to:

- Compare methods of injection: subcutaneous, intramuscular, intradermal, and intravenous.
- Demonstrate the procedures given.

A knowledge of the various kinds of injections, why each is used, and how each is administered should precede any attempt at giving an injection. Considerable skill is required to perform an injection satisfactorily.

The attitude of the nurse is an important consideration in giving injections. Being a patient is an experience which requires an adjustment, and the anticipation of multiple injections is not pleasant. The nurse, although sympathetic and understanding, must maintain a professional attitude regarding medications and treatments.

PREPARING AN INJECTION

Before studying how to administer an injection, the student must have practice in handling the syringe and needle without contaminating certain parts, and withdrawing solutions from vials and ampules. Ease in handling the equipment will make the preparation and the administration of the injection an easier process. The nurse can approach the patient with confidence; this confidence is felt by the patient and explanations are more readily accepted.

It is suggested that each procedure be read through first. Then, study and practice of the steps should take place.

Preparing the Syringe and Needle

The nurse must work in an uncluttered area. The counter should be free of unnecessary equipment. Work close to the counter to avoid dropping items on the floor.

1. Wash the hands thoroughly.
2. Select the proper syringe and needle. A 2 cc syringe with a 3/4 inch, 25 gauge needle is suggested.
3. Disposable syringe-needle units are already assembled. Peel off the outer covering and remove the unit; leave the sheath over the needle. Nondisposable syringes and needles must be assembled so that none of the critical parts are contaminated. If the syringe and needle have been boiled (as in some home cases) sterile forceps must be used throughout the process to maintain sterility of the parts, and to avoid burning the fingers. If the unit has been autoclaved and is packaged in a sterile pack, open the pack away from the body.

Section 3 Administration of Medications

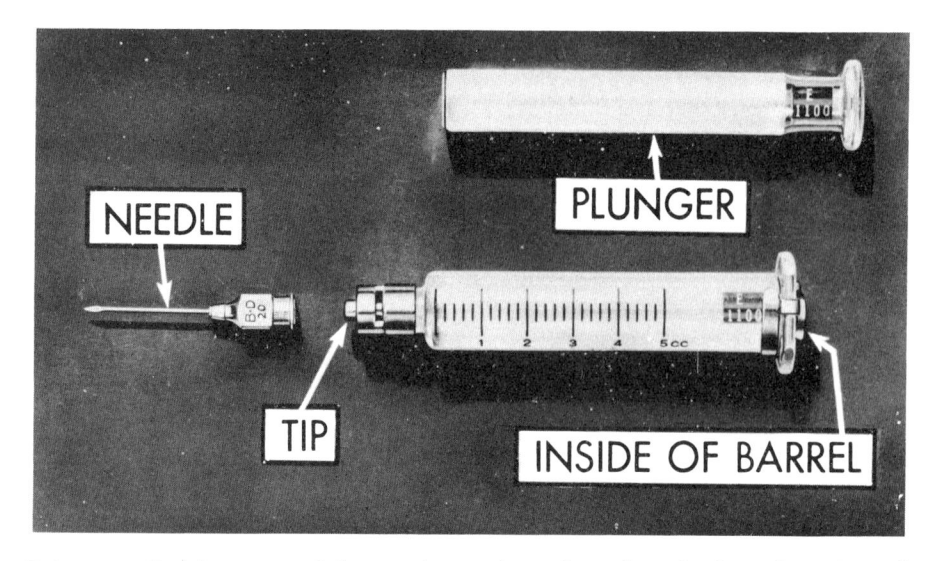

[Photo showing syringe components labeled: NEEDLE, TIP, PLUNGER, INSIDE OF BARREL]

4. Using sterile forceps, pick up the syringe barrel and place between thumb and fingers of the left hand. Pick up the plunger and insert in syringe barrel by using sterile forceps.

5. Pick up the needle by the square part of the hub and place on syringe tip by using sterile forceps. If using a separately packaged disposable needle, peel off the outer covering and place the needle on the separate sterile syringe, handling it in the same way. Study figure 17-1.

Withdrawing the drug

Check the name of the medication on the medicine card against the label of the container (vial or ampule) from which the medicine is to be obtained.

1. If using a vial, cleanse the top of the rubber-capped vial with cotton or gauze sponge containing 70% alcohol.

2. Draw up enough air in the syringe equivalent to the amount of ordered medication. Be careful not to touch the side of the plunger as you draw back on it. Inject the air through the sterile needle into the vial.

3. Withdraw the correct amount of medicine.

4. Replace the needle which was used for insertion in the vial with another sterile needle which will be used to administer the injection.

5. Protect the needle from contamination by surrounding it

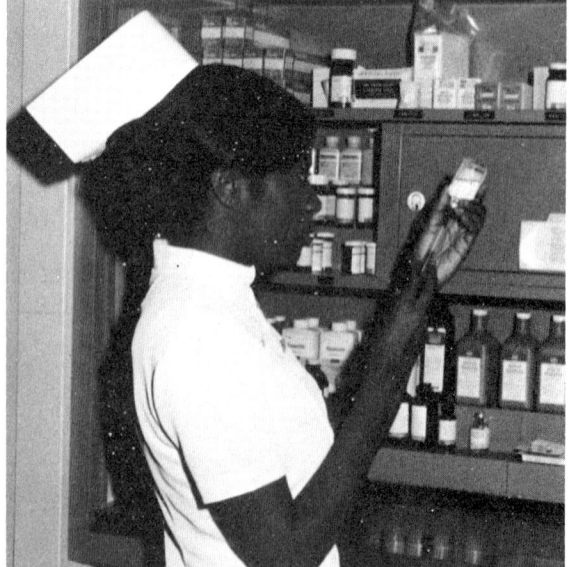

Fig. 17-2 Injecting air into vial and preparing to withdraw desired amount of drug

with a gauze sponge (or cotton) saturated with alcohol 70%. When using a disposable syringe, replace sheath on the needle. The injection is now ready to be administered.

6. Place the prepared syringe and needle with the medicine card.
7. When withdrawing medication from an ampule,
    a. air is not injected into the ampule
    b. the top of the ampule must be removed before it can be used and
    c. the needle used to withdraw the drug need not be replaced if it is still sterile and sharp.

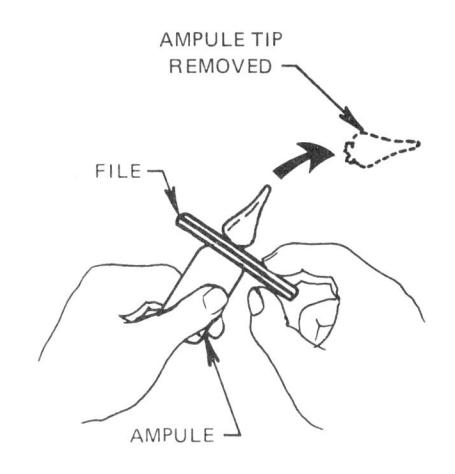

Fig. 17-3 Scoring an ampule

The top portion of the ampule must be scored with a file, figure 17-3. The tip is then broken off by gently tapping it with the flat end of the file. However, most of the medications packaged today are prescored and can be broken open without the use of a file.

Extreme care should be exercised to avoid contamination of the ampule and/or the needle as it enters the portion containing the drug.

GIVING THE INJECTION

Medication may be injected by subcutaneous, intramuscular, intravenous, and intradermal methods.

Subcutaneous Method

A subcutaneous injection is given just under the surface of the skin with a hypodermic needle and syringe. It may be given wherever there is subcutaneous tissue. However, the most frequent sites for this injection are the upper and outer part of the arm or the outer thigh.

Drugs are given subcutaneously for prompt action, for accuracy of dosage, to avoid loss of their effectiveness by digestive juices, and to avoid nausea from drugs which can be irritating to the stomach when taken orally. Examples of drugs used for this type of injection are morphine, insulin, and atropine.

There are certain drugs which may be ordered frequently but should never be used for subcutaneous injections because of the resulting pain and danger of tissue damage. These are the drugs put up in oil or the mercurial drugs. Penicillin is an example of a drug which should not be administered subcutaneously.

The amount of drug administered by a subcutaneous injection should be limited to 2 milliliters or cubic centimeters; more than this amount may cause discomfort and pain. If more than 2 cubic centimeters are ordered, the dose is made up by giving several injections at different sites.

Section 3 Administration of Medications

Administering a Subcutaneous Injection. After mastering the procedure for preparing a needle and syringe for injection, the student is ready to administer it.

1. On the tray, assemble the necessary equipment; the prepared syringe and needle, medicine card, cotton or gauze sponges and disinfectant for skin (alcohol 70%), extra needles in sterile containers (in case nurse contaminiates one), tray, and waste receptacle, figure 17-4.

2. Carry the tray to the bedside.

3. Check the patient's name on the wristband and compare it with the medicine card. Tell the patient what you plan to do.

4. Select the area of skin to be used for the injection and carefully cleanse it with alcohol 70%. Use a circular motion from the center out to about two inches beyond planned site of injection. Allow the skin to dry.

5. Pick up the prepared syringe, needle up, and expel any air, being careful not to lose any medicine and keeping the needle sterile.

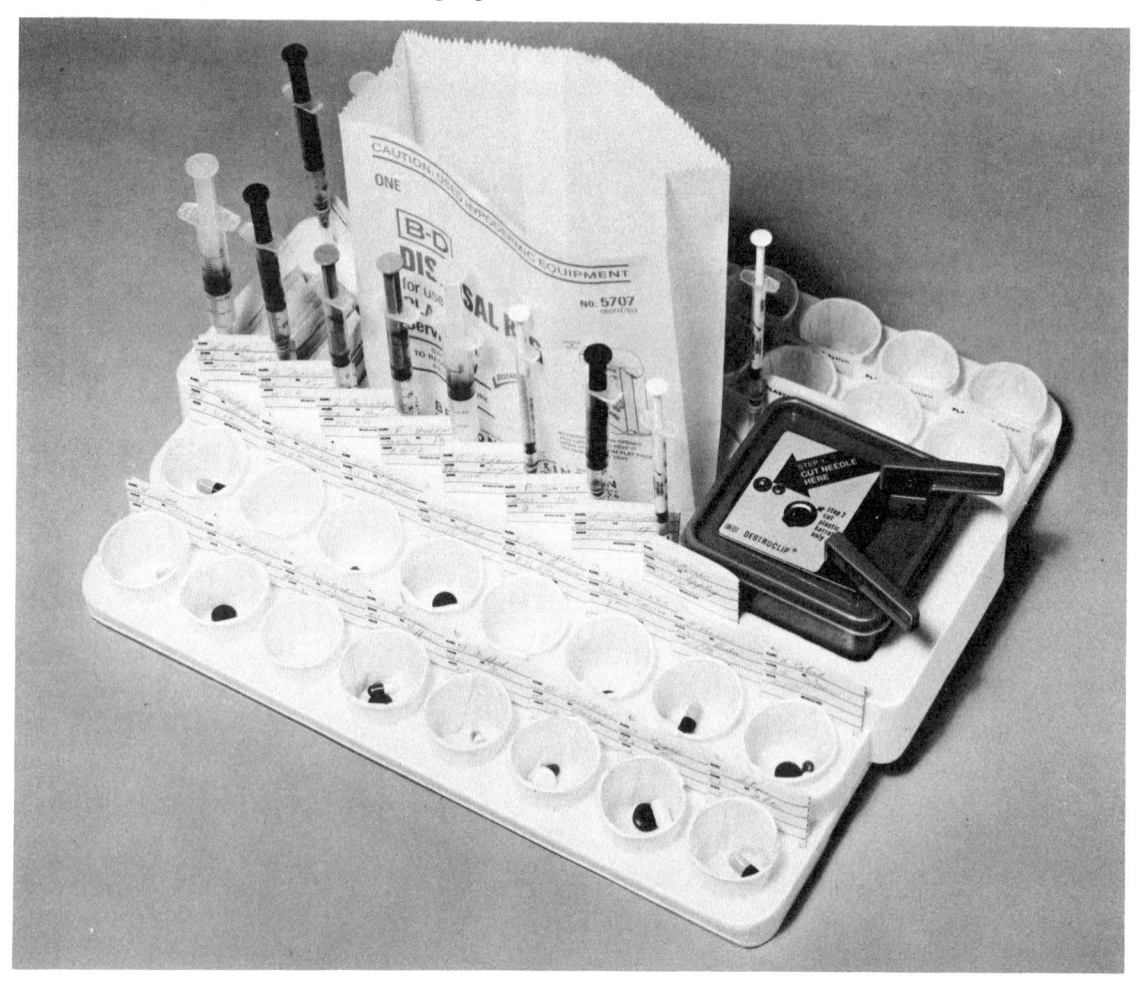

Fig. 17-4 PLASTIPAK Service Tray
(Courtesy Becton-Dickenson, Rutherford, N.J.)

6. Pinch the skin or press down firmly with your left hand and quickly insert the needle at a 45-degree angle from the skin, figure 17-5. Free the skin for a moment and draw back on the plunger slightly to be sure needle is not in a blood vessel. If blood should show when the plunger is drawn back, withdraw the needle. Prepare the medication again, using another syringe and needle, and choose another site for the injection.

   If no blood appears in the syringe when the plunger is withdrawn, firm the skin again and push the plunger with the thumb of your right hand until all the drug has been injected. With the cotton sponge in place, withdraw the needle quickly and massage the area gently.

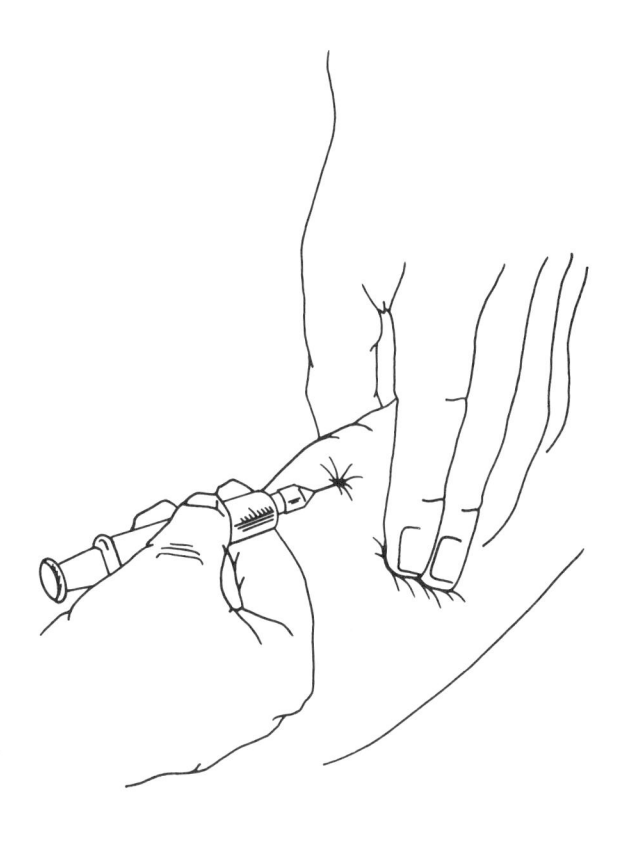

Fig. 17-5 Administering a subcutaneous injection

7. Chart the injection immediately.
8. Cleanse syringe and needle as quickly as possible.
9. Replace drugs to their proper storage center.
10. Cleanse and replace any other equipment which was used.
11. Return medicine cards to head nurse or to their proper location.

Intramuscular Injection

The intramuscular injection is given through the skin and subcutaneous tissue into the muscle tissue. The areas which may be used for the intramuscular injection are the:
- Gluteus medius. This is the upper outer quadrant of the gluteal region.
- Ventrogluteal. The anterior aspect of the gluteal region.
- Vastus Lateralis. The front of the thigh.
- Mid-Deltoid. The middle of the upper arm.

If the injection is not placed at the proper depth or is administered close to or into the large vessels and nerves, serious damage can result.

It is a method of injection that is used when a drug (such as liver extract) tends to be irritating to the upper layers of tissue. Some of the drugs favorably used for this injection are antibiotics, certain narcotics, and hypnotics. The rate of absorption by this method is comparatively rapid.

Section 3 Administration of Medications

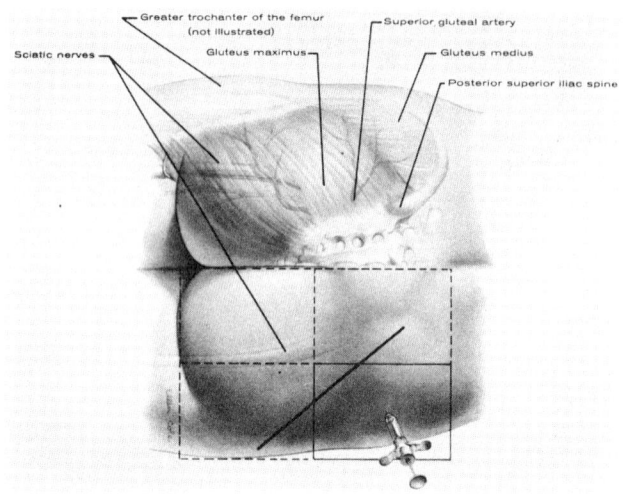

Fig. 17-6 Intramuscular injection in the Gluteus Medius. Patient should be lying flat in a toe-in position. Note the Sciatic Nerve and the blood vessels near it. Avoid this area.
(Courtesy Wyeth Laboratories, Philadelphia, Pa.)

The gluteal region and the buttock are not exactly the same thing. The buttock refers to the fleshy prominence. The gluteal region extends beyond the buttock, forward to the anterior superior spine of the iliac bone. The buttock (gluteus maximus) is *NOT* used for injection. The gluteus *medius* is used, figure 17-6. The ventrogluteal site may also be used.

Administering the Intramuscular Injection in the Gluteus Medius. As a rule, the amount of medication administered for one injection will not exceed 5 cc. If more than 5 cubic centimeters are ordered, several injections are given at different sites to make up the dose.

1. Select and assemble the necessary equipment as previously explained for the subcutaneous injection. Observe sterile technique throughout. Needle sizes for injection into the gluteal region range from 20 to 22 gauge and may be 1 1/2, 2 or 2 1/2 inches in length, depending on the thickness of the gluteal musculature. The syringe size is determined by the amount of fluid to be injected.

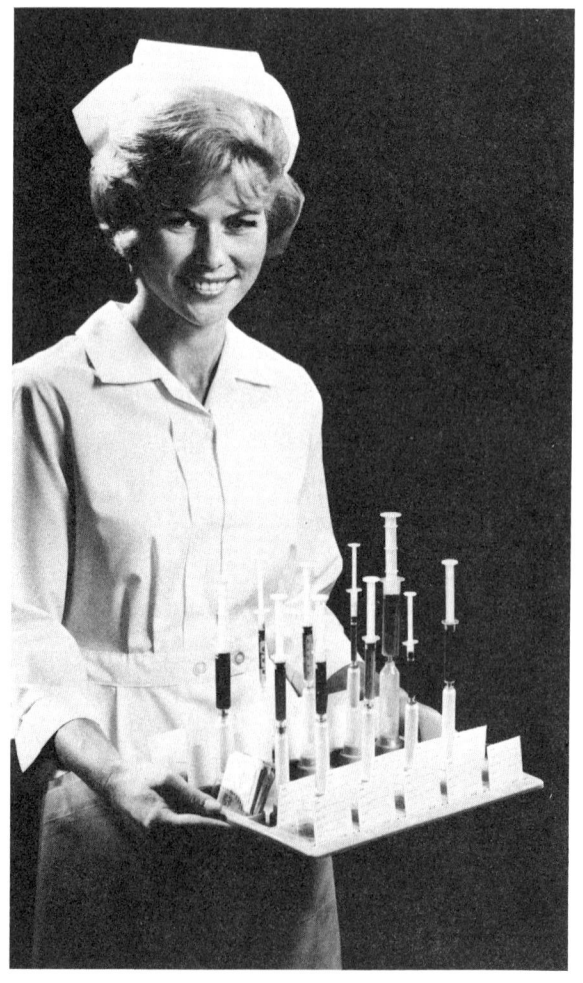

Fig. 17-7 Nurse carrying a tray with injectable medications

2. Fill the syringe with the amount of ordered dosage. Change to a new needle after filling the syringe.
3. Prepare the medicine tray.
4. Check the patient's name on the wristband and compare it with the medicine card.
5. Tell the patient what you plan to do.
6. Place the patient in a prone position. Encourage him to toe in as this will relax the muscle for injection.
7. Prepare the area for injection by cleansing it with cotton saturated with alcohol or other antiseptic ordered. The site for injection is the upper and outer quarter of the gluteal region, figure 17-8. By using this area the nurse will avoid hitting the

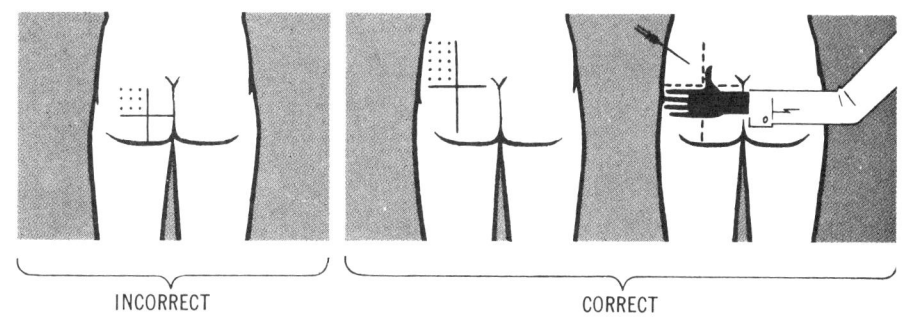

INCORRECT   CORRECT

Injection Site: Inject medication into the upper outer quadrant of the gluteal region.

Needle: Inject medication deep into the muscle. A 2-2½ inch, 20-22 gauge needle should be used. Obese patients may require a longer needle. Use one needle to withdraw the medication from vial and another needle for injection. Allow 0.5 ml (0.5cc) of air in syringe before injecting.

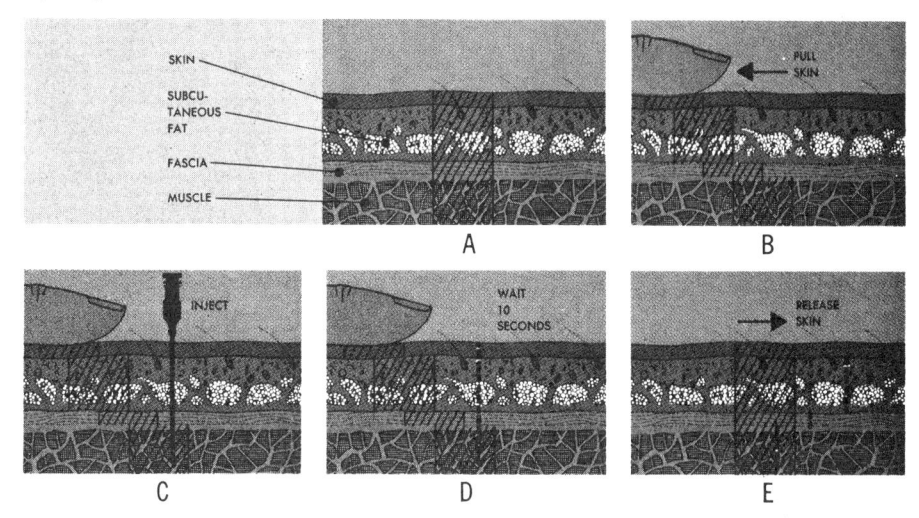

Z-Track technique: This injection technique is recommended to avoid leakage of medication into the subcutaneous tissue. Displacing the skin firmly to one side prior to injection and then releasing it after injection, seals off the medication and helps prevent staining due to leakage.

Position of the Patient: The patient should lie down in a prone or lateral position. Standing is not advisable. However, if the patient must stand, he should bear his weight on the leg opposite the injection site.

Fig. 17-8 Administering an intramuscular injection (Gluteus Medius)

Section 3 Administration of Medications

sciatic nerve. If she injects too far out, she may hit small blood vessels. Stand on the opposite side of the patient while he lies prone and face down, and flatten the tissue of the buttock by exerting pressure.

8. Hold the syringe firmly in the right hand between index, middle finger and thumb. Be sure there is no drug on the surface of the needle because it may irritate the skin. Plunge needle straight (vertically) into the buttock to approximately one-half the desired depth with a firm, bold pressure, figure 17-9. Complete pushing the needle to the desired depth with a light pressure.

9. Gently pull back the plunger to be sure the needle is not in a blood vessel. If not, proceed with the injection. If blood appears, change the site of the injection. Use another sterile syringe and needle.

10. Inject the medication slowly.

11. Use the Z-track technique as shown in figure 17-8 for medications which are irritating to the tissues, for example, the iron preparation, Imferon.

12. Place the cotton-alcohol pledget (compress) against the needle as you withdraw it rapidly. (except for Z-tract injections)

13. Chart the medication immediately and replace the medicine card.

14. Cleanse the syringe and needle, and cleanse and replace other equipment.

15. Return drug to storage center.

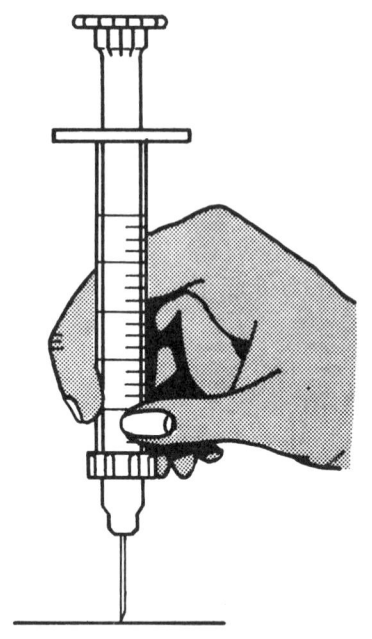

Fig. 17-9 Syringe held vertically

Giving the Intramuscular Injection in the Ventrogluteal Area. The ventrogluteal region is frequently used. The patient should be exposed well enough to assure that the exact site is identified. The nurse should find the greater trochanter, the anterior superior iliac spine and the iliac crest, see figure 17-10. The palm of the hand should rest on the greater trochanter, the index finger on the anterior superior iliac spine and the middle finger is spread as far from the index finger as possible. The injection is made in the center of the triangle (between the index and middle finger).

The illustrations on page 113 show how the intramuscular injection is given, using the Tubex Closed Injection System (Reprinted with permission of Wyeth Laboratories Philadelphia from "Intramuscular Injections", Division of American Home Products Corporation, copyright 1973.

Administering an Intramuscular Injection in the Deltoid Muscle. The upper arm or deltoid area is

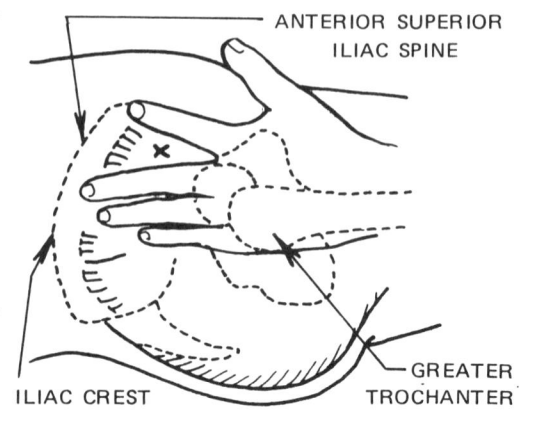

Fig. 17-10 Finding the site for ventrogluteal injection

112

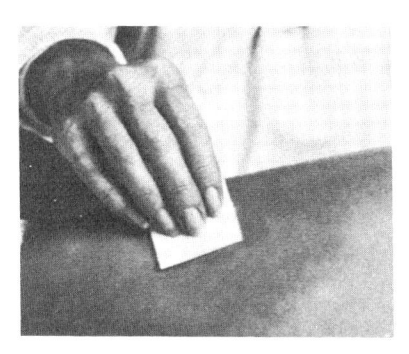

Unit 17 Administration of Medications by Injection

1. Using an alcohol sponge or swab, cleanse an area approximately two inches square around the proposed injection.

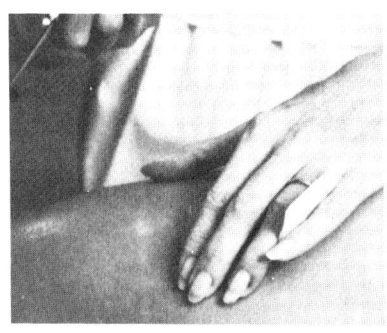

2. With the index and thumb of the left hand spread or tense the skin in the injection area.

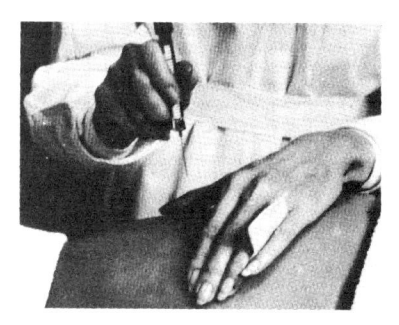

3. Holding the barrel of the syringe in the right hand in a dart or pencil grip, introduce the needle into the skin with a quick thrust.

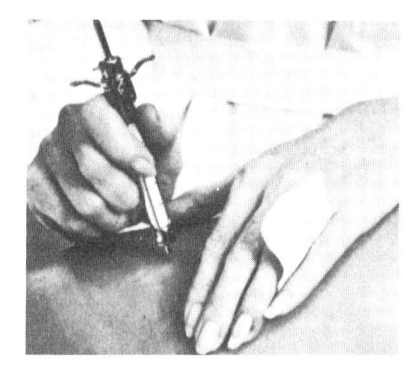

4. Once the surface of the skin has been punctured by the needle, the remainder of the penetration of the needle through the skin and into the muscle should be with a firm and steady pressure. In the case of average or heavy patients it is preferable to retain the pressure on the skin around the injection site with the thumb and index fingers of the left hand for the entire time the needle is being inserted. In thin patients, on the other hand, it is often preferable to release the pressure of the left hand once the puncture has been made, and change to a slight pinching grip in order to firm the injection site and avoid the possibility of going too deep and striking a bone, nerve or blood vessel.

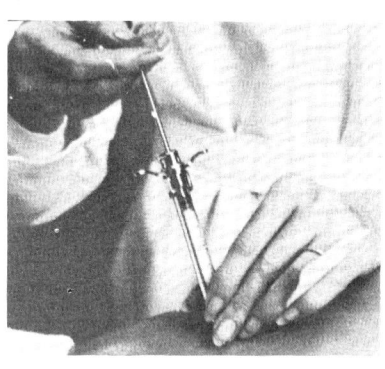

5. Once the desired depth of insertion has been reached, steady the syringe tip with the left hand and with the right hand pull back or out on the plunger approximately one-quarter inch for a few seconds, to see if any blood can be aspirated back into the syringe. Should blood appear in the syringe, the needle should be withdrawn and a new injection site selected.

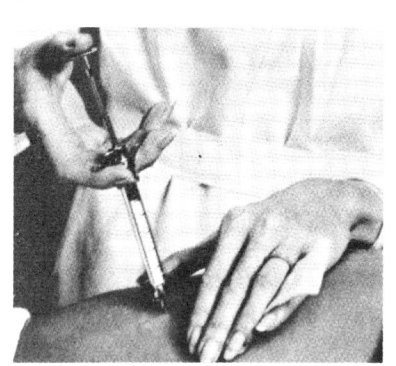

6. If no blood appears, the position of the fingers on the right hand can be shifted so that the thumb covers the head of the plunger and the index and middle fingers are hooked under the side grips on the syringe barrel. With a firm pressure on the thumb move the plunger downward into the syringe as far as it will go. (The small air bubble that is last to disappear is an important part of the injection, since it helps to spread the medication, clear the medicine from the needle, seat the injection site and prevent tracking of the medication as the needle is withdrawn).

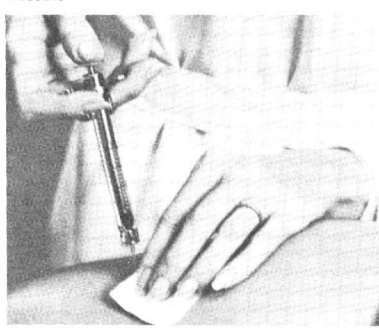

7. After the medication has been injected, apply pressure against the injection site with the alcohol sponge in the left hand as the needle is withdrawn by the right hand; this reduces the risk of medication leaking into the subcutaneous tissues and possibly forming abscesses.

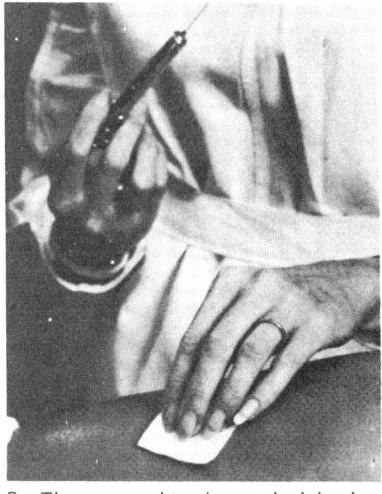

8. Then proceed to cleanse the injection site, by massaging the area with the sponge to remove any blood or medication that might be present. If rapid absorption is desired, the massaging should be continued for about two minutes.

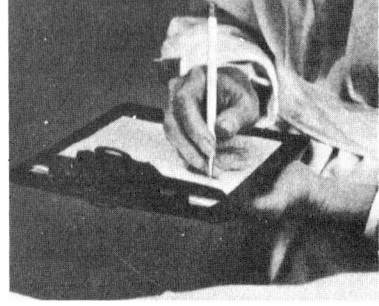

9. After the injection has been given, it is important that all the information be recorded on the patient's chart. This should include: the hour of injection, name of the medication, amount and strength, method of administration, specific site including which side of the body, any unusual reaction and your signature. No injection is complete until this has been done.

Fig. 17-11 Giving the intramuscular injection in the ventrogluteal area
(Courtesy Wyeth Laboratories, Philadelphia, Pa.)

Section 3 Administration of Medications

another site for an intramuscular injection. Although the muscle is fairly large, the area recommended for an intramuscular injection is small as there are major nerves, bones and blood vessels in the area. Intramuscular injections should not be repeatedly given in the mid-deltoid area as it cannot tolerate large quantities of medication or repeated drugs.

1. Assemble and prepare equipment as previously described. The needle most frequently used for this injection is a 1 1/2-inch 22-gauge. Syringe size will depend upon the amount of fluid to be injected. Observe sterile technique throughout.
2. Fill the syringe with amount of ordered dosage.
3. Prepare the medicine tray.
4. Check the patient's name on the wristband and compare it with the medicine card.
5. Tell the patient what you plan to do.
6. Prepare the site of injection as for a gluteal injection.
7. Face patient so that thick, central part of the deltoid muscle faces you.
8. With your free hand, grasp the muscle just below the shoulder, squeezing it between the thumb and forefinger.

    This helps to increase the muscle bulk, makes the skin taut for easier penetration, quards against striking the bone and keeps the injected area steady.
9. Thrust the needle in at an angle of about 90 degrees with the arm. Study figures 17-12 and 17-13. The proper position of the needle is shown in figures 17-8 and 17-9.
10. Pull back the plunger very slightly. If blood appears, change the site of injection. Use another sterile syringe and needle.

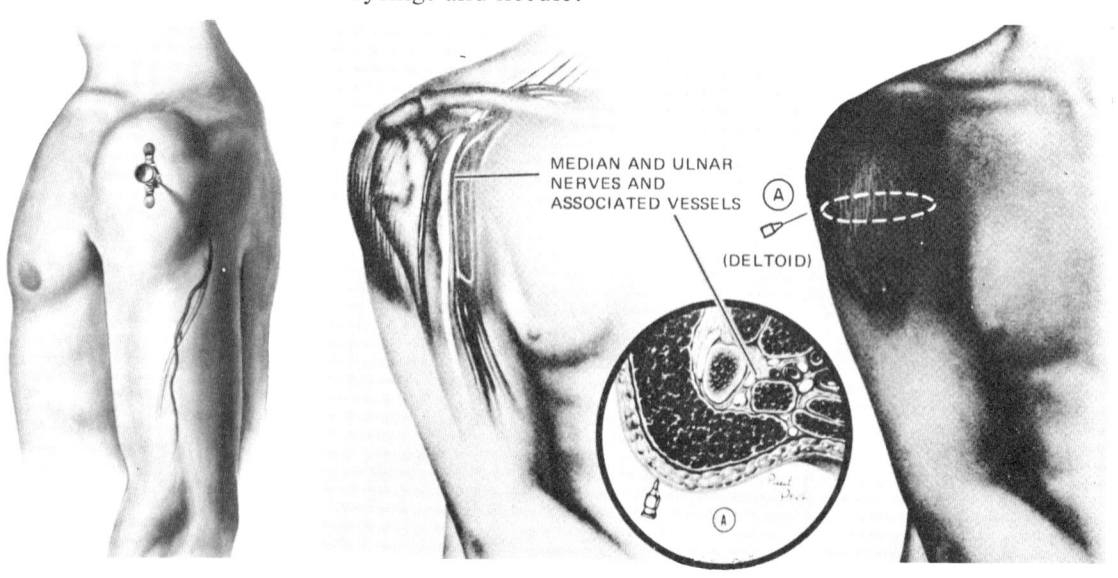

Fig. 17-12 Lateral View of Injection Site in Deltoid Muscle

Fig. 17-13 Area for Administering an Intramuscular Injection into Deltoid Muscle

11. Inject the medication slowly.
12. Withdraw the needle rapidly with the cotton pledget placed against it.
13. Massage the injection site for a few moments to help in the dispersion of the medication.
14. Chart the medication immediately and replace the medicine card.
15. Cleanse syringe and needle and cleanse and replace other equipment which was used.

Intradermal Injections

The intradermal or intracutaneous injection is given into the area between the skin and the subcutaneous tissue. An area is selected where the skin is thin and hair is scant, such as the inner part of the forearm. This type of injection is primarily used for diagnostic tests and for administering vaccines (immunizing agents). The Mantoux or tuberculin test, the Dick test for scarlet fever and the Schick test for diphtheria are administered by this method.

Preparing and Administering an Intradermal Injection

1. Select and assemble the syringe and needle. A tuberculin-type syringe with a 26-gauge, 3/8- or 1/2-inch needle is usually used for this method of injection. Observe sterile technique throughout. Fill the syringe with the amount of ordered dosage.
2. Prepare necessary items for the injection as was done for a subcutaneous injection.
3. Check the patient's name at the bedside and compare it with the medicine card.
4. Tell the patient what you plan to do.
5. Determine where the injection is to be given. The site of injection should have firm and tight skin. Carefully cleanse the site of injection with alcohol 70% and allow to dry.
6. Spread the skin with one hand at the site of injection and insert the needle into the layers of the skin (to about 1/8 inch depth), bevel side up, at an angle of about 10 to 15 degrees, figure 17-15. (Held at this angle it will not readily penetrate into the subcutaneous tissue.) When the needle is in the proper position, the opening of the bevel will be visible through the skin.

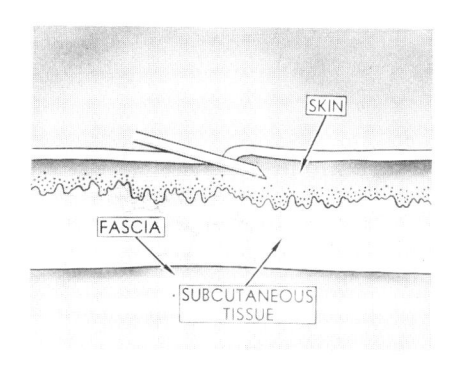

Fig. 17-14 Intradermal injection

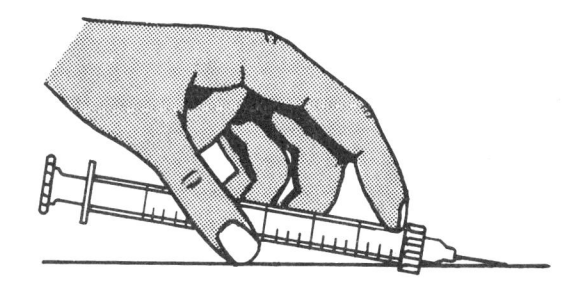

Fig. 17-15 Syringe held at a 10° to 15° angle for intradermal injections

Section 3 Administration of Medications

7. Slowly inject the drug by means of the plunger. A *wheal* (raising of the skin) will become evident as the drug is administered.
8. Remove needle, but *do not* massage area.
9. Carefully wipe off skin with sterile cotton or gauze.
10. Chart the injection immediately.
11. Cleanse the syringe and needle.
12. Return drug to refrigerator.
13. Cleanse and replace other equipment which was used.
14. Return medicine card to its proper location.

Preparing an Intravenous Injection

The intravenous injection is given into a superficial vein, usually one which is located in the arm. The most rapid effects are produced by this method. An intravenous injection is administered by a doctor or a health team member who is trained especially for intravenous work. The intravenous medications are given well diluted and slowly. The practical nurse will not be required to give an intravenous injection; she may be assigned to help the doctor and to watch the patient during the treatment. This assistance would include setting up for the intravenous, tying the tourniquet, wiping the injection site with an antiseptic, observing the patient during the treatment, and, finally removing the needle after the medication has been given. The same principles for sterile technique that were taught for other procedures (such as changing surgical dressings) are followed. Aseptic technique guards against infection.

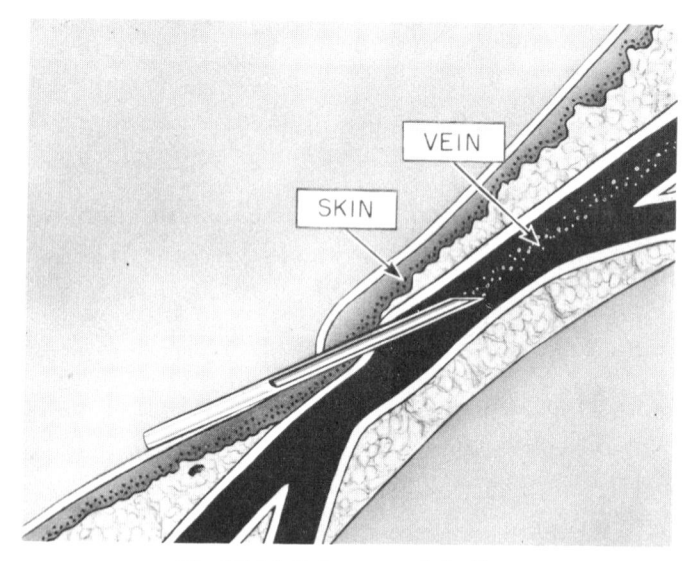

Fig. 17-16 Intravenous injection

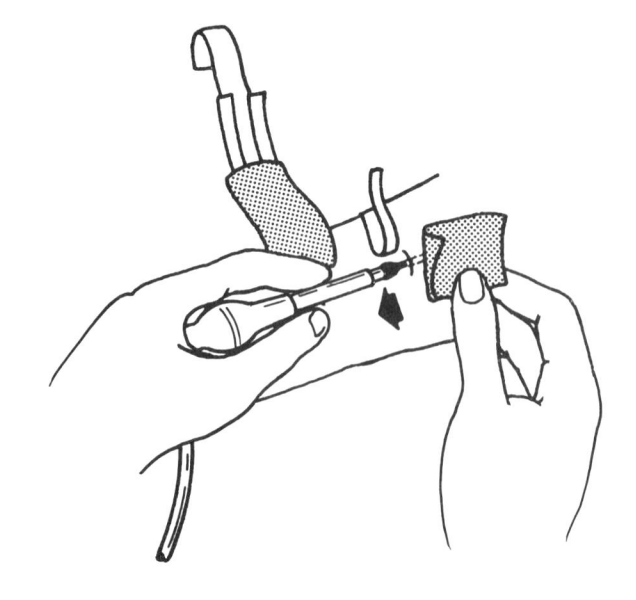

Fig. 17-17 Removing the intravenous needle upon completion of injection or infusion

Before an intravenous injection is done, the following should be on hand: the medication and I.V. setup; gauze sponges or cotton pledgets to be saturated with alcohol 70% before insertion of the needle; strips of adhesive tape; dry gauze sponges; tourniquet and/or blood pressure kit. (Sometimes the physician will use the blood pressure cuff in place of the tourniquet)

When an intravenous infusion is discontinued the nurse first clamps off the tubing. The tape which was stuck to the needle and the patient's skin is gently loosened from the skin but not removed from the needle. Holding the sterile gauze over the needle, it is withdrawn, gently, with the hub of the needle still kept close to the skin. The nurse applies pressure to the injection site with the sterile gauze sponge until bleeding stops. The patient is asked to flex his arm and the sterile gauze sponge may be left against the needle site until bleeding has stopped., figure 17-17.

SUGGESTED ACTIVITIES

- Observe a nurse who is giving an intramuscular injection at the hospital or other facility with which you are associated. Prepare a report on the procedure and discuss the procedure in class. Include medication, site of injection, reaction of patient and charting along with the technique itself.
- Practice assembling and disassembling a hypodermic syringe. Be able to identify the parts and state what parts should be kept sterile and why.
- Under supervision, practice giving injections subcutaneously, intramuscularly and intradermally.
- Role play a nurse assisting a physician start and finish administration of medication by intravenous method.

REVIEW

1. Name five drugs which are often administered by injection.

2. List three types of syringes and give an example of what they may be used for.

3. List the responsibilities of a nurse who is assigned to help a physician give an intravenous injection.

Section 3 Administration of Medications

4. The doctor has ordered codeine sulfate 60 mg by hypo (s.c.). Explain the steps in preparing and giving the medication.

EXTENDED STUDY

Learn the meaning and proper use of the following terms:

counterirritant	nasal catheter
desensitizer	plaster
douche	poultice
hyperbaric	systemic effect
inhalation	local effect
irrigation	suppository
inunction	

Unit 18 Administration of Drugs by Inhalation and Local Application

OBJECTIVES

After studying this unit, the student should be able to:
- Describe the conditions for administering drugs by inhalation and local application methods.
- List some common drugs given by each method.
- Perform the procedures for administering drugs by each method.
- State the safety precautions to be taken when oxygen is administered.

There are times when oral and injection methods for giving a medication are not possible or effective. The drug must be given by some other means such as by inhalation or by local application to the skin or body cavity.

Regardless of the route of administration, a drug may have a local effect and/or a systemic effect. A drug has a local effect when the drug action is desired at the site of application. The drug usually functions as a desensitizer, an astringent, antiseptic or counterirritant. A drug with systemic effect acts on the body systems and affects the whole body. For example, a lotion may be applied to the skin to relieve itching; it has a local effect. The same is true if a hemorrhoidal ointment is applied to the rectal area to relieve the pain; it has a local effect.

On the other hand, a drug can be applied locally, be absorbed, and produce a systemic effect. An example would be an aminophyllin suppository; it is given locally (by rectum) and yet, relieves difficult breathing due to asthma.

ADMINISTERING DRUGS BY INHALATION

The *inhalation* technique is used for the purpose of providing cold or warm air, usually in the form of medicated steam or aerosol therapy for the patient to breathe at intervals prescribed by the doctor. Drugs administered by this method produce either a local or systemic effect; they are given by inhalation for three reasons:
- To provide local treatment of infections of the respiratory tract when these areas can be treated only by vapor.
  For example, steam (moist) inhalations are used to relieve inflammations due to colds. The steam may or may not contain a drug.
- To provide systemic treatment for serious respiratory infections. For example, when oxygen is forced under pressure through a nebulizer containing penicillin or another antibiotic, fine particles of the drug are carried into the respiratory tract. The medium is the cold air.
- To supply a medication which can be absorbed into the bloodstream through the lungs, producing a rapid system effect. An example is the use of aromatic spirits of ammonia or smelling salts (ammonia gas). The inhaled fumes (dry inhalations) act as an emergency heart and respiratory stimulant.

Section 3 Administration of Medications

Adrenalin, 1:1000 solution, is commonly used as an antispasmodic to overcome asthmatic attacks, or it may act as a heart stimulant. Oxygen is used in the treatment of emphysema, cancer of the lung, pneumonia and other respiratory ailments. It is also used for heart conditions.

A mixture of 80% Helium and 20% Oxygen may be used at the physician's discretion in emphysema, bronchiectasis and some types of asthma. The mixture is 1/3 as heavy as air and can be breathed with less effort than oxygen or air. Helium is noninflammable, diffuses rapidly, and is only slightly soluble in the body fluids.

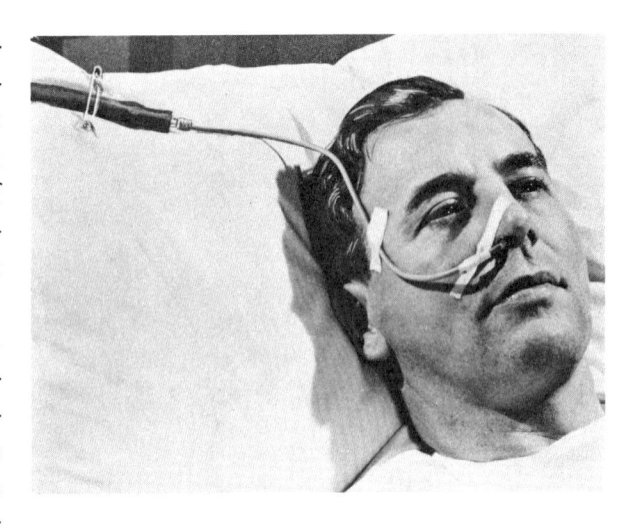

Fig. 18-1 Administering oxygen by use of a nasal catheter

Tetanus is treated by the administration of oxygen in the hyperbaric chamber. Its effect is to ease the effort of respiration. Antiseptics such as menthol, tincture of benzoin and oil of eucalyptol are used with steam to relieve coughing.

INHALATION METHODS

Certain drugs may be administered by aerosol therapy. An atomizer converts the medication, which is in liquid or powder form, into a fine mist. The nebulizer is a device which produces a very fine spray of liquid droplets. Oxygen is furnished to transport the vapor to the mucous membranes of the respiratory passages. The liquid used may be distilled water or a prescribed medication. In cases of nasopharyngeal and bronchial infections, warm moist inhalations are provided by an electric vaporizer.

Administration of Oxygen

Oxygen may be administered by several methods: by use of a nasal catheter, a nasal cannula, an oxygen mask, or an oxygen tent. The mode of administration and the dosage are determined by the physician on the basis of the patient's needs. The nasal catheter has advantages over other methods in that it permits the patient freedom of movement. A nasal cannula is often used but it is felt that some oxygen can be lost by this method.

There are two techniques for administering oxygen by catheter: the deep catheter technique and the shallow catheter technique. In the first, the catheter is inserted so that its tip is visible directly behind the uvula in the patient's mouth. In the second, the catheter is inserted only as far as the nasopharynx and then withdrawn one-half inch.

Administering Oxygen by Nasal Catheter (Deep Catheter Method)

When administering oxygen by catheter, it is very important to prevent excessive drying of the mucous membranes of the nose and throat. For this reason the oxygen flow is humidified before it reaches the patient.

1. Assemble equipment: tray with nasal catheter, lubricant in gauze, strips of adhesive tape, paper bag, tissue wipes, tongue depressor, flashlight.
2. Take equipment to bedside. Explain the procedure to the patient.
3. Measure the length of the catheter from tip of the patient's nose to the ear lobe. This will give the distance to insert it.
4. Lubricate the catheter with a water soluble lubricant such as K.Y. jelly. Do not use oil because there is danger of aspirating it and might cause lipid pneumonia.
5. Insert carefully through nostril, along septum and into nasopharynx or other area ordered.
6. Ask patient to open mouth. Depress the tongue with a tongueblade in order to see the tip of the catheter with the aid of a flashlight.
7. Start flow slowly until ordered liters per hour are reached on gauge.
8. In changing a catheter, turn off oxygen flow.
9. Disposable catheters are discarded after use. Remove "used" catheter gently with tissue wipe. Place it in paper bag.
10. Connect newly inserted catheter to glass connecting rod and tubing from oxygen cylinder. Check position of catheter with flashlight.
11. Fasten new catheter in place with adhesive tape. Resume oxygen flow slowly until previous rate is reached. Remove old adhesive tape with benzene or acetone and then wash with soap and water.
12. Change catheter every 8 hours.

> - Oxygen supports combustion. There is extreme danger of a fire starting when it is used. Ignition can be caused by friction, static electricity, or by a lighted cigarette. When oxygen is being administered, a sign should appear at the room door or ward entrance stating "Oxygen in Use – No Smoking."
> - Cotton blankets should be used rather than woolen ones because static electricity is less apt to be generated. Nylon uniforms are prohibited in some hospitals for this same reason when administering oxygen.
> - The nurse should check the patient in oxygen frequently as to the following items: amount of oxygen entering the tent, fullness of tank, ice content, electrical current, and connections.

Administering Oxygen by Tent Method

1. Assemble equipment: Clear plastic canopy, cylinder of oxygen or "piped-in" oxygen, refrigerating system, and air circulating motor system.
2. Check the canopy for holes before putting it over patient.
3. While the patient is in the tent, do nothing which will cause friction. If back care must be given while in the tent, pat the back instead of rubbing it.

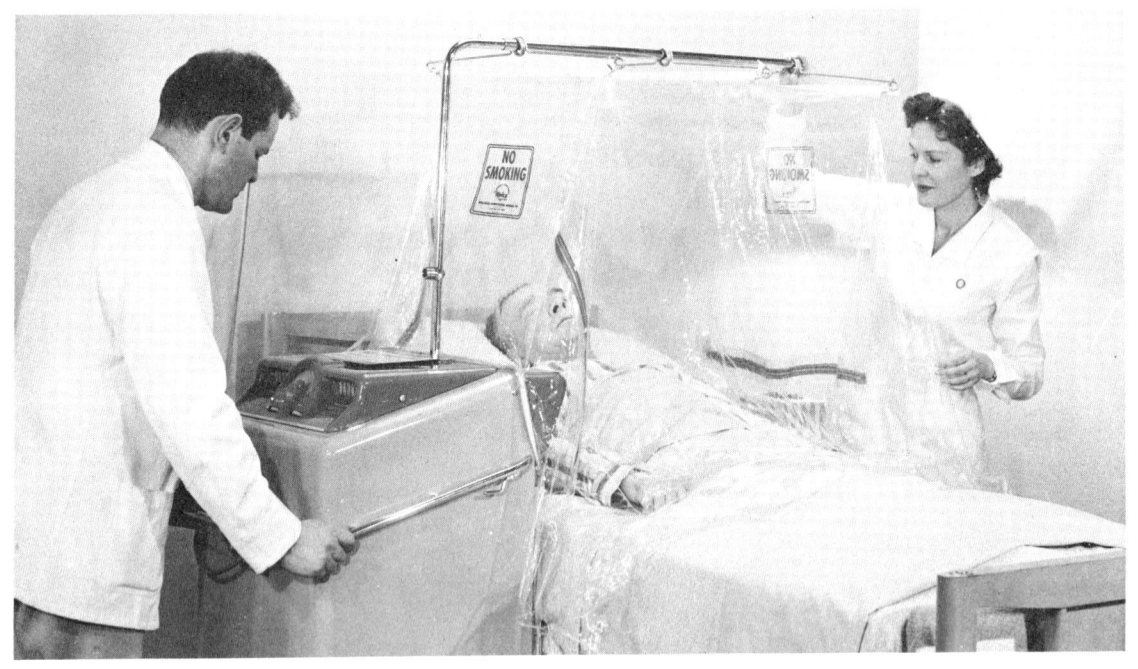

Section 3 Administration of Medications

Fig. 18-2 Administering oxygen by use of an oxygen tent

4. Take patient "out of oxygen" while electrical appliances such as X-ray suction or electrocardiographic machines are in use.
5. Use cotton blankets rather than wool.
6. Tuck in bed linens and the canopy on three sides. The lower part of the canopy should be placed between the folds of a drawsheet and must be tucked securely over lower portion of bed, figure 18-3.
7. Keep ice chamber filled with ice cubes, above a quarter full. Empty drainage pail as frequently as necessary.

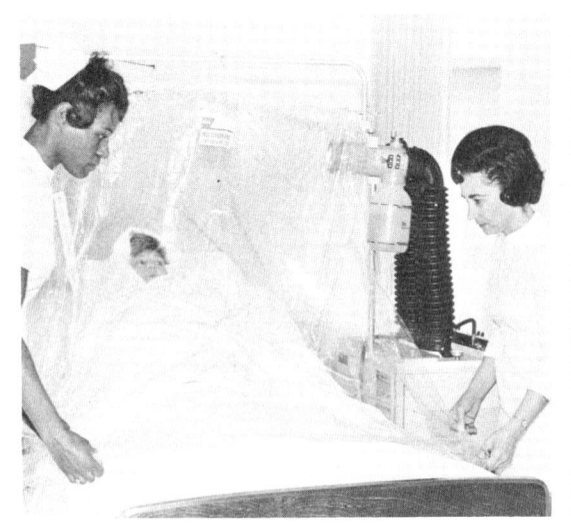

Fig. 18-3(A) Place sheet over patient. Unfold canopy before folding sheet over it.

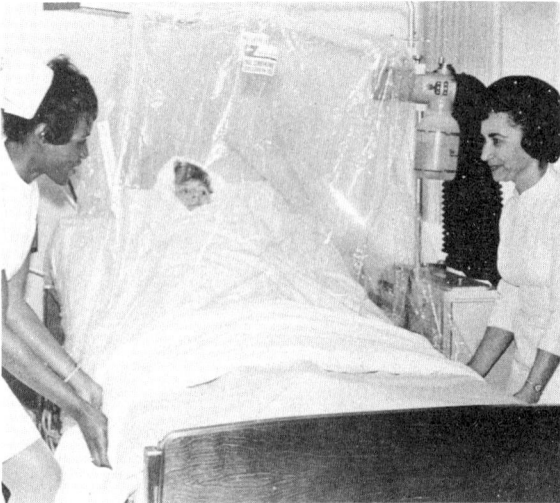

Fig. 18-3(B) Place the edge of the canopy between the folds and tuck the sheet under the mattress.

Unit 18 Administration of Drugs by Inhalation and Local Application

8. A thermometer placed within the tent will help the nurse keep a comfortable temperature within. She will not have to "feel" the temperature within the tent. A temperature of 18° to 21°C (65° - 70°F) and oxygen concentration of 50% make a comfortable situation for the patient.
9. Flood the tent with oxygen flowing at 12-15 liters for 20 minutes at the time the patient is first put into the tent. Then reduce the flow to 8-12 liters a minute depending upon the patient's condition.
10. When bathing and caring for the patient, tuck the canopy around the patient's neck and shoulders until you have finished and bed is made. Watch the patient's condition closely. Increase the oxygen flow temporarily until the desired concentration has been reached.
11. Check the wall plug and electrical current frequently to see that it has not been accidentally pulled out of the wall socket.

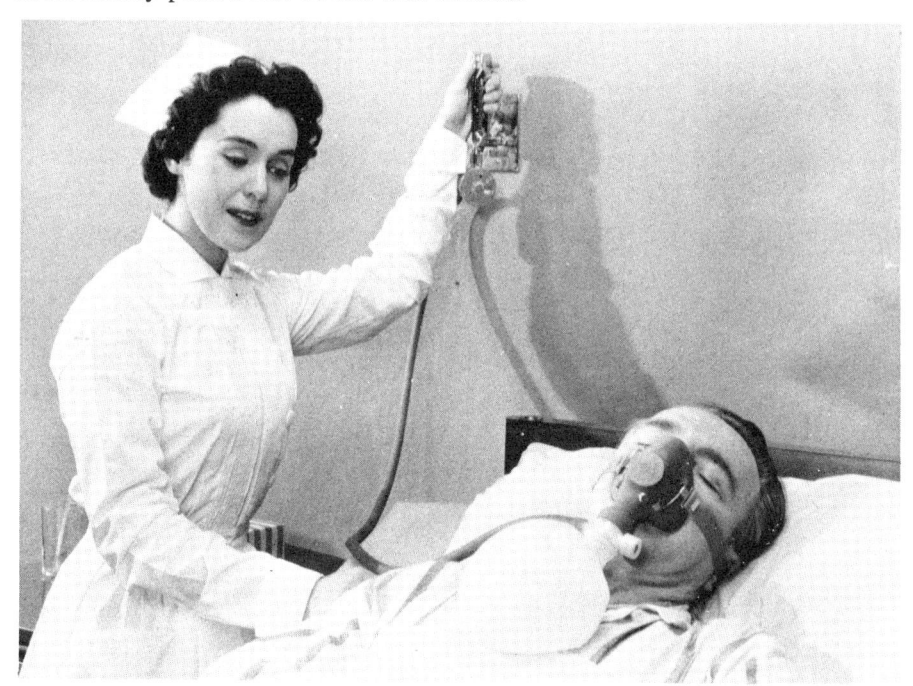

Fig. 18-4 Administering oxygen by mask

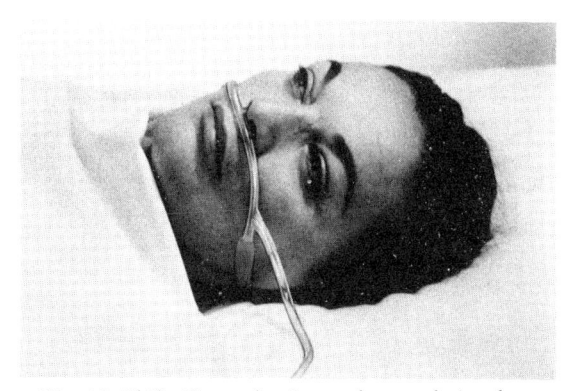

Fig. 18-5(A) Clear plastic nasal cannula in place

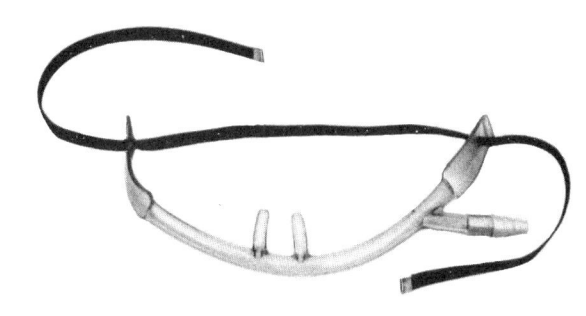

Fig. 18-5(B) Clear plastic nasal cannula

Section 3 Administration of Medications

12. If moisture appears inside the tent, this is usually caused by excess Carbon Dioxide (CO_2). Remove immediately and check the oxygen supply concentration, and tent.

ADMINISTERING DRUGS BY LOCAL APPLICATION

Drugs which are commonly used for application to the skin are directly applied. Ointments, lotions, liniments, wet medicated dressings, poultices and plasters are all applied onto the skin.

Drugs commonly used for local application to the mucous membrane of body cavities are administered by irrigation, instillation and insertion into the body openings.

Application to the Skin

Ointments are applied directly to the skin, or they may be applied as a dressing by spreading the medication on a piece of gauze. When the drug is directly applied by rubbing it into the skin, the method is called *inunction*. Ointments are used to relieve irritations and skin diseases of various kinds. Zinc oxide is an example of an ointment used for local application.

Lotions are drugs which are swabbed on the skin for antiseptic and/or astringent effects. Itching, dryness, and irritations caused by inflammation and diseases of the skin are relieved. Calamine lotion is an example of such a drug.

Liniments are drugs which usually have a counterirritant effect; they are rubbed on the skin quite vigorously to relieve soreness of muscles and joints. The psychological effect of massage is an important factor in the application of liniments. Camphor liniment and chloroform liniment are examples.

> - Avoid excessive rubbing of drugs which are counterirritants into skin because blistering may result.
> - When applying ointments and lotions to infected areas, use extreme care not to aggravate the infection. Apply medication as directed. Use rubber or plastic disposable gloves if there is any danger of infection to oneself, or if the drug may produce allergic reactions.

Medicated or wet dressings may be used for local treatment of skin disorders; they are gauze sponges, saturated with a drug in solution. The drug may act as an antiseptic or an astringent. Neomycin is an example of a drug which can be prepared as a solution and used as an antiseptic for local application.

> When medicated wet dressings are applied, the dressings must be changed frequently in order to produce the maximum desired effect.

Poultices and plasters are counterirritants applied to the skin for relieving pain and congestion in the deeper tissues. Mustard plasters and flaxseed poultices are examples of such medications.

> Care must be taken to remove plasters in time to avoid skin burns. Check frequently for reddening of skin.

Application to Body Cavities

Medications are applied to various body cavities to treat inflammation and infections in 3 ways: (1) *irrigation,* a flushing of the mucous lining with a solution for the purpose of removing secretions and soothing the tissues; (2) *instillation* which is an introduction of a drug, usually in liquid form, (nose drops, ear drops, eye drops) into the body cavity for temporary retention, and (3) *insertion* which refers to placing a suppository, tablet or powder in the cavity for local treatment.

Special equipment is used to irrigate the infected organ or wound and permit the solution to flow through it. Open cavities which are treated by irrigation (or instillation) are the nose, mouth, ear, throat, bladder, vagina and rectum. Commonly used solutions are saline for the nose and throat irrigations, and normal bicarbonate and hydrogen peroxide solutions for ear irrigations. Other irrigations (douches) and instillations require special strengths of solutions and medications.

> The temperature of all irrigations and douches must be moderate, about 39° to 40°C (103° to 105°F) to avoid burning the patient.

Drugs may be inserted rectally or vaginally when a patient is nauseated by oral intake of the drug, or if the patient is mentally ill or unconscious. Drugs are also given by this method when the doctor wishes sustained local action.

Suppositories are commonly inserted into the vagina and rectum in order to obtain general systemic effects; for example, sedatives, hypnotics, narcotics and anti-infective agents affect body systems to bring relief from pain, and to combat infections. Other drugs, such as tannic acid in cocoa butter, are used for local effect of soothing the rectal membrane. Vaginal suppositories and tablets are often prescribed for *vaginitis*, an inflammation of the mucous membrane which lines the vagina. Powders may be blown into a body cavity by using an *insufflator*, an instrument used to blow powdery substances into a nose or other cavity. Sprays are also used for local applications.

Administering a Suppository

Assemble the following items on a small tray: suppository from refrigerator, lubricant, (optional), tissue wipes, and disposable plastic or unsterile rubber gloves.

1. Screen the patient and explain what is to be done and how it is to be done.
2. Have the patient empty the bladder.
3. If a vaginal suppository is to be inserted, the patient should lie on her back with the knees flexed.
    a. Use plastic gloves or clean, unsterile rubber gloves. The one gloved hand is used to expose the vaginal opening; the other is used to hold and insert the suppository.
    b. Insert the suppository well into the vagina past the posterior cervix.
4. If a rectal suppository or tablet is to be inserted, have the patient turn on side.
    a. Put on plastic gloves or clean, unsterile rubber gloves. Lubricate the tip of the suppository with lubricant on a tissue wipe.
    b. Insert the rectal suppository well beyond the sphincter, pushing it in gently with your gloved forefinger.

Section 3 Administration of Medications

5. After slowly withdrawing your finger, press the folded tissue against the opening until the urge to expel the suppository subsides.
6. Pull off disposable gloves at the wrists and discard. Wash and sterilize the rubber gloves.
7. Replace equipment.
8. Chart medication. Observe patient for results and chart the effects.

> Drugs given in suppository form, particularly to mentally ill and unconscious patients, may be easily expelled, especially from the rectum. The patient should be kept under close observation to see that the suppository is retained.

SUGGESTED ACTIVITIES
- Write a report on the reasons for the increase in the number of cases of emphysema, the possible causes, and what happens to the alveoli of the lungs. Include an explanation of how the administration of oxygen relieves the oxygen-starved tissues, and the amount of oxygen used for the patient with emphysema.
- From drug literature and library references, study the various medicines available for local application, for rectal and vaginal use, and for inhalation. Prepare a list of medications for each method and submit for class discussion.
- Observe a nurse giving oxygen to a patient. Note the method used, the procedure which was followed and the precautions that were taken. Prepare a report of your observations.
- Under supervision, practice the procedures you have studied in this unit.

REVIEW
1. Under what circumstances would the following methods be used in the administration of drugs?

    a. Rectal — *FOR UNCONSCIOUS PATIENTS, ~~AND~~ NAUSEATED PATIENTS*

    b. Local Application — *TO RELIEVE LOCAL IRRITATIONS AND INFECTIONS*

    c. Inhalation — *TO PROVIDE LOCAL TREATMENT OF INFECTIONS OF THE RESPIRATORY TRACT, TO PROVIDE SYSTEMATIC TREATMENT FOR SERIOUS RESPIRATORY INFECTION*

2. Helium (80%) and oxygen (20%) mixtures are now used in the treatment of some cases of dyspnea. Name two medical conditions where this mixture might be ordered, and indicate why it might be preferred.

A. EMPHYSEMA AND BRONCHIECTASIS
B. IT MIGHT BE PERFERRED BECAUSE ITS LIGHTER.

Unit 18 Administration of Drugs by Inhalation and Local Application

3. Give an example of a drug which is administered by each of the following methods. Include its purpose and effect.

   Inhalation — SPIRITS OF AMMONIA IS A RESPIRATORY AND HEART STIMULANT; REVIVES THE PATIENT

   Rectal — ANUSOL SUPPOSITORY TO RELIEVE PAIN FROM HEMORRHOIDS; SHRINKS BLOOD VESSELS

   Local Application — CALAMINE LOTION RELIEVES ~~ITCHING~~; HAS ASTRINGENT ~~EFFECT~~

4. Explain why oxygen by nasal catheter, especially, should be humidified.

   PREVENTS EXCESSIVE DRAINAGE OF MUCOUS MEMBRANES OF THE NOSE AND THROAT

5. Give three reasons why nasal and oral care are very necessary in preventing infection and in making the patient more comfortable. — FOR CLEANLINESS, LUBRICATION, PREVENT IRRITATION, KEEPS ITS MUCOUS MEMBRANES IN GOOD CONDITION

6. Name the precautions which must be taken when administering oxygen.

   NO SMOKING SIGN, COTTON BLANKETS, CHECK FLOW OF O_2, CHECK TEMPERATURE OF O_2 TENT

EXTENDED STUDY

Learn the meaning and proper use of the following terms:

radioactive substances	radiation
tracer elements	radioactive
alpha rays	radioactive isotopes
beta rays	radiologist
gamma rays	tracer elements
nuclear medicine	half-life

127

Unit 19 Administration of Radioactive Substances

OBJECTIVES

After studying this unit, the student should be able to:

- Describe how radioactive substances are utilized in nuclear medicine.
- Describe the methods of administering radioactive treatments.

Radioactive substances first came into use with the discovery of radium by Becquerel in 1896 and by the Curies' research. Other radioactive substances were discovered thereafter.

The first use of these substances in the field of medicine was in the treatment of cancer. Since then, they have also come into use as tracer elements in medical research and for diagnosing certain illnesses. Radioactive substances are used to treat skin growths as well as malignant conditions of the body.

Tracer studies are revealing many of the secrets of nature. Radioactive carbon compounds can be used to follow the passage of certain types of food through the body. By following the path of sugar (a carbon) through the body, a better knowledge of sugar metabolism can be obtained as well as a better understanding of the causes of diabetes.

RADIOACTIVE SUBSTANCES AND THEIR EFFECTS

A *radioactive substance* is one which has the property of giving off a special type of energy. This energy is in the form of rays, invisible to the eye, which have varying degrees of penetrating power. The rays are termed or classified as alpha rays, which have very little penetrating power; beta rays, which are more penetrating; and gamma rays, which are very penetrating.

Alpha, beta and gamma rays are used for their power to produce chemical changes in tissues. The principal artificial sources for this form of energy are radium, thorium, and cobalt. As the rays are emitted, the metal becomes less radioactive. In respect to radioactive substances, *half-life* refers to the length of time in which the value of a given amount of radioactive material decreases by one half. Cobalt has a considerably shorter half-life than radium, but it is less expensive to prepare and use. Skin reactions from radioactive cobalt are usually less serious than those from radium.

For purposes of treatment, the beta and gamma rays are most frequently used. Beta rays are used for superficial treatments such as for unsightly skin growths. They may cause reaction of the skin but do not penetrate deep enough to reach the vital organs. The gamma rays penetrate deeply and may, therefore, be used for deep therapy. Very often, gamma rays are used in the treatment of serious malignant conditions. The effects of treatment with radioactive substances result in skin reactions of varying degrees.

> Exposure to gamma rays must be kept at a minimum; otherwise incurable skin reactions will result.

ADMINISTERING RADIOACTIVE TREATMENTS

Nuclear medicine is a highly specialized field; therefore, all procedures are carried out in a special unit. Radioactive substances are usually administered in the radiology department. Treatments may be given (1) by applying radioactive rays to parts of the body by means of special equipment, or (2) in the form of medications administered by mouth or by intravenous injection. Radioactive iodine is an example of a radioactive medicine given by mouth. It is used for the treatment of cancer of the thyroid gland. Any such medications must be ordered by the radiologist. Special orders are written for each case.

The nurse will probably not be directly involved in the administration of radioactive substances. However, there may be times when the nurse will be in contact with a patient who is to receive and/or has been given radioactive treatments. As a result, the patient may be emitting radioactive rays.

PREPARATION OF THE PATIENT

The patient who is to undergo treatment of a condition which requires the use of radioactive substances requires more understanding and patience than the "average" patient. Whether the condition is a benign skin tumor or a malignancy, the patient will be anxious about the treatment and its effects. The nurse should be tolerant of any irritability and anxiety, and try to help the patient accept the treatment. This can be done by maintaining a cheerful, reassuring attitude. Do not alarm the patient in any way. Provide any necessary comforts and follow special orders carefully. Meeting the patient's needs may include special diets and other restrictions. Knowing about the patient's likes and dislikes and relating these to the dietitian is one example of what nursing is all about. These patients do not have good appetites and proper nourishment is essential.

Explaining the treatment to the patient also helps reduce the anxiety. Patients do not know what will be going on when they reach the radiology department; sometimes, they anticipate that the procedure will be a painful one.

SAFETY PRECAUTIONS

The patient is usually placed in an area where his needs may be met, but where the disintegrating radioactive substances will not harm others. The area is posted Radioactive. The nurse meets the needs of the patient, but spends no more time in the room than is necessary. All excreta, towels, etc. discarded by the patient are placed in a specially designated area in covered lead-lined containers. A special squad collects this material. The purpose of this special care is to protect others from exposure to the radioactive rays.

There are many hazards associated with overexposure to radiation which may not be apparent at the time. Bone marrow may be damaged, thus interfering with nature's process of making red blood cells. Nurses, doctors, radiologists, and others working in or near radiation units are checked frequently for blood disorders.

Most radiation units are enclosed in thick walls lined with lead. There is also a lead partition between the therapist and the patient. Lead blocks the rays, thus protecting others in the hospital who are outside the unit.

Section 3 Administration of Medications

GOVERNMENT REGULATIONS

The government has wisely set up certain regulations to guard nurses, doctors, and other allied health personnel against the hazards of radioactive substances used in hospitals. Hospitals must be approved by the Federal Atomic Energy Commission before handling radioactive substances. These approved hospitals must have areas for handling and disposing of the substances. Medical and nursing personnel and other employees working in the area are frequently checked for complete blood counts and general physical condition. They must wear a badge which changes color when they have been exposed to the amount of radiation which is considered the maximum for safety.

SUGGESTED ACTIVITIES

- Refer to current medical publications and write or give an oral report on the applications of radioactive substances in the field of medicine.
- Report on how patients receiving radioactive treatments are cared for by the practical nurse in the hospital where you are obtaining clinical experience. Include pretreatment preparation of the patient.
- Make arrangements to visit a hospital where radioactive elements are used in therapy. Before the visit, study references to prepare for a report which will cover the following observations. As a result of the visit, include the following in the report.
  a. Safety measures used in constructing this specialized unit.
  b. Care taken by the radiologist during radiation therapy.
  c. Protective clothing worn by the radiologist and assistants during treatments.
  d. Advantages of using cobalt radiation as contrasted with radium radiation in cancer therapy.
  e. Investigate the process by which the following elements may be made radioactive: Cobalt, phosphorus, gold, calcuim, iodine, thorium, and carbon.
  f. Be able to explain how radioactive carbon, phosphorus and calcium act when used as tracer elements, and in formulating diagnoses.

REVIEW

1. Name two instances when radioactive substances may be used in the field of medicine.

2. How is a patient prepared for a radioactive treatment?

3. What does the term *half-life* mean in respect to radioactive substances?

EXTENDED STUDY

Learn the meaning and proper use of the following terms:

antibiotic	fungicide
antiseptic	fungistatic
anuria	germicide
bactericidal	hemolytic anemia
bacteriostatic	intestinal flora
blood dyscrasia	leukopenia
broad spectrum	narrow spectrum
chemotherapeutic	oliguria
crystallization	phagocyte
dermatitis	sulfonamide
disinfectant	tinnitus

Achievement Review 3

Section 3 Administration of Medications

A. In the space provided before each statement, mark (T) for those which are true, or (F) for those which are false.

_____ 1. Aerosol therapy is a method of administering a drug by inhalation.

_____ 2. When oxygen is being administered to a bed patient, wool blankets are preferred to cotton blankets.

_____ 3. The greatest danger in administering oxygen is that an overdose may be given.

_____ 4. Drugs which show a change in color should be discarded.

_____ 5. Some radioactive treatments may be given by intravenous injections.

_____ 6. A patient who has had radioactive treatments may transmit radioactivity to others.

_____ 7. If a patient responds to a drug favorably, it is not necessary to report it.

_____ 8. Any medication may be obtained from the hospital pharmacy upon a written order from the nurse in charge.

_____ 9. A medicine which is ordered s.c. is given orally.

_____ 10. The liquid in a medicine glass is measured at the highest part of the liquid's surface.

_____ 11. The medicine card is primarily used as the record of a medicine that has been administered to the patient.

_____ 12. A precipitate may result when mixing medicines.

_____ 13. Angina is a drug used in the treatment of a heart condition.

_____ 14. Emphysema is a disease of the arteries.

_____ 15. Hypodermic syringes are graduated in the metric scale.

_____ 16. Prepackaged sterile disposable hypodermic sets are rapidly displacing Pyrex syringes and steel needles.

_____ 17. A 27-gauge hypodermic needle indicates that its diameter is a small size.

_____ 18. When giving oral medications, the label on the bottle should be checked against the medicine card.

_____ 19. Penicillin is given subcutaneously.

_____ 20. Diagnostic tests are often given by intradermal injections.

Achievement Review

B. Give the meaning of the following abbreviations and symbols.

q.i.d. _____   p.r.n. _____

q. 4h _____   p.o. _____

q.d. _____   b.i.d. _____

a.c. _____   p.c. _____

R̥ _____   gtt.(s) _____

t.i.d. _____   q.n. _____

ml _____   mg _____

℥ⅱ _____   ℥ⅳ _____

C. From Column II, select the drug which best describes the item in Column I. Place the letter before the appropiate description.

Column I	Column II
_____ 1. Drug mixed with a liquid but not dissolved	a. emulsion
_____ 2. Drug which causes an external irritation	b. solution
_____ 3. Drug which usually represents 10% of the drug agent	c. mixture or suspension
_____ 4. Drugs of concentrated strength dissolved in alcohol	d. syrup
_____ 5. Drug which is usually sweetened and flavored, with alcohol used as the solvent	e. elixir
	f. tincture
	g. spirit
_____ 6. Drug which is sweetened and flavored, with water used as the solvent	h. fluidextract
	i. lotion
_____ 7. Drug which is easily vaporized	j. liniment
_____ 8. Drug which is usually made with oil as the solvent and administered with an atomizer.	k. spray
	l. capsule
_____ 9. Drug which functions to soothe and moisten the skin	m. precipitate
_____ 10. Drug dissolved in water, giving clear appearance	
_____ 11. Combination of oil and water giving a milky appearance	

133

Section 3 Administration of Medications

D. Complete the following statements by filling in the blank spaces with the appropriate word or words.
 1. The three general sources of drugs are _____.
 2. Cortisone is obtained from the _____ glands.
 3. Insulin is used in the treatment of _____.
 4. Of the three sources for drugs, sulphur, a nonmetallic element, is an example of a _____.
 5. Drugs containing sulphur are used in the treatment of _____.
 6. A drug manufactured by chemically compounding ingredients is called a _____ drug.
 7. Drugs are standardized in order that a doctor may be assured of their _____ and _____.
 8. Two sources for listings of standardized drugs are _____ _____ and _____.
 9. The _____ dose is given after the initial dose has reached the desired effect.
 10. In the metric system of measure _____ and _____ are terms used for fluid measure.
 11. Examples of the classification of the principal drugs used for selective action are the _____ and _____.
 12. Medicine bottles should always be stoppered when not in use to prevent _____ of the medicine.
 13. An injection given just under the skin is termed a _____ injection.
 14. When the drug action is desired at the site of application, the drug is applied _____.
 15. Drugs which are rubbed into the skin to obtain counterirritant action are _____.
 16. Four ways in which oxygen may be administered are _____ _____.

E. Briefly answer the following questions.
 1. By whose authority is a medication given?

 2. If a medicine order is not understood by a practical nurse, what should be done to clarify its interpretation?

3. List the items found on a patient's order sheet which would refer to the ordered medication.

4. Why is it important that a medicine be administered at prescribed intervals?

5. When should the medication which is administered be charted?

6. What should the nurse do with unused medications?

7. In the event that a patient should react unfavorably to a drug, what are the responsibilities of the nurse?

8. When may a nurse take medicines from the medicine cupboard for her own personal use?

9. The label on a medicine bottle should be read three times. List each time that it should be read.

10. List five devices used for measuring medications.

11. When may a patient administer a medication?

12. List the six correct steps of accuracy.

F. Select and underline the appropriate word or words which will complete each statement correctly. (Some questions may have more than one answer)
1. Enteric-coated pills: (a) dissolve easily; (b) will dissolve when they reach the intestines; (c) dissolve in the stomach.
2. Suppositories are classified as drugs for: (a) internal use; (b) external use; (c) both.

Section 3 Administration of Medications

  3. A hypodermic tablet is: (a) not dissolved readily; (b) dissolved in alcohol; (c) dissolved in a special solution; (d) dissolved easily.

  4. Drugs are primarily used to: (a) cure diseases; (b) change the function of body cells; (c) change activity of body cells; (d) bring about an abnormal state in the body.

  5. The action of a drug which affects a pathogenic organism is termed: (a) remote action; (b) specific action; (c) selective action.

  6. Drugs should not be used beyond their expiration date because: (a) they become contaminated; (b) they often deteriorate; (c) their storage becomes a problem; (d) new varieties of drugs are available by that time which are more effective.

  7. Certain medications which must be kept refrigerated are: (a) hormone products; (b) antibiotics; (c) vitamins in oil; (d) drugs affected by light; (e) insulin; (f) narcotics.

  8. The superscription includes the: (a) date; (b) amount of drug; (c) directions for giving the drug; (d) doctor's registration number; (e) symbol R_x.

G. Rearrange the following steps for giving an intramuscular injection in the deltoid muscle so that they are in their proper sequence. Number each in the space provided. (1-17)

_____ Face the patient so that the thick, central part of the muscle is facing you.

_____ Fill the syringe with the amount of ordered dosage.

_____ Prepare the site of injection.

_____ Tell the patient what you plan to do.

_____ Chart the medication.

_____ Inject the medication slowly.

_____ Assemble and prepare equipment.

_____ Cleanse syringe and needle.

_____ Pull back plunger slightly. If blood appears, change the site of injection, using another sterile syringe and needle.

_____ Check the patient's name on the wristband and compare it with the medicine card.

_____ With your free hand, grasp the muscle just below the shoulder, squeezing it between the thumb and forefinger.

_____ Thrust the needle at an angle of about 90° with the arm.

_____ Prepare the medicine tray.

_____ Return medicine card to its proper location.

_____ Return medicine to storage center.

_____ Withdraw needle rapidly.

_____ Massage the injection site.

Section 4 Drugs and Related Substances

Unit 20 Drugs Used to Counteract Infections

OBJECTIVES

After studying this unit, the student should be able to:

- Select an antiseptic or disinfectant appropriate for use in a given situation.
- Describe the characteristic action of antibiotics on microorganisms.
- State uses of common antibiotics.
- Describe the characteristic action of sulfonamides upon microorganisms.

Antiseptics, disinfectants, and antibiotics are used to counteract infections. In using anti-infectives, it must be remembered that their use on the skin and other body tissues in such strength as to kill microorganisms may also harm the tissues. Lesser concentration may be applied to inhibit bacterial growth without injuring the tissues. Figure 20-1, on page 138, lists antiseptics and disinfectants, substances prepared in different strengths; note that in many instances, the same drug may be used as an antiseptic or a disinfectant; that is, they may have bacteriostatic or bactericidal action. *Bacteriostatic* action refers to the slowing down or inhibition of bacterial growth. *Bactericidal* describes the destruction of bacteria. *Antiseptics* are substances which slow down and discourage the growth of bacteria; they have bacteriostatic action. Antiseptics can be safely used on living tissue. *Disinfectants* and *germicides* are substances, usually of chemical origin, which kill microorganisms; they have bactericidal action. *Fungicides* are substances which kill fungi.

ANTISEPTICS AND DISINFECTANTS

The effectiveness of antiseptics and disinfectants depends upon (1) the strength of the solution and (2) the time of exposure to the antiseptic or disinfectant.

Phenolics

Phenol was the first antiseptic. Other antiseptics are compared with phenol to measure their effectiveness; this measurement is known as the phenol coefficient (P/C). Many antiseptics contain phenol and related compounds and are called the phenolics.

Cresol is a phenolic compound which is soluble in soap. It is a potent disinfectant and is used in many disinfectant preparations. Lysol and Staphene are examples. In a 2% to 5% solution, they are used to disinfect utensils and excreta.

Section 4 Drugs and Related Substances

Substance	Strength	Action	Comments

Alcohol
  ethyl
  isopropyl
	70%
	full strength
		Antiseptic
		germicide
			astringent; toxic by mouth; useful on surgical instruments

Benzalkonium-chloride (Zephiran)	1:750 to 1:10,000	antiseptic	nonirritating to skin; soap must be rinsed off before using; inactivated by presence of soap

Phenolics
  (Cresol)
  (Lysol)
  (Amphyl)
  (Staphene)
	2% to 5%
	
	2 1/2%
	1/2%
		disinfectant
		
		disinfectant
		antiseptic
			disinfects contaminated objects such as linens, basins, and bedpans; action not affected by organic material
			footbath for athlete's foot; prolonged use may be injurious to tissues

Gentian violet	1:100 to 1:1000	antiseptic; fungicide	used on skin and mucous membrane for fungus infections (thrush, impetigo)
Iodine (solution or tincture) (Wescodyne) (Betadine)	2% iodine and detergent	antiseptic fungicide antiseptic	effective when used on small wounds, abrasions; hand-rinse; kills organisms sensitive to iodine
Merbromin, (solution or tincture) (Mercurochrome)	2%	bacterio-static	used as skin antiseptic and for urinary infections; 1% solution for bladder irrigation; 5% for skin preparation
Hydrogen peroxide	3%	antiseptic	cleans wounds of pus and dead tissue. Diluted with 1 to 4 parts of water
Zinc undecylenic acid (Desenex) soap	2%	fungicide	for fungus infections of skin: athlete's foot and ringworm, exclusive of nails and hairy areas.
Formalin (Cidex)	0.5 to 0.9% 6 to 12 hours	disinfectant	effective against viruses, spores; irritating to tissues
Potassium permanganate	1% 1:5000	antiseptic antiseptic	strong oxidizing chemical used for vaginal and urethral irrigations
Green soap (solution or tincture)	1:10	antiseptic	handwash
Silver nitrate	1:1000 1 to 2% (eye drops) 1:10,000	antiseptic antiseptic antiseptic	astringent prevents gonorrheal conjunctivitis bladder irrigations

Fig. 20-1 Antiseptics and Disinfectants

Alcohol

Ethyl alcohol is a very commonly used antiseptic. It is used to prepare the skin for injections and the taking of blood specimens. It is also used to prevent infection from minor abrasions. The most effective solution is 70%.

Isopropyl alcohol (99%) is a germicide used full-strength for the disinfection of instruments. It may also be used in a 75% solution for the disinfection of oral thermometers.

Iodine

Iodine is a germicide and fungicide. It is available in a tincture and a solution of 2 percent. It is effective when used on small wounds and abrasions. In solution with alcohol, iodine kills the tubercle bacilli.

Like phenol, iodine is combined with cleansing agents for disinfection. An example of iodine and detergent is Wescodyne. Wescodyne is used as a handrinse after scrubbing and as an antiseptic to kill microorganisms sensitive to iodine. It is also effective against the tubercle bacillus.

Organic Formalin Complexes

Formaldehyde is used in various solutions to disinfect instruments and other articles which cannot be sterilized by heat.

Formalin is a 37% solution of formaldehyde. Cidex is a commercial preparation of formalin. This germicide is effective against viruses as well as spores. A .5% solution will destroy all microorganisms in 6 to 12 hours. Because it is irritating to tissues, it is not used as an antiseptic.

ANTIBIOTICS

All through nature we find that some plants and animals give support to each other. This constructive relationship is called *symbiosis*. Other plants and animals destroy each other. This destructive relationship is called *antibiosis*.

Antibiotic drugs get their name from the fact that they are chemical substances produced by microscopic yeasts and molds which destroy or inhibit the growth of other microorganisms. Some antibiotics may now be partially or completely manufactured by synthetic means, but they retain the name "antibiotic" because of their characteristic action of "attacking" microorganisms. Antibiotics have been responsible for such wonderful cures that they have frequently been called miracle drugs. These drugs have altered the entire field of medicine.

- Narrow-spectrum antibiotics are those effective against only a few microorganisms. Examples of narrow-spectrum drugs are: Penicillin, Streptomycin and Bacitracin.

- Broad-spectrum antibiotics are those effective against many microorganisms. Examples of the broad-spectrum antibiotics are: Tetracyclines, Chloramphenicol, Neomycin, Kanamycin and Erythromycin.

The penicillins and tetracyclines are the most extensively used and also the most effective antibiotics.

In administering antibiotics, both the initial dose and the maintenance doses must be potent. The dosage must be strong enough so that the patient may recover rapidly before the pathogen develops a resistance to the antibiotic and the drug becomes ineffectual in fighting the infection. However, unnecessarily large doses may lead to toxic reactions in the patient. Microorganisms sometimes develop resistance to antibiotics. Anti-infectives other than antibiotics should be given for minor infections so that antibiotics will not encounter resistant organisms in severe conditions. Strains of staphylococci resistant to antibiotics have developed frequently in hospitals.

A good antibiotic must be harmless to the blood and blood-forming organs, the liver, and the kidneys. The antibiotic must remain in the body tissues for some time. Therefore, low toxicity of the antibiotic is an objective.

Penicillin

Penicillin was discovered by Sir Alexander Fleming in England in 1928. It is derived from certain strains of molds such as Penicillium Notatum and Penicillium Chrysogenum. The penicillins which have been developed are F, G, K, O. V, and X. Penicillin G is the most commonly used. Penicillins O and V also have some therapeutic applications. Penicillin G is the only penicillin completely synthesized to date; others have been partially synthesized.

Penicillin is effective in treating pneumonia, gonorrhea, syphilis, bronchitis, and bacterial endocarditis. Generally, it has no toxic effects even in large doses unless the person is hypersensitive to it. A discussion of anaphylactic shock, a severe reaction which may occur in hypersensitive individuals, will be detailed in Unit 30. Penicillin is most effective when given intravenously and intramuscularly. It is excreted rapidly by the kidneys. It enters body tissues easily with the exception of the bone marrow, brain, and spinal fluid, and the humors of the eye. The drug passes easily from the maternal blood to the blood of the fetus.

Types of Penicillin. Penicillin G is available in several forms. Potassium penicillin G and sodium penicillin G are crystalline. Therefore, they dissolve in water and are absorbed rapidly in the body. They are used for severe infections which require prompt treatment. Noncrystalline penicillin, on the other hand, is slowly absorbed and has a prolonged action. Examples include benzathine penicillin G and procaine penicillin G. Methicillin and oxacillin are semisynthetic penicillins which may be ordered for staphylococcal infections that do not respond to penicillin G. Ampicillin, also a semisynthetic penicillin, has the same uses as penicillin G, but it is also effective against organisms causing types of influenza, pyelitis, and diarrhea.

Dosages of Penicillin. The U.S.P. specifies a wide range of dosages: 200,000 to 1,000,000 units orally four times a day, 300,000 to 2,000,000 units intramuscularly daily, and 6,000,000 to 40,000,000 units intravenously daily. Only penicillin marked for intravenous use is given intravenously.

Streptomycin

Streptomycin is not well absorbed from the intestinal tract, and so it is administered intramuscularly. It passes poorly into the cerebrospinal fluid and is excreted slowly from the kidneys. Damage to the eighth cranial nerve, shown by vertigo and deafness, is a serious toxic effect. The chief use of streptomycin is in the treatment of tuberculosis. In tuberculosis the best results are obtained with a combination of streptomycin, para-aminosalicylic acid (P.A.S.), and isonicotinic acid hydrazide (isoniazid or I.N.H.). The dosage is 1 Gm daily.

Bacitracin

Bacitracin (Baciguent) is derived from a type of bacteria. This antibiotic is bactericidal, and its antibacterial effect is similar to that of penicillin. Patients seldom become hypersensitive to it and, therefore, it can be used for conditions when the patient is allergic to other antibiotics. Because it is toxic to the kidneys, its use is generally limited to topical application. It is available in aerosol mist, ophthalmic drops, and ointments as well as in powder and soluble tablets for injection.

The Tetracyclines

The tetracyclines are similar to each other and have identical functions. They are called broad-spectrum antibiotics because they are effective in several infections such as pneumonia, urinary tract infection, rickettsial infections, and amebiasis. They may be administered intravenously, intramuscularly, and orally. Continued use over long periods of time may alter the intestinal flora. Normal bacterial organisms of the intestine are destroyed by the antibiotic so that pathogenic organisms, formerly controlled by normal flora, flourish and cause complications. The average dosage is 250 mg q.i.d. Drugs in the tetracycline group include:

>   Oxytetracycline (Terramycin)
>   Tetracycline (Achromycin)
>   Demethylchlortetracycline (Declomycin)
>   Doxycycline (Vibramycin)
>   Methacycline (Rondomycin)

Chloramphenicol

Chloramphenicol (Chloromycetin) is a broad-spectrum antibiotic. It is effective against many infections especially those caused by rickettsial organisms, typhoid fever, and lymphogranuloma. It may be administered intravenously, intramucularly, and orally. A serious side effect is depression of bone marrow, resulting in blood dyscrasia. For this reason its use is limited. The average dosage is 250 mg q. 6h.

Neomycin Sulfate

Neomycin (Mycifradin) is a broad-spectrum antibiotic. If injected, it is toxic to the kidneys and may damage the eighth cranial nerve, resulting in hearing loss and dizziness. It is not absorbed from the intestines and is administered orally in preoperative situations to cause a local sterilization in the bowel. Concentrations of it will accumulate in the intestines, thus sterilizing it for surgery. It is irritating when given parenterally. The dosage is 0.5 to 2 Gm q.i.d. orally and 0.5% in ointment or solution, topically. The preoperative dose for bowel sterilization is 1 Gm q. 4h for 24 to 72 hours.

Kanamycin

Kanamycin (Kantrex) is similar to neomycin and streptomycin when taken orally. It is effective against some staphylococcus infections, urinary tract infections, respiratory tract infections, and some cases of tuberculosis. Side effects include kidney damage because it is entirely eliminated by the kidneys. For this reason a high fluid intake should accompany its administration. Damage to the eighth cranial nerve, numbness and tingling of the arms and hands and pain at the injection site are other adverse reactions. Patients should be observed for tinnitus and deafness. The usual preoperative dose for bowel sterilization is 1 Gm every hour x 4 doses, then 1 Gm q. 6h for 36 to 72 hours.

Erythromycin

Erythromycin (Erythrocin) is similar to penicillin. It is given when the pathogen has developed a resistance to penicillin and in cases of hypersensitivity to penicillin. Although it is well-absorbed from the gastrointestinal tract, it is destroyed by gastric secretions. Therefore, when given orally, it is prepared in enteric-coated tablets or nonsoluble preparations. Mild gastrointestinal side effects may accompany its use. Oral dosage is 250 mg q.6h.

Novobiocin Sodium

Novobiocin (Albamycin) is used mainly in the treatment of staphylococcal infections. It is effective in the treatment of urinary tract infections. It may be considered as having a moderate (rather than broad or narrow) spectrum. Because of its serious side effects, it is reserved for use in serious infections when the patient may be allergic to other drugs. Side effects include skin rashes, fever, and yellowing of the sclera of the eye as in jaundice. It is rapidly absorbed from the intestinal tract and so is administered orally. It may be administered intravenously at a very slow rate. The average dosage is 250 mg every 6 hours or 500 mg every 12 hours.

Triacetyloleandomycin

Triacetyloleandomycin (TAO, Cyclamin) is effective chiefly against staphylococcus infections. It is completely absorbed from the intestinal tract. The side effects are mild, such as anorexia, nausea, loose stools and skin irritations. Preparations include 125-250 mg capsules p.o., oral drops 100 mg per ml, and suspension 25 mg per ml.

Antifungal Antibiotics

Most of the antibiotics are ineffectual against mycotic (fungus) infections. Therefore, several synthetic drugs and antibiotics have been produced for this special purpose.

Amphotericin B. Amphotericin B (Fungizone) is effective against a broad spectrum of deep-seated fungi and yeast infections. Side effects include phlebitis at the site of injection, chills, fever, vomiting, and respiratory distress. Kidney function tests should be done frequently. The dosage is based on body weight; initially 0.25 mg/kilogram of body weight, then 1 mg/kg, 2 or 3 times a day. Slow intravenous infusion is recommended over a period of 5 to 6 hours.

Nystatin. Nystatin (Mycostatin) is fairly effective against many yeast and mold infections. It is poorly absorbed from the intestinal tract. Local administration is used in resistant anal and vaginal monilial infections. It is also used in the treatment of thrush. There are mild side effects such as gastric upsets. The dosage is 500,000 to 1,000,000 units three times daily in oral suspension or tablets for gastrointestinal moniliasis, and 100,000 unit tablets or suppositories inserted once or twice a day for vaginal moniliasis.

Griseofulvin. Griseofulvin (Fulvicin, Grifulvin) is a fungistatic antibiotic; that is, it prevents the infection from spreading. Following absorption upon oral administration, it becomes part of the keratin of the hair, nails, and skin. Thus, as the new cells develop, they are fungus-free. Griseofulvin is effective in the treatment of ringworm of the scalp, body, and feet.

Side effects may include headaches, gastric upset, diarrhea, and skin eruptions. Frequent blood tests must be done because of the possibility of leukopenia. Preparations include 250- and 500-mg tablets. Adult dosages vary, according to the severity of the infection, from .5 Gm to 2 Gm daily. The dosage for children is 10 mg per pound of body weight, given in divided doses.

Cephalosporins

Cephalothin (Keflin) and cephaloridine (Loridine) are members of a family named cephalosporins after the fungus from which they are derived. They are semisynthetic, broad-spectrum antibiotics used for patients who have infections caused by more than one microorganism. They are poorly absorbed from the gastrointestinal tract and are usually administered intramuscularly, although the intravenous route is used in serious conditions. The oral preparation is available under the trade name of Keflex.

Cephalothin is used in treating infections such as pneumonia, bacterial enteritis, osteomyelitis, bacterial endocarditis, and infections of the kidneys and bladder. A side effect of cephalothin may be pain with soft tissue damage following intramuscular injection. For this reason deep injection into a large muscle mass (such as the gluteus medius) is recommended. The adult dosage is .5 Gm to 1 Gm, I.M., 4 to 6 times daily. A false positive reaction for glucose may occur with Clinitest tablets but not with Tes-tape.

Cephaloridine is ordered for serious infections of the respiratory tract, genito-urinary tract (including gonorrhea in the male), bones and joints, bloodstream, soft tissue, and skin. It is toxic to the kidneys and is contraindicated for patients with renal impairment.

Lincomycin (Lincocin) is unrelated structurally to other antibiotics. It is used in streptococcal and staphylococcal infections. Since it is quickly absorbed from the gastrointestinal tract, lincomycin is administered orally. The usual dose is 500 mg q. 8h p.o.; 600 mg daily I.M.; and 600 mg q.12h.

Patients Allergic to Penicillin. Cephalosporins are sometimes given *with great caution* to patients who are hypersensitive to penicillin as the cephalosporins have many of the penicillin properties and have a broader antibacterial spectrum; also, they are easier to tolerate. Patients who are allergic to penicillin may tolerate cephalosporins but should be watched carefully, especially if the medication is given over a period of time or in large doses.

With the discovery of more and more antibiotics, the medical profession now has the opportunity to use other antibiotics when a patient is allergic to penicillin. But as nurses, we are in a position to pick up information from the patient (such as an allergy to penicillin) which he may not have told the physician or the physician may have forgotten. *If a patient is placed on a drug belonging to the cephalosporin group and the patient is allergic to penicillin,* the nurse must be sure that the physician is aware of this fact as well as all other staff members. If the patient continues on the drug, the nurse helps the physician and the patient by *close observation of the patient and the laboratory reports.* Severe reactions, including death from anaphylaxis, have been reported in some instances when penicillin-sensitive patients received these drugs.

SULFONAMIDES

Sulfonamides were discovered in Italy in 1935 by Domagk, a college research student. His product was a dye called Prontosil which was later found to have anti-infective qualities. The sulfonamides are prepared synthetically to act directly against pathogenic microorganisms, and so they are classified as chemotherapeutic agents. They are especially effective against specific infections of the urinary and intestinal tracts. They tend to be more toxic to human tissues than the penicillins and other antibiotics.

The sulfonamides inhibit the growth of susceptible bacteria. They mimic a substance which certain microorganisms use for food. These microorganisms cannot use the drug, and are weakened so that they cannot grow. By its action the drug makes the susceptible bacteria subject to the action of the phagocytes, our second line of defense against disease.

Many of the sulfonamides are well-absorbed from the gastrointestinal tract and can be administered orally. The sulfonamides diffuse easily into body tissues, including the spinal fluid, and so they are useful in treating meningitis. They are able to reduce bacterial growth in the intestines and colon. They are excreted through the urinary tract. Fluids must be forced to dilute the urine.

Sulfonamides may be administered in combination with an antibiotic, or two or three different sulfonamides may be prescribed. Generally, these drugs are low in cost. The incidence of toxicity in the combined sulfonamides drugs is comparatively rare. When toxicity does occur, it is usually due to renal disturbances or hypersensitivity. Signs and symptoms of toxicity include nausea, vomiting, dizziness, headache, mental depression, and/or dermatitis. Severe side effects may include jaundice, hemolytic anemia, oliguria, and even anuria.

Sulfisoxazole

Sulfisoxazole (Gantrisin) is used chiefly in urinary tract infections. It is easily absorbed and has little tendency to cause crystalluria in the kidneys. The dosage is 4 Gm initially, and then it is reduced to 1 Gm every 4 to 6 hours.

Sulfamethoxypyridazine

Sulfamethoxypyridazine (Kynex, Midicel) is a newer, long-acting sulfonamide. It is excreted slowly from the urinary tract, thus limiting damage to the kidneys. Because it is readily absorbed and diffused into the spinal fluid, it has antibacterial action in that area.

Sulfadiazine

Sulfadiazine is especially effective in the treatment of meningitis. It is also the most effective of all the sulfonamides. It is readily absorbed from the gastrointestinal tract. The dosage is usually 1 Gm by mouth every 4 hours.

Other Sulfonamides

The nurse should be familiar with the following drugs and their special avenues of attack.

- Triple Sulfa (Methamerdizine, Sulfatriazine, Terfonyl, Trionamide, Tripazine, Tri-sulfameth, Tri-sulfazine): a sulfonamide mixture with equal parts sulfadiazine, sulfamerazine, and sulfamethazine.
  Dosage: Oral .5 Gm tablets
- Sulfadimethoxine (Madribon, Madriqid): easily absorbed from gastrointestinal tract, less effective than sulfadiazine. An advantage of the drug is that it can be given less frequently than other sulfonamides.
  Dosage: Oral .5 Gm – 1.0 Gm every 24 hours
- Succinylsulfathiazole (Sulfasuxidine): used to suppress the growth of bacteria in the large bowel.
- Phthalylsulfathiazole (Sulfathalidine): an effective intestinal antiseptic.
- Nitrosulfathiazole: used in treatment of ulcerative colitis. It is administered rectally.
- Salicylazosulfapyridine (Azulfidine): used in the treatment of chronic ulcerative colitis. It is administered orally.

The drugs included in this unit are but a sampling of the most common antibiotics and chemotherapeutics now available, and new drugs are being introduced every year.

SUGGESTED ACTIVITIES

- Select a microbiology text and review the types of pathogens and their respective characteristics. Prepare a chart for easy reference.
- Assume that you have been assigned to prepare a hospital unit for a new patient. The previous patient was discharged early in the morning. The diagnosis was tuberculosis. From study of the antiseptics and disinfectants in this unit, what steps would be taken to:
  a. destroy bacilli on bed linen?
  b. sterilize the oral thermometer?
  c. sterilize the bedpan?
  d. disinfect the bed, table, and chairs?
  e. clean the mattress?
  f. sterilize nondisposable rubber goods?
  g. use as an antiseptic rinse after handwashing?
- Observe the Penicillium Notatum under the microscrope. Draw and label its parts.

Section 4 Drugs and Related Substances

REVIEW

1. What strength of silver nitrate eye drops will the nurse hand the obstetrician for use on the newborn?   *1 TO 2% (EYE DROPS)*

2. Explain the characteristic action of an antibiotic upon microorganisms.
   ANTIBIOTIC DRUGS GET THEIR NAME FROM THE FACT THAT THEY ARE CHEMICAL SUBSTANCES PRODUCED BY MICROSCOPIC YEASTS AND MOLDS

3. Why are certain drugs called *antibiotics*?
   THEY INHIBIT THE GROWTH OF MICROORGANISMS

4. Give an example of a broad-spectrum antibiotic and a narrow-spectrum antibiotic.
   BROAD SPECTRUM - TETRACYCLINES
   NARROW SPECTRUM - PENICILLIN

5. Name the five antibiotics which make up the tetracyclines.
   OXYTETRACYCLINE   DOXYCYCLINE
   TETRACYCLINE   METHACYCLINE
   DEMETHYLCHLORTETRACYCLIN

6. Which of the penicillin group has been synthesized to date?
   PENICILLIN - G

7. Name the characteristics of a good antibiotic.
   A GOOD ANTIBIOTIC MUST BE HARMFUL TO THE BLOOD & BLOOD FORMING ORGANS, THE LIVER, AND THE GOOD KIDNEYS. IT MUST REMAIN IN THE BLOOD STREAM FOR A LONG PERIOD OF TIME

8. A patient who is on daily doses of sulfonamides should be told of symptoms which should be reported to the physician. What are those symptoms?
   NAUSEA, VOMITING, DIZZINESS, DERMATITIS

9. If the patient is unable to reach the physician but shows some of the above symptoms, what advice would the nurse give him?
   DISCONTINUE USE

10. What factor in the taking of sulfonamide products might produce precipitation of the drug in the renal tubules?
    IT HAS A TENDENCY TO CRYSTALLIZE

Unit 20 Drugs Used to Counteract Infections

11. What advice must be given to a patient on sulfonamide therapy to prevent complications? *2 TO 3,000 CC OF WATER A DAY*

12. What is the characteristic action of a sulfonamide upon microorganisms? *THE SULFONAMIDES WE THEIR SO THAT THE MICROORGANISMS CAN EAT THEM. THEY WEAKEN AND THE PHAGOCYTES COME AND EAT THE MICROORGANISMS*

13. Complete the following chart:

Antibiotic	Source	Effective Against	Toxicity
Penicillin	MOLD	STAPH, STREP, PYOGENES	HYPERSENSITIVITY
Tetracyclines	MOLD	PNEUMONIA, URINARY TRACT INFECTIONS	DIARRHEA, ABDOMINAL DISCOMFORT
Streptomycin	MOLD	TB	DIZZINESS, DEAFNESS 8TH CRANIAL
Erythromycin	MOLD	SAME AS PENICILLIN	SAME

14. Match the items in Column II with the appropriate items in Column I.

__K__ 1. sulfonamides
__J__ 2. broad-spectrum antibiotic
__H__ 3. penicillin
__B__ 4. fungicide
__G__ 5. symbiosis
__I__ 6. narrow-spectrum antibiotic
__A__ 7. chemotherapeutic agent
__E__ 8. phenol coefficient
__D__ 9. streptomycin
__C__ 10. antibiosis

a. Prepared synthetically
b. Substances which kill fungi
c. Destructive relationship between plants and animals
d. Administered I.M. – poorly absorbed from intestinal tract
e. Measure used to rate drug effectiveness
f. Formula of a drug
g. Plants and animals which give support to each other
h. Discovered by Alexander Fleming
i. Effective against a few microorganisms
j. Tetracycline is an example
k. Discovered by Domagk in 1935

147

Section 4 Drugs and Related Substances

EXTENDED STUDY

Learn the meaning and proper use of the following terms:

antimetabolite	malignant
benign	metastasize
cytotoxin	neoplasm
leukemia	polycythemia
leukopenia	remission
lymphoma	chemotherapeutic

Unit 21 Drugs Used in Malignant Diseases

OBJECTIVES

After studying this unit, the student should be able to:

- Differentiate between benign and malignant tumors.
- Explain the action of the antimetabolites.
- Explain why these drugs are highly toxic.

Cancer is a disease in which the cancer cells multiply wildly and invade normal cells and tissues. These are *malignant* growths, virulent growths which tend to become progressively worse. The transfer of the disease from one part of the body to another is referred to as *metastasis*. An example of a malignant tumor is a *lymphoma*; it involves the lymph nodes and metastasizes quickly to other organs.

Other tumors may grow to be very large but they do not invade and destroy normal tissues. These are called benign growths; they can usually be completely removed with benefit to the patient.

Therapy for cancer consists of radiation, surgery, and chemotherapy. The chemotherapeutic drugs are effective against cells that multiply rapidly. These include not only the malignant cells but also blood cells and cells of the gastrointestinal tract. It is difficult to administer large doses of anti-cancer drugs since these same doses actually destroy normal healthy cells. Therefore, many chemotherapeutic drugs give temporary relief from symptoms or *remission* from the malignancy. Only early diagnosis, surgery, and radiation can really cure the condition.

Leukemia is a blood disorder which is an uncontrolled proliferation of white blood cells; it, therefore, can be considered a kind of malignant neoplasm in that these cells multiply, growing beyond their limits without any control over regrowth. Chemotherapy is the treatment for acute or chronic leukemias. It is not unusual to find that the white cell counts in leukemias may range from 100,000 to 1,000,000 per cubic millimeter; the normal white cell count ranges between 5,000 – 10,000.

A lymphoma is a tumor of lymphatic tissue; it usually originates in lymph nodes and grows and spreads to other lymphoid tissues. Hodgkin's disease, lymphosarcoma, multiple myeloma are examples of lymphomas. Some lymphomas are treated by X ray and/or chemotherapy. Corticosteroids have been used and proven effective for a time.

Polycythemia vera refers to excessive formation of red blood cells which cannot be controlled.

When chemotherapeutic drugs are given for cancer, the blood and blood-forming organs are frequently affected. As there may be an abrupt drop in the leukocyte count (leukopenia), a decrease in the hemoglobin level and in the platelet count, the nurse should observe the patient for signs of bleeding such as bruises and bleeding gums. The patient should be handled gently and undue pressure on parts of the body should be avoided or relieved to prevent bruising. Since the patient is prone to infection, strict medical asepsis must be maintained. A bland diet is usually ordered to alleviate nausea and vomiting. Frequent blood tests are usually ordered and the nurse should study the lab reports.

Because toxicity is a problem in the administration of large doses of chemotherapeutic drugs, an effort is being made to give drugs to a specific area of the body by local injection into the artery. By this method the local circulation can be stopped as the solution is injected into the artery. These are limited cases, however, and the problem of toxicity continues, especially in the gastrointestinal tract.

The drugs used for cancer therapy are classified as follows: antimetabolites, cytotoxic or alkylating agents, antibiotics, and hormones, figures 21-1 through 21-4. The action of the antimetabolites is similar to that of the sulfonamides. The antimetabolite is ingested by the malignant cell as if it were a proper element necessary for cell metabolism. Since it cannot function normally without the presence of the element which the antimetabolite replaces, the cell dies. Cytotoxic agents, as their name implies, are toxic to cells. Study the charts which describe each group.

Medication	Action	Uses	Results
4-aminopteroylglutamic acid sodium (Aminopterin)	attacks tissues in rapid growth	acute leukemia lymphosarcoma Hodgkin's disease	temporary remission
Methotrexate	as above	choriocarcinoma acute leukemia Hodgkin's disease advanced breast cancer	some complete cures in choriocarcinoma only temporary remission
6-mercaptopurine (Purinethol)	attacks nucleus of cells	acute leukemia	temporary remission
Azathioprine (Imuran)	as above	acute leukemia human homotransplants	prolongs life of transplanted tissue
5-fluorouracil	as above	carcinoma of breast, bowel, rectum, ovary and bladder	temporary remission
Vincristine sulfate (Oncovin)	unknown; may affect cell division (mitosis)	acute leukemia of childhood	remission
Vinblastine sulfate (Velban)	as above	Hodgkin's disease, leukemia, carcinoma of breast	probable cures remission

Fig. 21-1 Antimetabolites

Unit 21 Drugs Used in Malignant Diseases

Medication	Action	Uses	Results
Nitrogen mustard (Mustargen)	DNA is vulnerable drug; prevents cell division	Hodgkin's disease, chronic leukemia, carcinoma of lung	temporary control and remission
Chlorambucil (Leukeran)	see nitrogen mustard	see nitrogen mustard	see nitrogen mustard
Triethylene melamine (TEM)	as above	as above	as above
Busulfan (Myleran)	as above	chronic myelogenous leukemia	as above
Melphalan (Alkeran)	as above	multiple myeloma	as above
Triethyleneophosphoramide (Ethylenimine) (Thiotepa)	as above	Hodgkin's disease cancer of ovary chronic leukemia lymphosarcoma	as above
Cyclophosphamide (Cytoxan) (Endoxan)	as above	Hodgkin's disease lymphoma, lymphosarcoma, chronic lymphocytic leukemia	as above

Fig. 21-2 Nitrogen Mustards and Alkylating Agents

Medication	Uses	Results
ACTH (Corticotropin) (Acthar) (Cortrophin Solacthyl)	acute leukemia, multiple myeloma, mycosis fungoides	short remission
Cortisone (adrenal steroid) and derivatives	acute leukemia, lymphosarcoma, Hodgkin's disease, multiple myeloma, mycosis fungoides	short remission
Estrogens (Female hormones)	carcinoma of prostate, carcinoma of female breast after menopause	palliative only Note: if given before cessation of menstruation, may increase possibility of breast cancer
Androgens (Male hormones)	carcinoma of breast	palliative only

Fig. 21-3 Hormones

Section 4 Drugs and Related Substances

Medication	Action and Use	Results
Actinomycin D (Sanmycin) (Cosmegen) (Dactinomycin)	antibiotic which blocks cell division. Hodgkin's disease, lymphomas, Wilm's Tumor	remission
Ethyl carbonate (Urethan)	interferes with cell division. chronic myelogenous leukemia multiple myeloma	remission
Sodium Phosphate p^{32} Solution (Phosphotope)	radioisotope which ejects electrons in cell. Polycythemia vera Chronic myelogenous leukemia Chronic lymphatic leukemia	Used extensively for polycythemia; longer remission
Hydroxyurea (Hydrea)	anticancer chemical. Melanoma Chronic myelocytic leukemia	Some remissions in virulent melanoma.
Procarbazine (Matulane)	A monoamine oxidase inhibitor advanced Hodgkin's Disease	remissions
L-asparaginase	Chemical that acts on biochemical difference between cancer and normal cells. Acute leukemia Lymphoma	(+ On clinical trial) remission.

Fig. 21-4 Other Antineoplastic Agents

The patient should be spared as much discomfort as is possible while undergoing treatment; therefore, whenever toxic symptoms appear, they should be reported immediately. Some drugs which are useful in controlling the toxicity of the anticancer agents are Leucovarin (a preparation of folinic acid); Thymodine, and Sodium thiosulphate.

Special nursing care directed to the patient's emotional needs and that of the family must be always present. Not only does this care provide the persons involved with emotional support, but often helps the patient to tolerate the unpleasant effects of drug therapy.

SUGGESTED ACTIVITY
- Assume that you are assigned to take care of a patient with a terminal disease. After researching and reading articles in nursing periodicals and texts, write a report explaining how you would care for the patient and deal most effectively with his mental and emotional adjustment and needs. List the reference articles at the end of the report.

REVIEW
1. Explain the difference between a benign tumor and a malignant one.

2. List four adverse drug reactions to chemotherapeutic drugs used for cancer therapy.

3. Explain why these chemotherapeutic drugs are so toxic.

4. Based on your understanding of terms relating to this unit, match the definition in Column II with the appropriate word in Column I.

Column I

___ 1. antimetabolite
___ 2. remission
___ 3. benign growth
___ 4. neoplasm
___ 5. leukemia
___ 6. leukopenia
___ 7. lymphoma
___ 8. malignant growth
___ 9. metastasis
___ 10. polycythemia vera

Column II

a. a substance which competes with material needed by a cell
b. another word for tumor
c. excessive formation of red blood cells
d. temporary relief from symptoms
e. transfer of disease from one part of the body to another
f. virulent growth which tends to become progressively worse.
g. decrease of white blood cells
h. tumor which involves lymph nodes
i. growth which does not invade and destroy normal tissue
j. disease of the blood, with abnormal increase of white blood cells

EXTENDED STUDY

Learn the meaning and proper use of the following terms:

adrenergic
allergen
anaphylactic shock
antihistamine

eczema
histamine
rhinitis
urticaria

Unit 22 Antihistamines and Motion Sickness Drugs

OBJECTIVES

After studying this unit, the student should be able to:
- Describe an allergic reaction.
- State the causes and treatment of anaphylactic shock.
- Differentiate between the contributing and physiological causes of motion sickness.
- List the conditions for which antihistamines and motion sickness drugs are given and their common side effects.

Individuals sensitive to foreign substances have received great relief from the antihistamine drugs. These persons may be sensitive to any one or several of the following: foods, cosmetics, pollens, soaps (detergents), synthetic fabrics, wool, and animal hair. The substance to which they are allergic is called an allergen. An exposure to an allergen to which a person is sensitive causes the release of histamine from body cells and the manifestation of the allergic symptoms. This is called an *allergic reaction.* Common symptoms to an allergic reaction include rhinitis (inflammation of nasal mucosa), hay fever, asthma, eczema, contact dermatitis, nausea, vomiting, and urticaria. *Contact dermatitis* refers to a skin rash caused by contact with an allergen; for example, animal fur. *Urticaria* is an itchy skin condition marked by transient eruption of wheals; it is often referred to as hives. Most of these allergic reactions respond to the antihistamine drugs.

ANTIHISTAMINES

In addition to the treatment of allergies, the histamine-antagonizing drugs may be used in the treatment of motion sickness, morning nausea, Meniere's disease, nausea following middle ear surgery, mild insomnia, and urticaria. The antihistamines become effective in approximately 15 minutes following oral administration because they are easily absorbed from the gastrointestinal tract. Some antihistamines cause drowsiness, but this is usually a limited type of action. These drugs may also produce allergic responses of their own, especially skin reactions.

ANAPHYLACTIC SHOCK

The injection of certain sera of animal origin, and certain other drugs and conditions to which the person is sensitive may produce a severe response called anaphylactic shock. This allergic reaction is first indicated by the rapid swelling at the site of injection, and it soon becomes generalized. General symptoms include hypotensive shock and collapse and extreme respiratory difficulty. Unless epinephrine (Adrenalin) is administered by intramuscular injection very soon, the patient may expire. This reaction can be avoided by administering a sensitivity test before giving the injection.

Epinephrine, (Adrenalin)

Epinephrine is the drug usually administered intramuscularly to counteract the effects of histamine poisoning in anaphylactic shock. It relaxes the bronchial tubes and constricts the arterioles which dilate in anaphylactic shock due to the freeing of histamine in the body. Dosage is 0.2 to 1 ml of 1:1000 solution.

Epinephrine is a potent adrenergic drug. That is, it produces the effect of stimulating the sympathetic nervous system. Accordingly, it constricts the arterioles of the viscera and skin while dilating the arterioles of the brain and skeletal muscles; it increases heart action, blood sugar, and blood clotting and usually raises the blood pressure. Because it stimulates the sympathetic nervous system, it causes the patient to become anxious and restless.

Other drugs used to treat anaphylactic shock are levarterenol, ephedrine, phenylephrine, metaraminol, and methamphetamine.

MOTION SICKNESS DRUGS

Some antihistamines and the motion sickness drugs are effective in preventing and relieving motion sickness. Physiologically, motion sickness is caused when the nerve in the labyrinth of the middle ear stimulates the vomiting center in the medulla of the brain.

Medication	Action	Administration and Dosage	Adverse and/or side effects
Diphenhydramine hydrochloride (Benadryl hydrochloride)	moderately antispasmodic; antihistamine	p.o. 25-50 mg 3-4 times daily; parenteral and topical as ordered; I.V. 10-50 mg	drowsiness
Tripelennamine hydrochloride (Pyribenzamine hydrochloride)	antihistamine; less likely to cause drowsiness	p.o. 50 mg 3 times daily; topical as ordered s.c., I.V., I.M.	gastrointestinal irritation
Chlorpheniramine maleate (Chlor-trimeton maleate) (Teldrin)	antihistamine enteric-coated tablet prolongs action	p.o. 8-12 mg (enteric-coated tablet), 2-8 mg every 8 hours (regular tablet); parenteral 5-10 mg	mild drowsiness
Promethazine hydrochloride (Phenergan hydrochloride	antihistamine; relieves motion sickness; also used as tranquilizer; fairly long sedative action suitable for surgical and OB patients; antiemetic	p.o. 12.5-25 mg 3-4 times daily; parenteral 1 mg per Kg of body weight	drowsiness
Brompheniramine (Dimetane)	antihistamine in therapeutic doses	p.o. 4 mg 3-6 times daily	mild drowsiness

Fig. 22-1 Antihistamines

Section 4 Drugs and Related Substances

Medication	Action	Administration and Dosage	Adverse and/or side effects
Dimenhydrinate (Dramamine)	antihistamine; similar to (Benadryl) controls nausea and vomiting in motion sickness; alleviates vertigo caused by Meniere's disease radiation sickness, and middle ear surgery	**p.o.** 50 mg 1/2 hr. before departure, then up to 100 mg q. 4h as needed; rectal 50-100 mg suppositories; I.M. 50 mg	drowsiness
Cyclizine hydrochloride (Marezine hydrochloride)	antihistamine; antiemetic; controls nausea and vomiting in motion sickness	**p.o.** 50 mg before departure and 50 mg 3 times daily before meals; dosage tapered off according to need; rectal 50-100 mg suppositories; I.M. as cyclizine lactate 50 mg	blurred vision and drowsiness in large doses
Trimethobenzamide hydrochloride (Tigan hydrochloride)	mild antihistamine; effective antiemetic controls nausea and vomiting in motion sickness, radiation sickness, infection and as effect of other drugs; effective in 20-40 minutes; action may be prolonged for 3-4 hours	**p.o.** 100-250 mg capsules; I.M. vials, ampules of various potency; rectal 200 mg suppositories	dizziness, diarrhea, irritation at site of injection
Meclizine (Bonine)	antihistamine especially useful in treatment of nausea, vomiting, and motion sickness action may be prolonged up to 24 hrs	**p.o.** 25 mg tablets b.i.d.	blurred vision, dryness of mouth drowsiness

Fig. 22-2 Motion Sickness Drugs

Vertical movements of a plan or ship contribute to motion sickness. Susceptible persons may get car sick. The labyrinth of the middle ear responds more to the up-and-down (vertical) movements of the vehicle than to side-to-side (horizontal) movements. Some symptoms of motion sickness are: increased salivation, pallor, profuse perspiration, and chilliness followed by nausea and vomiting.

Due to the sedative side effects of some motion sickness drugs, they must be taken with caution by the operators of vehicles. *All adverse and side effects should be reported*, as they may precede or represent toxic situations.

SUGGESTED ACTIVITIES

- Prepare a report on Meniere's disease, giving its causes, symptoms, and treatment. State why motion sickness drugs and antihistamines are used in this condition. Include reading references at the end of the report.
- Prepare a report on one of the following allergic conditions: asthma, eczema, or hay fever. Include its causes, symptoms, and treatment. Document your findings with a reading list.

REVIEW

1. Describe anaphylactic shock, including its causes, symptoms, and the action of epinephrine in its treatment.

2. Explain what occurs when an individual is exposed to an allergen to which he is sensitive.

3. Name four conditions which are treated with antihistamines.

4. Name the common side effects of antihistamines.

5. Explain the contributing causes of motion sickness.

6. Explain the physiological reactions which bring about motion sickness.

7. Why are motion sickness drugs frequently administered by suppository?

EXTENDED STUDY

Learn the meaning and the proper use of the following terms:

hypervitaminosis	catalyst
hypovitaminosis	electrolyte
intrinsic factor	cation
vitamin	anion
intracellular	extracellular
mineral	homeostasis

Unit 23 Vitamins and Minerals

OBJECTIVES

After studying this unit, the student should be able to:
- Name deficiency diseases resulting from the lack of vitamins.
- List common symptoms of vitamin deficiency.
- Describe the contribution of a well-balanced diet to good health.
- Differentiate between fat-soluble and water-soluble vitamins.
- Describe the functions of specific minerals.

Vitamins are chemical compounds which regulate body processes necessary for the proper functioning of the body. The Latin word for life is *vita*, a term which explains the importance of these substances. All of the known vitamins occur naturally in food; therefore, a well-balanced diet is one of the best contributions we can make toward the maintenance of our health.

VITAMINS

Both plants and animals are sources of vitamins. These are essential to the functioning of our bodies. Vitamins are found in most natural foods but refining and cooking processes frequently remove much of the vitamin content.

The large, three-lobed liver of the salt water fish is an example of a vitamin source. It is a rich source for vitamin A and D. Vitamin D is the sunshine vitamin which helps to prevent rickets in growing children.

An example of a vitamin source is the carrot. It is a rich source of carotene, a portion of which is

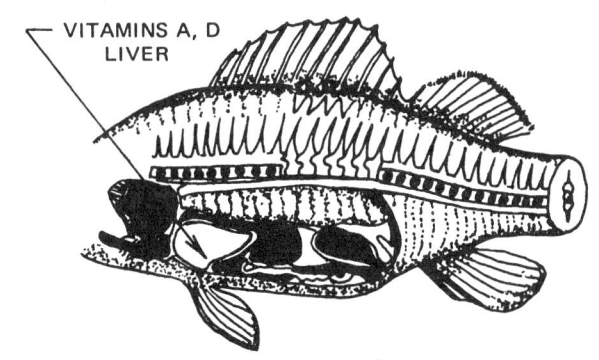

Fig. 23-1 Aquatic Animal Vitamin Source

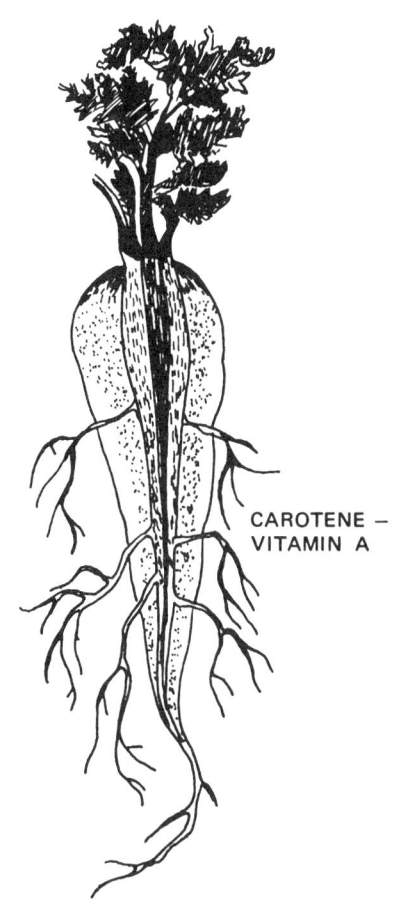

Fig. 23-2 Vegetable Drug Source

159

Section 4 Drugs and Related Substances

converted into vitamin A in our digestive system. It is essential to growth and is used in the treatment of the condition known as night blindness.

Some terms which are often used when the place of vitamins in health is discussed are:

- Hypervitaminosis: a condition which may develop due to the consumption of too large doses of vitamins. Excessive doses of vitamin A may produce toxic effects in children, and a large intake of vitamin D may have adverse effects on both adults and children.

- Hypovitaminosis: a state of vitamin insufficiency, usually due to an inadequate diet. This state manifests itself by fatigue, lack of energy, and pains and aches throughout the body; it can be corrected by diet.

- Conditioned Avitaminosis: caused by inadequate vitamin absorption.

- M.D.R.: minimum daily requirement.

USES OF VITAMINS

Vitamins are organic substances which are necessary for normal growth and development. They are important for enzyme secretion; they act as catalysts (cat-a-lists) in the metabolism (building up and breaking down) of carbohydrates, fats and proteins. A *catalyst* is a substance which does not itself enter into a chemical reaction but aids or changes the speed of the reaction.

Vitamins can be synthesized or made by the intestinal flora. They are sensitive to heat and light so they should be kept in a cool place and in dark bottles. Comparatively small amounts of vitamins are needed to keep a person well.

Some vitamins are fat soluble; others are water soluble. The fat soluble vitamins are: A, D, E, and K. The water soluble vitamins are: the B-complex vitamins and C. The deficiencies of fat soluble vitamins appear more slowly than those of the water soluble vitamins.

FAT-SOLUBLE VITAMINS

The fat-soluble vitamins are stored in the liver and fatty tissues. The minimum daily requirement shown in the following descriptions refers to adults unless stated otherwise.

Vitamin A

Vitamin A is essential for growth in the young and for health at all ages.
Sources: Dairy products, fish liver oils, animal liver, green and yellow vegetables.
Stored: In the liver.
Deficiency symptoms: Retarded growth, susceptibility to disease, skin lesions, night blindness.
Hypervitaminosis: Anorexia, loss of hair, pain in long bones, fragility of bones, dry skin, and pruritis.
M.D.R.: 5000 units (1500 for infants; 3000 for children)
Commercial sources: Vitamin A capsules, halibut liver oil, B.P., cod liver oil

Vitamin D

Vitamin D (calciferol) is known as the sunshine vitamin. Its best source is the sunshine (ultraviolet rays); it is synthesized in the body by exposure of the skin to sunlight.

Sources: Ultraviolet rays, dairy products, fish liver oils.

Deficiency symptoms: If in childhood, the deficiency disease is called rickets. Signs of rickets include poorly formed arms, legs, skull and enlarged abdomen.

Hypervitaminosis: Demineralization (softening) of bone and calcium deposits in soft tissue.

M.D.R.: 400 units

Commercial sources: Drisdol, Dical-D, cod liver oil.

Vitamin E

It is thought that vitamin E may promote normal reproduction. Although signs of deficiency have not been shown in man, a deficiency of the vitamin causes sterility and abortions in laboratory animals.

Sources: Leafy green vegetables and seed-germ oils such as wheat germ.

Deficiency symptoms: Sterility in rats.

M.D.R.: Undetermined.

Commercial sources: Epsilan-M, Eprolin.

Vitamin K

Vitamin K (antihemorrhagic vitamin) is essential in the formation of prothrombin in the liver which is necessary for normal blood clotting. It is synthesized in the body by bacterial action in the intestines.

Sources: Leafy green vegetables, cauliflower, soybeans, pork liver, and alfalfa from which the vitamin is synthesized by the intestinal flora.

Deficiency symptoms: Poor blood clotting, and even hemorrhage.

M.D.R.: Unknown because it is synthesized by the intestinal flora.

Commercial sources: Menadione, Hykinone, Synkayvite, Mephyton (vitamin K).

WATER-SOLUBLE VITAMINS

The water-soluble vitamins are of two types: those which help make red blood cells (such as folic acid and vitamin B_{12}), and those which aid in the release of energy from foods (such as thiamine and riboflavin). There is very little storage of these vitamins in the body. Excessess are usually excreted in the urine.

Thiamine (Vitamin B_1)

Thiamine is essential for the release of energy from carbohydrates, and is essential for nerve conduction.

Sources: Yeast, wheat germ, lean meats, pork, peas, and whole-grain enriched products.

Indications of Deficiency: Beriberi, in which there is inflammation of peripheral nerves, edema, and congestive heart failure.

M.D.R.: 1 to 2 mg.

Commercial source: Sold as thiamine hydrochloride.

Riboflavin (Vitamin B_2)

Riboflavin is essential for cellular oxidation and the storage of energy.

Sources: Organ meats and meat, milk, vegetable greens, eggs, fowl, and yeast.

Deficiency symptoms: Skin and lip lesions, malfunctioning of eyes and inflammation of cornea, lack of vigor.

M.D.R.: 1.5 mg for women, 1.7 mg for men.

Commercial source: Riboflavin.

Niacin (Nicotinic acid)

Niacin is the antipellagra vitamin.

Sources: Meat, fowl, fish, legumes, whole grain and enriched products.

Indications of Deficiency: Pellagra, the symptoms of which are insomnia, loss of appetite, irritability, dizziness, skin and mucous-membrane lesions.

M.D.R.: 20 mg.

Commercial sources: Sold as nicotinamide, niacinamide.

Pyridoxin (Vitamin B_6)

Pyridoxin is necessary for the metabolism of amino acids and fatty acids.

Sources: Muscle meats, liver, yeast, molasses, and whole grain cereals.

Deficiency symptoms: Skin lesions, anemia, hypochromic anemia, and possibly convulsions in infants.

M.D.R.: 2 mg.

Commercial source: Pyridoxine

Folic Acid

Folic Acid is necessary for the synthesis of amino acids and DNA.

Sources: Liver, yeast, green leafy vegetables from which vitamin may be synthesized.

Indications of deficiency: Macrocytic anemia, which is a type of anemia in which the red blood cells do not mature normally. Because of their increased size they transport less oxygen to the tissues. Folic acid is contraindicated in treating pernicious anemia because it masks the symptoms of this condition.

M.D.R.: 0.15 mg is recommended. There is no definite dosage because the vitamin is synthesized by the flora of intestines.

Commercial source: Folvite

Vitamin B_{12} (Cyanocobalamin)

Vitamin B_{12} is called the "extrinsic factor." The absorption of this vitamin from food will not take place unless a substance called the intrinsic factor is produced by the cells of the stomach. In pernicious anemia, vitamin B_{12} is injected because lack of the intrinsic factor makes it unable to be absorbed orally.

Sources: Liver, kidney, milk, fish, muscle meats.

Indications of deficiency: Pernicious anemia.

M.D.R.: 3 to 5 mcg (micrograms).

Commercial source: Rubramin.

Vitamin C (Ascorbic acid, Cevitamic Acid)

Vitamin C prevents scurvy and promotes healing of wounds. This vitamin is easily destroyed by air and heat. Canning and cooking destroy it.

Sources: Citrus fruits, tomatoes, melons, fresh berries, raw vegetables.

Indications of deficiency: Scurvy, the symptoms of which are sore and puffy gums (gingivitis), tendency to bruise easily, slow healing of wounds, and subcutaneous bleeding (petechiae).

M.D.R.: 70 mg.

Commercial sources: Cevalin, Ce-Vi-Sol.

MINERALS

Minerals are nonorganic substances which are supplied in a varied or mixed diet of animal and vegetable products. Minerals play an important part in maintaining the water balance in the body.

The body's weight is 60% to 70% water. All cells are bathed by a watery solution which brings nourishment to the cells and removes wastes. *Electrolytes* are suspended in this aqueous solution; they are particles which result from disintegration of compounds. They are found dissolved in body fluids as ions which carry electrical charges. Those with positive charges are called *cations*. Those with negative charges are called *anions*. The normal fluid state in which positive and negative ions are in balance is called *homeostasis*.

Cations

Among the chief *cations*, the positively charged metallic ions are sodium, potassium, calcium and magnesium.

Sodium is responsible for intracellular and extracellular pressures. Loss of great amounts of sodium may lead to shock. Great excesses may be a factor in causing edema in congestive heart failure and some types of kidney disease. Good sources are salt, meat, fish, fowl, tomato juice, etc.

Potassium deficiency may affect skeletal as well as cardiac muscles. Good sources are meat, fish, fowl, cereals, fruit beverages, tea, cola.

Calcium ions are important in normal heart rhythm, blood clotting, muscle contraction, and nerve irritability. Good sources are milk, cottage cheese, ice cream, shrimp, broccoli, etc.

Magnesium ions are important in maintaining muscle and nerve irritability. Best sources are milk and cereals.

Anions

Among the chief *anions*, the negatively charged non-metallic ions are chlorides, iodides, phosphates and bromides.

Chlorides are responsible for osmotic pressure in the cells. Good sources are salt, milk, eggnog.

Iodides are responsible for maintaining our metabolism; they are stored in the thyroid gland as protein compounds. Good sources are sea food, iodized salt, etc.

Section 4 Drugs and Related Substances

Phosphates are important in our buffering system; they metabolize fats, transport fatty acids, metabolize carbohydrates, and help build bones and teeth. Good sources are milk, egg yolk, whole grains, etc.

Bromides have been used in the past as sedatives and hypnotics but are less frequently used now.

Chief Cations and Anions

The extracellular fluid refers to fluid which is outside the cells. The intracellular fluid refers to fluid *inside* the cell.

- Sodium is the chief cation in the extracellular fluid.
- Chloride is the chief anion in the extracellular fluid.
- Potassium is the chief cation in the intracellular fluid.
- Phosphate is the chief anion in the intracellular fluid.

SUGGESTED ACTIVITIES

- Review the basic four food groups. Make a chart which lists the food sources for each vitamin studied in this unit and the basic food group to which each belongs.
- Plan a day's menu from the basic four food groups; supply the minimum daily requirements for each vitamin.

REVIEW

A. Match the two columns by placing the letter of the word or phrase from column II in the most suitable space in column I.

Column I

F 1. Vitamin A
K 2. Vitamin B$_1$
D 3. Vitamin B$_6$
J 4. Niacin
H 5. Vitamin B$_{12}$
I 6. Vitamin C
G 7. M.D.R.
C 8. Vitamin E
B 9. Vitamin K
E 10. Vitamin B$_2$

Column II

a. Secondary anemia
b. Aids in the coagulation of blood
c. Antisterility vitamin
d. Skin lesions and hypochromic anemia
e. Skin and lip lesions, malfunctioning of eyes and inflammation of cornea
f. Prevents night blindness and promotes health of mucous membranes
g. Minimum daily requirement
h. Administered intramuscularly for treatment of pernicious anemia
i. Prevents scurvy
j. Prevents pellagra
k. Prevents beriberi

B. Answer the following questions.
1. What is the function of the *intrinsic factor* in the absorption of vitamin B_{12}?
   THE ABSORPTION OF VITAMIN B_{12} WILL NOT TAKE PLACE UNLESS THE INTRINSIC FACTOR IS PRODUCED BY THE CELLS OF THE STOMACH

2. What are vitamins. Why are they essential in our diets?
   ORGANIC SUBSTANCES ESSENTIAL FOR NORMAL GROWTH AND DEVELOPMENT

3. Name the general symptoms of hypovitaminosis.
   FATIGUE, LACK OF ENERGY, DRY SKIN

4. a. List the water-soluble vitamins. Where are they stored in the body?
   FOLIC ACID AND B_{12}, THIAMINE AND RIBOFLAVIN. THEY HAVE VERY LITTLE STORAGE. EXCESSES ARE SECRETED IN THE URINE

   b. List the fat-soluble vitamins. Where are they stored in the body?
   A, D, E, K. THEY ARE STORED IN THE LIVER AND FATTY TISSUES

5. Name the methods of preparing food that destroy vitamin C.
   IT IS DESTROYED BY AIR AND HEAT, ALSO BY CANNING, & COOKING

6. Explain how vitamins play a part in enzyme secretions.
   THE ACT AS CATALYSTS IN THE METABOLISM OF CARBOHYDRATES

7. Name two vitamins which are synthesized in the body. Explain how each is synthesized.
   VIT. K IS SYNTHESIZE BY BACTERIAL ACTION IN THE INTESTINE.
   VIT. D IS SYNTHESIZE BY EXPOSURE OF THE SKIN TO SUNLIGHT

8. Define minerals. Explain what relationship exists between water balance of the body and minerals.
   NON ORGANIC SUBSTANCES WHICH ARE SUPPLIED IN A VARIED OR MIXED DIET OF ANIMAL AND VEGETABLE PRODUCTS.

Section 4 Drugs and Related Substances

C. Match Column I with Column II.

Column I

- __J__ 1. electrolyte
- __G__ 2. vitamins
- __I__ 3. cation
- __E__ 4. chlorides
- __H__ 5. sodium
- __D__ 6. calcium
- __L__ 7. homeostasis
- __C__ 8. catalyst
- __A__ 9. nonorganic substances
- __B__ 10. anion

Column II

a. Substances found in animal and vegetable products.

b. Negatively charged non-metallic ion

c. A substance which aids or changes the speed of a chemical reaction.

d. Factor in heart rhythm, blood clotting, muscle contraction and nerve irritability.

e. Factors in osmotic pressure of cell.

f. Found only in iodized salt

g. Organic substances necessary for normal growth

h. Factor in intracellular and extra-cellular pressures.

i. Positively charged metallic ions.

j. Particle resulting from the disintegration of compounds.

k. Found only in beef products.

l. A normal fluid state in which positive and negative ions are in balance.

EXTENDED STUDY

Learn the meaning and the proper use of the following terms:

acquired immunity
active immunity
antigen
antitoxin serum
gamma globulin

immune serum
natural immunity
passive acquired immunity
toxoid
vaccine

Unit 24 Serums, Vaccines, and Toxoids

OBJECTIVES

After studying this unit, the student should be able to:

- Differentiate between natural immunity, active acquired immunity, and passive immunity.
- Define antitoxins, vaccines, and toxoids.
- Give examples of methods of immunization for specific diseases.

In order to understand immunization agents such as vaccines and toxoids, it is necessary to understand what immunity is. *Immunity* means resistance to the harmful effects that might be caused by an infectious agent. *Antibodies* provide the resistance needed.

TYPES OF IMMUNITY

There are two types of immunity: natural and acquired.

There is only one kind of natural immunity. It refers to the production of natural antibodies present at birth.

There are two kinds of acquired immunity.

a. Active acquired immunity — antibodies are produced because the person has had the disease or has been given an injection of a substance which causes the growth of antibodies (an antigen).

b. Passive acquired immunity — animal or human serum which contains antibodies is administered to the person.

In other words, everyone is born with a natural immunity to certain diseases. There are antibodies present in the plasma that can provide resistance to invading bacteria.

On the other hand, active acquired immunity is present when the body has been exposed to a disease and produced antibodies against it, for example, smallpox or chickenpox.

Active immunity may also be acquired artificially by the injection of an antigen. An antigen is a substance which causes the growth of antibodies. It is made of a suspension of living microbes or a toxin made by the microorganism.

Passive acquired immunity is so called because the individual has had nothing to do with building antibodies. He has, in most cases, received the blood serum of an animal who has developed the antibodies from injections of the microbes. In some cases he may receive human serum with its antibodies already developed. This will give the person a period of immunity to the disease, but it will be temporary in nature.

IMMUNIZATIONS

Immune serum is obtained from an animal or human who has developed antibodies to a particular disease. *Immune serum globulin* (USP) is a sterile solution containing antibodies which are normally present in the human body. This immune serum is useful in the protection of those exposed to infectious hepatitis if it has been standardized for this disease. Human gamma globulin is obtained from the plasma of human blood. It is used for temporary protection against measles, poliomyelitis, pertussis, and some other communicable diseases.

Antitoxin serums are made in the bodies of animals who have been actively immunized by a specific toxin. Antitoxins are administered against certain diseases to neutralize their toxins. Examples of these are diphtheria antitoxin (USP), mixed gas gangrene antitoxin, tetanus antitoxin, and a mixed vaccine of tetanus and mixed gas gangrene antitoxins.

Vaccines are suspensions of either killed or attenuated organisms which are given for the prevention and/or treatment of infectious diseases. Many of these are grown in chick embryos. A vaccine must be in the body for a certain period of time before providing immunity to the disease. Some must be given in more than one dose, intervals apart.

Some examples of vaccines are:

- cholera vaccine (USP)
- influenza virus vaccine, Type A (Asian strain)
- influenza virus vaccine (USP)
- tuberculosis vaccine, (BCG)
- yellow fever vaccine
- German measles vaccine
- mumps vaccine
- rabies vaccine
- smallpox vaccine
- typhoid and paratyphoid vaccine
- typhus vaccine

The vaccine for poliomyelitis is available in two forms, the oral (live) vaccine developed by Albert Sabin, and the injectable (killed virus) developed by Dr. Jonas Salk.

Toxoids are made of toxins modified so that they are nontoxic, but still capable of producing antibodies in the body. These are prepared in precipitated products using alum or aluminum hydroxide and so they are slowly absorbed into the tissues, providing more favorable immunizing tendencies than plain toxoid. Examples of these are: diphtheria toxoid (USP), and tetanus toxoid.

IMMUNIZATION SCHEDULE

According to the U.S. Center for Disease Control, surveys show that there is "an alarming trend of declining immunization levels." It has been estimated that up to 10 million children between the ages of one and four are not protected against one or more of the major preventable diseases.

Children from one to four years of age should be immunized against diphtheria, tetanus, pertussis (whooping cough), measles, rubella (German measles), and polio. There

Unit 24 Serums, Vaccines and Toxoids

RECOMMENDED SCHEDULE FOR ACTIVE IMMUNIZATION OF NORMAL INFANTS AND CHILDREN

2 mo	DTP[1]	TOPV[2]
4 mo	DTP	TOPV
6 mo	DTP	TOPV
1 yr	Measles[3]	Tuberculin Test[4]
	Rubella[3]	Mumps[3]
1 1/2 yr	DTP	TOPV
4-6 yr	DTP	TOPV

[1] DTP — diphtheria and tetanus toxoids combined with pertussis vaccine.
[2] TOPV — trivalent oral poliovirus vaccine. This recommendation is suitable for breast-fed as well as bottle-fed infants.
[3] May be given at 1 year as measles-rubella or measles-mumps-rubella combined vaccines (see Rubella, section 9, and Mumps, section 9, for further discussion of age of administration).
[4] Frequency of repeated tuberculin tests depends on risk of exposure of the child and on the prevalence of tuberculosis in the population group. The initial test should be at the time of, or preceding, the measles immunization.

Fig. 24-1 Recommended schedule for active immunization and tuberculin testing of normal infants and children. Reprinted by permission of the American Academy of Pediatrics from its Report of the Committee on Infectious Diseases, ed. 17, 1974 (Red Book)

is a trend toward adding the mumps vaccine to the immunization schedule. A booster of combined immunization called DTP (diphtheria, tetanus, pertussis) is often given at 5-6 years of age. Figure 24-1 shows the recommended schedule for active immunization of normal infants and children. The nurse should study this information and make every effort to see that children receive the toxoids and vaccines required. Parents should be advised to contact their local health departments. The nurse can help by finding out the scheduled dates and encourage the parent to call and make an appointment with the department or their personal physician.

FEDERAL REGULATION

All vaccines are under Federal regulation and sale. Pharmaceutical firms must be licensed in order to prepare and distribute them. The National Institutes of Health of the U.S. Public Health Service licenses and supervises these firms. Since many vaccines are made from egg or horse inoculations, the individual to receive them must be tested for sensitivity to these products.

SUGGESTED ACTIVITIES

- Discuss why human-developed antisera or antitoxins have a marked advantage over animal-made antisera.

- Prepare a report on the production of gamma globulin and explain its advantages and disadvantages.

- Discuss a major role of the nurse in the education of the public concerning the need for a suitable and adqaute immunization plan against tetanus, diphtheria, smallpox, measles, and German measles.

Section 4 Drugs and Related Substances

REVIEW

A. Select the item which best completes each statement.

1. The kind of immunity which provides for protection is
   a. active acquired
   b. passive acquired
   c. natural
   d. none of the above

2. Active immunity may be acquired by the injection of
   a. an allergen
   b. chickenpox
   c. an antigen
   d. none of the above

3. Active immunity to the disease may be acquired from having
   a. influenza
   b. chickenpox
   c. pneumonia
   d. none of the above

4. Immune serums and vaccines are manufactured from
   a. injected chick embryos
   b. immunized people
   c. immunized animals
   d. all of the above

5. Poliomyelitis (live) oral vaccine was developed by
   a. Dr. Rene Dubos
   b. Dr. Howard Florey
   c. Dr. Albert Sabin
   d. Dr. Alexander Fleming

6. Poliomyelitis (killed) virus, administered by injection was developed by
   a. Dr. E. Kendall
   b. Dr. Jonas Salk
   c. Dr. Albert Sabin
   d. Dr. Howard Florey

B. From Column II, select the method(s) of immunization protection to match the items in Column I. Some items have more than one answer.

Column I	Column II
_____ 1. poliomyelitis	a. human immune serum
_____ 2. diphtheria	b. antitoxin serum
_____ 3. tetanus	c. vaccine
_____ 4. pertussis	d. toxoid
_____ 5. DTP	e. toxoid – vaccine combination
_____ 6. smallpox	

EXTENDED STUDY

Learn the meaning and proper use of the following terms:

agitation	electroshock therapy
antidepressant	insulin shock therapy
ataractics	psychotherapeutic agent
depression	tranquilizers

Unit 25 Psychotropic Drugs

OBJECTIVES

After studying this unit, the student should be able to:
- Identify common side effects of certain psychotropic drugs.
- Explain the purposes of ataractics and antidepressants.

Mental health emphasis and the development of new drugs have helped emotionally disturbed patients to function and cope with problems. Therefore, it becomes increasingly important for the nurse to know the recently developed drugs and how they affect the mind and body.

The mind and body are interrelated. Both the physical and mental state of all patients must be considered when giving nursing care. In psychiatric nursing, the nurse must especially understand that many factors contribute to the patient's distress.

Psychotropic agents are drugs which modify certain aspects of mental and emotional disorder. Their chief action is to tone down emotional overactivity.

Drugs which have had great impact on psychiatric care are the tranquilizers, which calm the patient. The newly developed psychic energizers may cause restlessness, while the psychostimulants cause excitement.

TRANQUILIZERS

Tranquilizers are also called *ataractics* (a-ta-rac-tics) and *selective depressants*. They are commonly used in medical practice, in general hospitals and, (usually in larger doses) in psychiatric hospitals. They help to calm patients who are anxious and under stress.

There are two main types of ataractics: rauwolfia products and phenothiazines. Phenothiazines act more quickly than rauwolfia products. Varying degrees of sedation are produced. They suppress anxiety, tension, and fear. Agitation in elderly persons and disturbed children may be controlled with these drugs. They are used with care in coronary heart disease and in cerebral arteriosclerosis. No serious side effects are recorded.

Most of the drugs in figures 25-1 through 25-3 can be given by mouth or intramuscularly. Some can be given intravenously or rectally. However, since oral administration is used so frequently, a column showing the range of the average dose, by mouth, has been added to the charts. This refers to *dosage for psychotherapeutic purposes*.

ANTIDEPRESSANTS

Antidepressants are drugs administered to patients suffering from depression to give them a feeling of energy, to restore alertness, and to revive normal interest. The following drugs may control abnormal behavior and lessen the patient's symptoms. These drugs should not be given late in the afternoon or evening which would lead to insomnia. It is important to be on the alert for possibility of suicide. Alcohol and barbiturates have their effects potentiated by antidepressants.

Section 4 *Drugs and Related Substances*

Medication	Action	Administration and Dosage	Adverse and/or Side Effects	Avg. Dose Range Daily
Rauwolfia Source Reserpine (Serpasil) (Rau-Sed) (Reserpoid) (Sandril)	relieves hypertension; reduces anxiety, worry; does not alter brain waves; reduces effect of outside stimuli; slow action to several weeks; effects persist after discontinuance	p.o. 0.5 to 5 mg daily in divided doses I.V., I.M.: 5 mg in 2 ml	low toxicity; nasal stuffiness, weight gain, diarrhea, gastric irritation, drowsiness	0.5 to 5 mg
Phenothiazines Chlorpromazine Hydrochloride (Thorazine)	acts on CNS to control agitation and anxiety; improves memory; used in manic phase of manic-depressive psychosis	p.o. tablets 10 to 100 mg, spansules 10 mg to 1 Gm (in three doses) I.M.: 25 mg/ml Rectal: 25 to 100 mg	dryness of mouth, dermatitis, photosensitivity, drowsiness, jaundice, blood dyscrasias	60 to 1600 mg
Trifluoperazine Hydrochloride (Stelazine)	similar to chlorpromazine, but more active	p.o. 1 to 40 mg, depending on severity of symptoms; 1, 2, 5, and 10 mg tablets	none	4 to 20 mg
Prochlorperazine (Compazine)	similar to chlorpromazine but more potent, is antiemetic	p.o. 50 to 150 mg I.M.: 10 to 20 mg rectal: 25 mg	dryness of mouth, disturbed vision	15 to 200 mg
Promazine hydrochloride (Sparine)	resembles chlorpromazine, effective antiemetic	p.o. 10 to 200 mg I.M., I.V.: 50 to 100 mg	drowsiness, drop in blood pressure, agranulocytosis convulsions	25 to 300 mg
Thioridazine hydrochloride (Mellaril)	mild tranquilizer	20 to 800 mg daily in 10, 25, 50 and 100 mg tablets	drowsiness	300 to 800 mg
Fluphenazine hydrochloride (Permitil) (Prolixin)	20 times more potent than chlorpromazine, more sustained action	initial dose p.o. or I.M. 2.5 to 10 mg and maintenance dose 1 to 20 mg daily	muscular rigidity, shuffling gait, masklike face, drowsiness	
Methaqualone (Quaalude) (Sopor)	tranquilizer	p.o. 150 mg	restlessness, dizziness, nausea and vomiting, depression, tachycardia	

Fig. 25-1 Major Tranquilizers

Medication	Action	Administration and Dosage	Adverse and/or Side Effects	Avg. Dose Range Daily
Other Ataractics				
Meprobamate (Equanil) (Miltown)	skeletal muscle relaxant; tranquilizer; relieves anxiety and tension; calms and quiets without dulling brain action	p.o. adult: 400 mg t.i.d., sustained-release capsules and tablets	urticaria, habituation	600 to 1200 mg
Chlordiazepoxide (Librium)	relieves anxiety; sedates patient; increases appetite; relaxes skeletal muscles	p.o. 15 to 40 mg t.i.d., I.V. ampules; 100 mg	(low in toxicity) drowsiness, ataxia, dizziness, confusion, mild hypotension	
Diazepam (Valium)	muscle relaxant; relieves mild to moderate depression, anxiety; has cumulative effect	p.o. 4 to 10 mg daily	drowsiness	

Fig. 25-2 Minor Tranquilizers

Medication	Action	Administration and Dosage	Adverse and/or Side Effects
Chlorprothixene (Taractan)	acts on CNS to control agitation and anxiety improves memory; used in manic-depressive psychosis	p.o. 30 to 600 mg in 24 hours, I.M. 75 to 200 mg in 24 hours	muscular rigidity shuffling gait, drowsiness
Haloperidol (Haldol)	controls hyperactivity of the manic phase	p.o. .5 mg to 2 mg (b.i.d. or t.i.d.) I.M. 2 to 5 mg	same as above

Fig. 25-3 Other Antipsychotic Drugs

Antidepressants are of two kinds: Monoamine oxidase inhibitors (psychic energizers) and Anticholinergic antidepressants (psychostimulants). Side effects of both types of antidepressants are: dizziness, drowsiness, anorexia, restlessness, nausea, tachycardia, dry mouth, and blurred vision.

MAO inhibitors (psychic energizers)	
Drug	Avg. Daily Dose
Isocarboxazid (Marplan)	10 to 30 mg
Nialamide (Niamid)	75 to 200 mg
Phenelzine (Nardil)	30 to 75 mg
Tranylcypromine (Parnate)	20 to 60 mg

Patients who are being treated with the above listed drugs should avoid the following foods: cheese (especially strong or aged), bananas, avocados, beer and Chianti wine, or they can have a hypertensive crisis whose symptoms are severe headache, stiff neck, nausea and vomiting; sweating, and chest pain.

Anticholinergic antidepressants (the psychostimulants)	
Drug	Avg. Daily Dose
Imipramine hydrochloride (Tofranil)	100 to 150 mg
Amitriptyline hydrochloride (Elavil)	75 to 150 mg

Fig. 25-4 Antidepressants

ADDITIONAL SIDE EFFECTS

Some antipsychotic drugs cause extrapyramidal side effects in some patients. These consist of mask-like face, tremor, rigidity, and a shuffling gait. There may be excessive salivation and bizarre movements of face, arms, and legs.

These side effects are often controlled by the use of antiparkinsonian drugs such as

Trihexylphenidyl hydrochloride (Artane)

Dosage: p.o. 1 to 2 mg   3 or 4 times daily

Benztropine mesylate (Cogentin)

Dosage: p.o., I.M., I.V.   Usually p.o.
0.5 to 2 mg   2 or 3 times daily

SHOCK THERAPY

With the introduction and use of psychotropic drugs, shock therapy is not used as frequently as it once was. However, some patients still receive this treatment. *Insulin shock therapy* is a method of treating mental illness through physical means. Patients are injected with doses of insulin. Only nurses who are prepared in this technique should work with these patients. Electroshock is probably the most convenient and practical form of shock therapy.

SUGGESTED ACTIVITIES

- Select a patient who is receiving a psychotropic drug. Submit a study of the patient, focusing on the drug, its generic and trade name, the diagnosis of the patient and its relation to reasons for the medication being ordered, side effects to watch for, action to take. In short, a comprehensive nursing care study with the drug as the central topic.
- Prepare a report about insulin shock therapy and present it to the class for discussion. Investigate how patients are selected for this treatment, how they are prepared, what medications are used before the treatment, the insulin coma, and the results of the treatment, and the follow-up care of the patient.

REVIEW

A. Answer the questions in the space provided.

1. A patient who is on reserpine therapy 0.25 mg t.i.d. begins to sneeze; her nose becomes stuffy. You are unable to reach the doctor. In your judgment what is advisable for you to do?

2. The word, *ataractic* comes from the Greek word which means peace of mind. Explain how this drug group brings about "peace of mind".

3. Name two kinds of antidepressants.

4. Give four examples of MAO inhibitors.

5. What foods should be avoided by anyone receiving MAO inhibitors? Explain why.

6. Name two drugs which may be ordered to control some side effects from antipsychotic drugs.

Section 4 Drugs and Related Substances

B. Match Columns I and II

Column I

_____ 1. tranquilizers
_____ 2. phenothiazines
_____ 3. MAO inhibitors
_____ 4. a rauwolfia drug
_____ 5. meprobamate
_____ 6. chlorpromazine
_____ 7. chlordiazepoxide
_____ 8. antidepressant
_____ 9. rauwolfia products and phenothiazines
_____ 10. psychotherapeutic agent

Column II

a. Act more quickly than rauwolfia products
b. Serpasil
c. Miltown, Equanil
d. Thorazine
e. Insulin shock therapy
f. Librium
g. Types of ataractics
h. Drug used to treat mentally ill patients
i. Electroshock therapy
j. Drugs which help to calm and relax apprehensive patients
k. Enhances the effects of alcohol and barbiturates
l. May produce a hypertensive crisis if certain foods are eaten

C. In the first column is a list of drugs. In the second column is a list of symptoms which might occur from the administration of the drugs when used for mental disorders. Indicate in the space before the drug, the letter or letters which reflect the symptoms which might result.

_____ Sparine
_____ Valium
_____ Thorazine
_____ Miltown
_____ Reserpine
_____ Ritalin
_____ Compazine
_____ Mellaril
_____ Librium

a. convulsions
b. urticaria
c. lowered blood pressure
d. increased alertness
e. mental depression
f. nausea and vomiting
g. habituation
h. dryness of mouth
i. ataxia
j. nasal congestion
k. disturbed vision
l. drowsiness

EXTENDED STUDY

Learn the meaning and proper use of the following terms.

analgesic
anticoagulant
corticosteroid
corticoid

curariform
cyanosis
edema

Achievement Review 4

Section 4 Drugs and Related Substance

A. Choose the phrase which best completes each statement and encircle the letter preceding it.

1. Disinfectants are anti-infective agents which
   a. kill all types of microorgansims
   b. kill spores only
   c. are safe for use on only metal instruments
   d. are unsafe for application on living tissue

2. Anaphylactic shock is a condition which
   a. causes a local allergic reaction
   b. raises the blood pressure
   c. is fatal if untreated
   d. increases heart action

3. Tetracycline is an example of a
   a. broad-spectrum antibiotic
   b. narrow-spectrum antibiotic
   c. sulfonamide
   d. depressant

4. A very serious adverse reaction to penicillin is
   a. damage to the eighth cranial nerve
   b. anaphylactic shock
   c. depression of bone marrow
   d. crystallization in kidney tubules

5. As it is slowly absorbed from the gastrointestinal tract, neomycin is often prescribed
   a. for severe kidney infections
   b. intravenously
   c. for local sterilization of the bowel
   d. topically only

6. Adverse drug reactions involving the kidneys may result from the use of the following antibiotics
   a. novobiocin, penicillin, streptomycin
   b. neomycin, kanamycin, bacitracin
   c. nystatin, griseofulvin, amphotericin B
   d. cephalothin, erythromycin, chloramphenicol

Section 4 Drugs and Related Substances

7. When chemotherapeutic drugs are administered for cancer,
    a. frequent blood tests are usually ordered
    b. strict medical asepsis is maintained
    c. a bland diet is usually ordered
    d. all of these

8. A common side effect of the antihistamines is
    a. damage to the eighth cranial nerve
    b. nausea
    c. anaphylactic shock
    d. drowsiness

9. Excessive doses of the following vitamin may cause adverse effects:
    a. vitamin A
    b. thiamine
    c. riboflavin
    d. vitamin C

10. An ataractic is used
    a. to stimulate activity
    b. to relieve anxiety and tension
    c. in shock therapy
    d. only in acute schizophrenia

11. Poliomyelitis live oral vaccine was developed by
    a. Dr. Rene Dubos
    b. Dr. Howard Florey
    c. Dr. Albert Sabin
    d. Dr. Alexander Fleming

12. Poliomyelitis killed virus, administered by injection was developed by
    a. Dr. E. Kendall
    b. Dr. Jonas Salk
    c. Dr. Albert Sabin
    d. Dr. Howard Florey

13. The newly developed psychostimulants tend to
    a. cause patient restlessness
    b. increase irritability in patient
    c. excite and energize the patient
    d. produce calmness and tranquility

14. Fat soluble vitamins stored by the body are
    a. A, D, E and K
    b. Vitamins K and D
    c. B group and C
    d. A, D, C and K

Achievement Review

15. Vitamins are important parts of our enzyme system because
    a. they keep the body in normal fluid balance
    b. they act as catalysts in metabolism of carbohydrates, fats and proteins.
    c. both of the above
    d. none of the above

B. Complete the following statements.
   1. A drug most often used in the treatment of anaphylactic shock is_____.
   2. Immunity which is obtained by injection of a substance which produces antibodies is called _____ immunity.
   3. A disorder caused by up-and-down movements, stimulating the vomiting center in the brain is called _____.
   4. The most common side effect from antihistamines is found to be _____.
   5. The substance produced by the body in response to a special allergen to which a person is sensitive is _____.
   6. The severe reaction to sera of animal origin and to some drugs and which requires immediate treatment is _____.
   7. The anti-infective agent which destroys pathogens on inanimate objects is a _____.
   8. The anticancer agent which is ingested by the cancer cell but cannot be used by it is called an _____.

C. Answer the following questions briefly in the space provided.
   1. Explain why it is important for an antibiotic to act quickly.

   2. How does griseofulvin act to combat fungus infections?

   3. How do tranquilizers and antidepressants differ in their action on the patient?

   4. What is the difference between a broad spectrum antibiotic and a narrow spectrum antibiotic? Give an example of each.

179

Section 4 Drugs and Related Substance

D. Select the items in Column II which describe the items in Column I and write the letter in the space provided.

Column I

_____ 1. antibiotic
_____ 2. rhinitis
_____ 3. sulfonamide
_____ 4. antihistamine
_____ 5. adrenergic
_____ 6. contact dermatitis
_____ 7. hypervitaminosis
_____ 8. antigen
_____ 9. toxoid
_____ 10. ataractic
_____ 11. allergen
_____ 12. metastasis
_____ 13. urticaria
_____ 14. electrolyte

Column II

a. drugs which relieve people sensitive to foreign substances
b. capable of stimulating sympathetic nervous system
c. transfer of a disease from one part of the body to another
d. weakened toxin capable of producing antibodies
e. another name for hives
f. substance which stimulates growth of antibodies
g. condition resulting from excessive intake of vitamins
h. skin rash caused by contact with an allergen such as animal fur, clothing material, plants, etc.
i. tranquilizer
j. chemical substance which destroys or inhibits growth of certain microorganisms
k. particle resulting from the disintegation of compounds
l. the substance to which one is allergic
m. condition resulting from low vitamin intake
n. chemical substance which mimics another substance bacteria need for food
o. inflammation of the nasal mucosa
p. destruction of bacteria

Section 5 Effects of Medications on Body Systems

Unit 26 Medications Used for Circulatory System Disorders

OBJECTIVES

After studying this unit, the student should be able to:

- Explain the action of digitalis products and diuretics in congestive heart failure.
- State the definitions and uses of hematinics, coagulants, anticoagulants, vasoconstrictors and vasodilators.
- Differentiate between exogenous and endogenous cholesterol.
- Explain the process of digitalization.

The function of the circulatory system is to maintain a stable composition of the fluid which bathes all cells, to supply these cells with a constant supply of nutrients and oxygen, and to remove the waste substances resulting from metabolism; namely organic salt, carbon dioxide, and ammonia. When the circulation does not continue to perform these functions even for a short time, cell changes occur.

The circulatory system is composed of the heart and the blood vessels, made up of arteries, veins and capillaries. Gases and dissolved substances pass to and from the cells through the tiny thin-walled capillaries. The heart may be viewed as a forceful pump and the blood vessels as a closed tube system.

There are several controls over the circulatory system:

- the rate and rhythm of the heartbeat.
- the force of contractions of the ventricles.
- the control of widening or narrowing of the lumen of the blood vessels.

Various medications may be used to alter the above factors. Some medications affect the cardiac muscle; others act upon the reflex area in the medulla, and others affect the brain centers controlling the heart rate.

DRUGS WHICH AFFECT HEART ACTION

The medications to be discussed may affect the heart in one or more different ways. They may (1) strengthen the heartbeat, (2) alter the rate of the heartbeat, (3) alter the rhythm of the heartbeat, or (4) increase or decrease the output of blood from the heart.

Section 5 Effects of Medications on Body Systems

Heart Failure

Heart failure may occur when the heart does not work well as a pump. It is frequently a late complication of a heart or blood vessel disease, such as rheumatic fever, arteriosclerosis, coronary insufficiency, or hypertension. Failure of the heart to beat efficiently can lead to lung congestion, dyspnea, and coughing. When there is this kind of circulatory failure and fluid accumulates in the lungs, it is called congestive heart failure. Digitalis products are ordered to improve cardiac function, and diuretics are given to rid the body of excess fluid. Diuretics are drugs which increase urinary output. They are discussed in Unit 29.

Digitalis products are used to treat heart failure and they are frequently called *cardiotonics* because of their ability to increase the muscle tone of the heart. Digitalis is obtained from the dried leaf of the Digitalis purpurea (purple foxglove). It strengthens the heart muscle (myocardium), increases the force of the systolic contraction, slows the heart, and improves the muscle tone (degree of vigor and tension) of the myocardium. Consequently, the ventricles empty more efficiently, allowing the auricles to take in increased amounts of venous blood and relieving congestion in the lungs.

Digitalis drugs are usually administered orally, but they may also be given intramuscularly and intravenously. They are well absorbed through the intestinal walls. The gastric mucosa is less irritated if digitalis is taken with the meal. The effects of digitalis products develop slowly. Repeated doses cause a cumulative effective in the body, and an excess accumulation will cause a toxic reaction. It is important that the nurse (1) takes the pulse before giving digitalis preparations (2) withhold the medication if the pulse is 60 or below and (3) notify the physician of the low pulse.

Even after the drug is discontinued, the effects continue for some time. When a patient is first started on digitalis, the aim is to *digitalize* him. This means that digitalis is given until the desired optimum effects have been gained. The heart beat is strengthened, breathing improves, and diuresis rids the body of the excess fluid. The amount of this dosage varies with the person. When the patient being digitalized shows symptoms such as nausea and vomiting, the patient is considered digitalized and is then put on a *maintenance dose*. This, too, varies with the person. Frequently, the patient must continue to take digitalis for the remainder of his life.

Arrhythmias

The rhythm and rate of the heart are under the control of the sinoatrial node (S-A) in the right auricle, figure 26-2. The node gives off electrical impulses to the muscle of the auricle, causing it to contract and force blood into the ventricles. The S-A impulse passes down to the atrioventricular node (A-V), down the bundle of His in the center of the heart, and is then transmitted to the muscles of the ventricle by nerves. The ventricles contract a second or so after the auricles.

Any change from the normal order of muscle action of the heart is called an *arrhythmia*. Sometimes the muscles of the heart do not work in cooperation with each other. Some contract more frequently than others; the ventricles beat less efficiently. Some node impulses may occur very rapidly at rates up to 250 per minute.

Three drugs which are used to treat arrhythmias are: quinidine sulfate, procainamide hydrochloride and propranolol.

Medication	Action	Administration and Dosage	Side Effects and/or Toxic Effects
Digitalis leaf	long acting; slows down and strengthens heartbeat in congestive heart failure increases force of contraction of heart to help relieve lung congestion	**p.o.** powder initial: 1.5 Gm in divided doses (for 1-2 days) Maintenance: 0.1 Gm daily	loss of appetite, nausea, vomiting, pulse below 60, irregular pulse has pronounced cumulative effects.
Digitoxin (Crystodigin) (Digitaline) (Nativelle) (Purodigin)	same as above	**p.o.** 1.0-1.5 mg initial; 0.1-0.2 mg maintenance I.V. 0.5 mg initial; 0.1 mg maintenance	same as above
Digoxin (Lanoxin)	same as above, but medium acting	Adult: **p.o.** initial: 0.5 to 2 mg maintenance: 0.5 mg Pediatric elixir: 0.5 mg/ml	same as above
Gitalin (Gitaligin)	see digitalis leaf	**p.o.** initial 6.5 mg maintenance .5 mg q.d. I.V. 2.5-3 mg	see digitalis leaf
Ouabain (Strophantin-G)	same as above	I.V. only, slowly 0.5 mg (0.25-1.0 mg/ml)	same as above
Lanatoside C (Cedilanid)	same as above	**p.o.** initial 8 mg maintenance 0.5-1 mg	same as above
Deslanoside (Cedilanid D)	same as above	I.V. only, slowly digitalize: 1.2-1.6 mg	same as above

Fig. 26-1 Digitalis Products

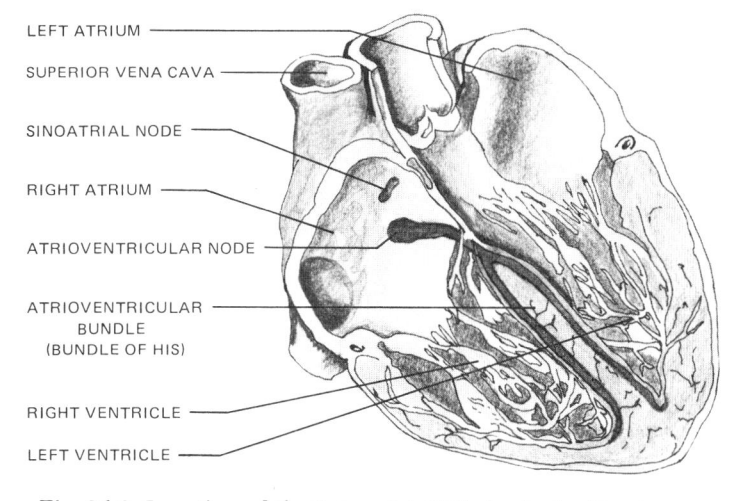

Fig. 26-2 Location of the S-A and A-V Nodes in the Heart

Section 5 Effects of Medications on Body Systems

Quinidine sulfate is used in the management of disorders of cardiac rhythm. Like quinine, it is obtained from the cinchona bark. The drug decreases the number of times the auricular muscle will contract. Therefore, it is used to treat *auricular fibrillation,* a condition in which the heart muscle quivers.

The patient may develop symptoms of hypersensitivity to the drug. These include asthmatic symptoms, depressed breathing, drop in blood pressure, fainting, dermatitis, and sometimes circulatory collapse.

Dosage: Oral, initial: 0.2-0.4 Gm q4h for 2-3 days

Maintenance: 200-600 mg daily

Procainamide hydrochloride (Pronestyl) decreases irritability of the ventricles of the heart. It is also effective in auricular fibrillation. It may be given orally or intramuscularly; it may also be given intravenously, in an emergency, under close and careful observation.

Dosage: Oral, capsules 250 mg q6h

Propranolol (Inderol) is given to prevent ventricular arrhythmias. It is sometimes also effective in the treatment of angina; the dosage must be individualized. The drug is contraindicated in cases of bronchial asthma, congestive heart failure and hypotension.

Dosage: Oral, 10-30 mg 3-4 times daily before meals and at bedtime.

Intravenous, 1-3 mg under careful monitoring.

Medication	Action	Administration and Dosage	Side and/or Toxic Effects: Nursing Action
Levarterenol (Levophed) (Nor-Epinephrine)	raises and sustains blood pressure: used in shock	I.V. 4 ml or 2% solution, one or more ampules added to 1000 ml of I.V. solution	elevation of blood pressure: remain with patient while drug is given; check blood pressure every 2-5 minutes
Phenylephrine (Neo-Synephrine)	raises blood pressure	p.o., I.M., s.c. 10 to 25 mg as ordered; I.V. 0.5 to 1 mg slowly; topical 0.25 to 1% solution	elevation of blood pressure: check blood pressure frequently
Isoproterenol (Aludrine) (Isuprel)	accelerates heartbeat; used in heart block	10 to 15 mg sublingual tablets; inhalant (1:100, 1:200, 1:400)	may produce tachycardia with precordial distress: use c̄ caution; check pulse
Metaraminol (Aramine) (Pressonex)	intense vasoconstriction action; elevates blood pressure	I.M. or s.c. 2 to 10 mg (0.2 per 1 ml solution)	rapid blood pressure rise: observe carefully; check B.P. frequently

Fig. 26-3 Vasoconstrictors

DRUGS WHICH AFFECT THE BLOOD VESSELS

There are many important drugs which act principally on the blood vessels. These medications fall into two general categories: vasoconstrictors and vasodilators.

Vasoconstrictors

Vasoconstrictors contract or lessen the lumen of the blood vessels and thus raise the blood pressure. These drugs are more valuable in the milder degrees of shock than in severe cases. Adrenalin (epinephrine) and ephedrine sulfate act as vasoconstrictors as well as heart stimulants.

Vasodilators

Vasodilators (hypotensives) are drugs used to dilate or widen the blood vessels; this lowers resistance to the circulating blood and lowers the blood pressure. In arteriosclerosis, for example, the blood vessels have become narrowed. Therefore, the circulation in the extremities and sometimes in the brain has become poor. Vasodilator drugs are given so that the blood pressure lowers and the blood vessels in the extremities dilate, bringing an increased supply of blood to the area.

Vasodilators are used chiefly in cases of hypertension (high blood pressure), a common disease of middle and older age groups. The disappointment in their use on a long-term basis is due to the fact that cardiovascular (heart and blood vessel) disease is now recognized as of renal (kidney) origin and that hypertension is but one manifestation of the disease.

The nitrites are temporarily effective in hypertension. The nitrite tablets are very rapidly absorbed through the mucous membrane of the mouth or stomach. Toxic effects from overdose ("the nitrite reaction") include flushing of the skin, a throbbing headache, dilation of the pupils, and a fall in blood pressure. Collapse may result if the nurse is not alert to report symptoms to the doctor.

ANTICHOLESTEROL DRUGS

Exogenous cholesterol is taken in the diet. Endogenous cholesterol is made in the body. The presence of cholesterol may lead to plaque formation. Plaques are white fatty substances which accumulate inside the arteries, narrowing the lumen and causing less circulation at the area of accumlation.

There has been an upsurge of interest in anticholesterol drugs. These drugs are given to lower the cholesterol levels in the blood as well as to reduce cholesterol deposits inside the arterial walls. These accumulated plaques contribute to such conditions as atherosclerosis, arteriosclerosis, angina pectoris, myocardial infarction, hypertensive heart disease, aneurysms, and cerebral vascular disorders. Exogenous cholesterol contributes to the plaque formation.

Drugs used to lower the blood cholesterol are listed in figure 26-5, on page 183.

DRUGS THAT AFFECT THE BLOOD

Coagulants, anticoagulants and hematinics are drugs which influence specific elements in the blood.

Section 5 Effects of Medications on Body Systems

Medication	Action	Administration and Dosage	Side Effects and/or Toxic Effects
Glyceryl Trinitrate (Nitroglycerin)	relieves pain of angina pectoris by dilating small arteries, capillaries and coronary vessels	sublingual 0.4 mg (1/150 gr.) may be repeated in 5 minutes for 2 times	flushing, severe headache, hypotension, nausea, vomiting
Isosorbide dinitrate (Sorbitrate) (Isordril)	decreases frequency and severity of attacks in angina pectoris, thus decreasing need for nitroglycerin	p.o. 5 mg q.i.d., sublingual; 5-10 mg q.i.d. or 1 sustained release tablet q.12h.	vascular headaches, dizziness, gastrointestinal disturbance to be used with caution for glaucoma patients.
Pentaerythritol Tetranitrate (Angicap) (Nitrolans) (Pentritol) (Peritrate)	prophylactic use: to prevent angina, reduce its severity	p.o. 10-20 mg q.i.d., or 1 sustained release tablet q.12h.	flushing, headache, nausea
Amyl nitrite	relieves pain of angina pectoris by dilating small arteries, capillaries and coronary vessels	inhalation (ampule) 0.3 ml (5 minims)	flushing, severe headache, nausea, vomiting
Hydralazine (Apresoline)	controls early hypertension by dilating blood vessels	p.o., I.M., I.V., 10-25 mg q.i.d.	headache, nervous tension, nausea, tinging of extremities, urticaria (hives)
Mecamylamine (Inversine)	hypotensive drug, duration 6-12 hrs.	2.5 mg daily initial dose to 25 mg maintenance in 3 doses	headache, flushing dizziness
Methyldopa (Aldomet)	decreases peripheral vascular resistance	p.o. 250 mg tablets twice daily	sedation, depression, edema, fever, nasal congestion
Phentolamine (Regitine)	blocks action of adrenal stimulation	p.o. 50 mg tablets q.i.d. I.M., I.V., ampules of 5 mg q.i.d.	palpitations, hypotension, gastrointestinal distress, weakness, dizziness, flushing
Cyclandelate (Cyclospasmol)	peripheral vasodilator	p.o. 100-200 mg tablets 2 to 4 times daily	tingling, flushing, sweating, dizziness, headache
Nylidrin (Arlidin)	relaxes smooth muscles of arterioles to relieve pain; improves peripheral circulation	p.o. tablets 3-6 mg t.i.d. or q.i.d. I.M., s.c. 2.5 to 5 mg 1 to 3 times daily	trembling, nervousness, dizziness, palpitations, nausea and vomiting

Fig. 26-4 Vasodilators

Medication	Action	Administration and Dosage	Side and/or Toxic Effects
Dextrothyroxine sodium (Choloxin)	increased oxidation and increased excretion of cholesterol	1-2 mg daily initially; maintenance 4-8 mg daily	may set off angina attack. Used with caution for diabetic patients; insomnia, palpitations, weight loss, enhanced effects of anticoagulants: Check for bleeding tendencies and elevated blood sugar.
Clofibrate (Atromid-S)	possibly blocks synthesis of blood lipids	p.o. 500 mg q.i.d.	gastrointestinal disturbances, urticaria, loss of hair
Sitosterols (Cytellin)	increases excretion of cholesterol; lowers blood cholesterol	p.o. 10 Gm daily in divided doses a.c. 20% suspension	none reported to date
Niacin (Nicotinic acid) (Nicotinamide)	reduction in blood lipids	p.o. 1-2 Gm t.i.d. with meals or antacid	severe gastrointestinal upset, flushing, pruritus, urticaria

Fig. 26-5 Anticholesterol Drugs

Medication	Action	Administration and Dosage	Side Effects and/or Toxic Effects
Fibrinogen (human)	coagulant	I.V. 2-6 Gm in 300 ml distilled water	possible viral hepatitis
Thrombin	coagulant; hemostatic: controls bleeding during surgery	topical: in solution or as powder; 100-2000 units per cc in solution; never given intravenously	none
Menadione (Vitamin K) (Hykinone)	encourages blood clotting; administered in dicumarol intoxication, liver conditions	p.o., I.M., s.c., I.V., 0.5 to 2 mg daily or based on prothrombin level in blood	none
Calcium salts	necessary for blood clotting	p.o. 1 Gm, I.V.	none
Gelatin sponge (Gelfoam)	absorbable; hemostatic	left in wound	no reaction
Gelatin film (Gelfilm)	surgical repair of membranes	left in membrane	no reaction
Fibrin foam	mechanical coagulation in surgery of brain, liver	left in wound	no reaction
Oxidized cellulose (Oxycel)	forms artificial clot	left in wound	no reaction

Fig. 26-6 Coagulants

Section 5 Effects of Medications on Body Systems

Medication	Action	Administration and Dosage	Side Effects and/or Toxic Effects: Nursing Care
Heparin (Liquaemin)	slows down clotting time	I.V., I.M.; dosage varies according to clotting time	chills, tendency to bleed from mucous membranes; allergic reaction: check clotting time frequently
Bishydroxycoumarin (Dicumarol)	as above	p.o.; dosage varies according to prothrombin time	tendency to bleed; check prothrombin time frequently
Warfarin (Coumadin)	as above	p.o., I.V.; dosage varies according to prothrombin time	hematuria, tendency to bleed: check prothrombin time and urine frequently

Fig. 26-7 Anticoagulants

Medication	Action	Administration and Dosage	Side Effects and/or Toxic Effects
Ferrous sulfate (Feosol)	used in iron deficiency anemias; hematinic in primary anemia	p.o. 200 mg t.i.d.	gastric distress dark or black stools
Crude liver	hematinic; contains large amounts of B_{12}	I.M. 1 unit daily	soreness at site of injection
Cyanocobalamin (Vitamin B_{12}) (Rubramin)	used in pernicious anemia to form red blood cells	p.o. USP 1 unit daily; p.o., I.M., 20 to 100 mcg as ordered	none
Folic acid (Folvite)	partial replacement for B_{12} deficiency	p.o. 5-15 mg daily; parenteral 10 mg daily	masks symptoms of pernicious anemia
Ascorbic acid	helps body absorb iron	p.o. 100 mg q.d. or t.i.d.	none
Iron dextran (Imferon)	hematinic	ampules 50 mg; give deep I.M. by Z-track method	skin discoloration if not given by proper method

Fig. 26-8 Hematinics

Coagulants

Coagulants (hemostatics) are drugs ordered by the physician for patients whose blood is slow to clot as in diseases of the liver and bile ducts. They are also used in treating hemorrhage.

Anticoagulants

Anticoagulants are drugs which are administered to slow down the clotting time of the blood, figure 26-7. These medications are ordered to prevent thrombosis and blood clotting in coronary arteries and elsewhere in the body. They are frequently ordered following coronary thrombosis.

Hematinics

Hematinics are medications which stimulate the production of red blood cells and hemoglobin to counteract anemia. The most common anemia is caused by iron deficiency.

SUGGESTED ACTIVITIES

- Prepare a report on the source of digitalis. How did the drug happen to be used to treat heart cases? What are some of the products of digitalis being administered to cardiac cases?
- Select three patients who have cardiac problems. State the diagnoses, drugs which are administered, and the changes which were evident following the use of the drugs. Present your observation to the class.
- Based on outside reading, investigate and discuss the different types of anemia. Explain the difference between microcytic or hypochromic anemia, and macrocytic or hyperchromic anemia.
- Explain the general action of each of the following drugs and the responsibility of the nurse in regard to their administration.
  - a. Adrenalin
  - b. Demerol
  - c. pituitrin
  - d. histamine
  - e. Neo-Synephrine
  - f. Serpasil

REVIEW

A. From Column II select the term which best fits each description in Column I. Place the appropriate letter in the blank provided.

Column I

- _G_ 1. an inhalant dilator
- _E_ 2. coronary dilator
- _F_ 3. decreases need for sublingual nitroglycerin
- _H_ 4. heart depressant; may restore rhythm to heart in arrythmias
- _B_ 5. makes heart beat faster; elevates blood pressure
- _C_ 6. lowers blood cholesterol
- _A_ 7. dilates walls of coronary and other arteries bringing about fall in blood pressure
- _D_ 8. stimulates heart action by slowing and strengthening the beat
- _K_ 9. placed in wound to stop bleeding

Column II

a. nitroglycerin
b. Adrenalin
c. Atromid-S
d. digitalis leaf
e. isosorbide
f. Sorbitrate
g. amyl nitrite
h. quinidine
i. mercuhydrin
j. pituitrin
k. Gelfoam

Section 5 Effects of Medications on Body Systems

B. Answer the following questions.
1. What is the difference between exogenous cholesterol and endogenous cholesterol?
   EXOGENOUS IS TAKEN IN THE DIET
   ENDOGENOUS IS MADE IN THE BODY

2. Which kind of cholesterol contributes more to the accumlation of cholesterol plaques?
   ANTICHOLESTEROL DRUGS - EXOGENOUS DRUGS

3. What are plaques? *WHITE FATTY SUBSTANCES WHICH ACCUMULATE INSIDE THE ARTERIES, NARROWING THE LUMEN AND CAUSING LESS CIRCULATION AT THE AREA OF ACCUMULATION*

4. Why are diuretics ordered in congestive heart failure? *IT RIDS THE BODY OF EXCESSIVE FLUIDS*

5. What is meant by the phrase "digitalize a patient"? *IT IS USED TO IMPROVE CARDIAC FUNCTIONS*

6. When should the patient be placed on "maintenance" therapy? *WHEN THE PATIENT HAS NAUSEA OR VOMITING*

EXTENDED STUDY

Learn the meaning and proper use of the following terms.

antispasmodic	inhalation
bronchodilator	internal respiration
cough depressant	parenteral
expectoration	respiratory stimulant
external respiration	tachycardia

Unit 27 Medications that Affect the Respiratory System

OBJECTIVES

After studying this unit, the student should be able to:
- Identify the action of respiratory stimulants, bronchodilators, and expectorants.
- Explain the two ways in which respiratory stimulants may affect respiration.
- Identify the active ingredient in selected cough preparations.

Respiration is necessary for life. As we inhale, the air is warmed, moistened and filtered. As we exhale we get rid of excess carbon dioxide and water vapor. There are two types of respiration which we should keep in mind: external respiration in which there is an exchange of oxygen and carbon dioxide between our bodies and the outside environment and internal respiration in which there is an exchange of oxygen and carbon dioxide between the tissue cells and the blood or lymph which form their fluid environment. The blood carries the respiratory gases (oxygen and carbon dioxide) to and from all tissues of the body.

Respiratory movements are involuntary. The respiratory center in the medulla of the brain is affected by the chemistry and temperature of the blood supplying it. The level of carbon dioxide in the blood stimulates the respiratory center to activity. The amount of oxygen in the blood does not affect the respiratory center, but affects chemoreceptors in the aorta and carotid arteries.

The organs of respiration include the nasal passages, pharynx, larynx, trachea, bronchi, and lungs. The thoracic cage, intercostal muscles and the diaphragm assist with respiration. Air flowing into the lungs passes through these areas until it reaches the *alveolar sacs*, which are thin layers of epithelial tissue richly endowed with blood capillaries, figure 27-1.

In cases of respiratory ailments, controlling rate and depth of respiration are of primary concern. This may be accomplished by the use of drugs which act to stimulate respiration.

Many kinds of medications, some of which you have studied in previous units, are used to treat disorders of the respiratory system. Inhalation therapy antibiotics, used

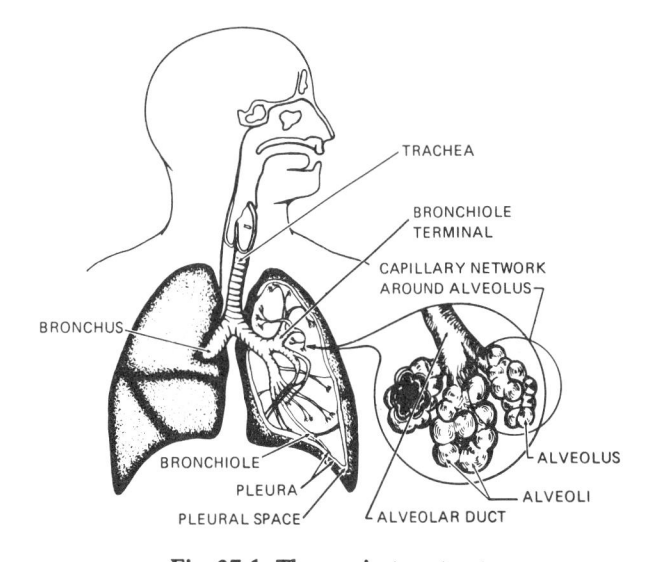

Fig. 27-1 The respiratory tract

Section 5 Effects of Medications on Body Systems

in treating diseases such as pneumonia and tuberculosis, and antihistamines, ordered for asthma, may be reviewed at this time.

RESPIRATORY STIMULANTS

Drugs which increase the rate and depth of respiration are respiratory stimulants. They may (1) affect the respiratory center in the brain through the bloodstream, or (2) affect sensory stimuli which reach the brain from the mouth, nose, throat, and skin. Examples may be seen in figure 27-2.

EXPECTORANTS AND COUGH DEPRESSANTS

Cough mixtures are medications used to induce expectoration (productive coughing). This is desirable in cases of bronchitis and some kinds of pneumonia and to relieve persistent coughs, figure 27-3.

Medications	Action	Administration and Dosage	Side and/or Toxic Effects
Carbon dioxide (95% oxygen 5% carbon dioxide)	stimulates respiratory center in brain	inhalation (mask) 7-8 deep inhalations, 4-10 liters per minute	marked increase in respirations
Spirits of ammonia (Smelling salts)	irritates mucous membrane to make patient gasp (reflex action)	inhalation, few whiffs	feeling of suffocation
Nikethamide (Coramine) (emergency drug)	stimulates respirations and elevates blood pressure	parenteral, 1.5 ml of 25% solution	sharp rise in blood pressure, anxiety, nausea, vomiting
Doxapram (Dopram)	increases depth of respiration; increases rate of respiration	I.V. 0.5 to 1.5 mg per kilogram of body weight comes in 20 ml vials	elevation of blood pressure and heart rate; increased salivation and body temperature; nausea and vomiting; contraindicated in hypertension
Caffeine	large doses stimulate the respiratory center	caffeine-sodium benzoate ampules 0.5 Gm	abdominal cramps due to increased flow of hydrochloric acid in stomach, also excessive irritability, insomnia, palpitations
Ethamivan (Emivan)	centrally acting respiratory stimulant	I.V. 100-500 mg ampules	signs of CNS irritation (restlessness, sneezing, coughing, twitching)

Fig. 27-2 Respiratory stimulants

Medications	Action	Administration and Dosage	Side Effects and/or Toxic Effects
Elixir of terpin hydrate	decreases bronchial secretions	**p.o.** 4 ml	none
Syrup of ipecac	stimulates secretion of mucus; emetic	**p.o.** 1-8 ml for adults 5 minims for 1 yr old infant	nausea and vomiting
Ammonium chloride	increases bronchial secretions by irritation	**p.o.** 0.3 Gm q.i.d. c̄ full glass of water	nausea and vomiting (large doses)
Benzonatate N.F., (Tessalon)	relieves cough without depressing respirations cough suppressant	**p.o.** 50 and 100 mg capsules Dosage: 100 mg every 4 hours	no serious side effects. drowsiness, nasal congestion, tightness in chest
Noscapine N.F. (Nectadon)	depresses cough reflex is opium alkaloid	**p.o.** 15 to 30 mg t.i.d. also syrup, 2 mg per ml	minimal, nausea
Codeine (narcotic)	cough depressant	**p.o.** .03 - .06 Gm; parenteral .008 to .06 Gm	drowsiness, constipation, addiction

Fig. 27-3 Cough Mixtures

Expectorants are of two types. The *stimulating expectorant* tends to induce healing of the bronchial mucosa by decreasing the amount of mucus secretions which are in the respiratory tract. An example of the stimulating expectorant is elixir of terpin hydrate. The *sedative expectorant* usually depresses the cough and, in some cases, may cause nausea, as in the use of syrup of ipecac. The sedative expectorant (cough depressant) causes an increased secretion of mucus, thus soothing the bronchial mucosa. The increase in the mucus secretions tends to decrease the coughing spasms. Examples of the sedative type of expectorant are ammonium chloride and the iodides. Codeine is not ordered as a cough depressant in tuberculosis because expectorating is desirable here.

Because most cough mixtures are given to relieve local irritation, they are administered without water unless directed otherwise by the physician. The patient needs adequate hydration, however, and fluids are given at other times since this helps to liquefy the secretions.

Section 5 Effects of Medications on Body Systems

ANTISPASMODICS

Antispasmodics are drugs which decrease muscle contractions. Antispasmodics which relax spasms of the bronchi are called bronchodilators. Bronchodilators also reduce swelling and congestion of the mucous membrane, figure 27-4.

Medication	Action	Administration and Dosage	Side Effects and/or Toxic Effects
Aminophylline (Theophylline)	dilates bronchi and coronary arteries; relaxes smooth muscles in bronchi	p.o. 100-200 mg tablets daily, I.V. and rectal suppositories, 100-500 mg	fall in blood pressure, headache, dizziness
Epinephrine (Adrenalin)	relaxes smooth muscles of bronchi, inhibits bronchial secretions, constricts pulmonary blood vessels	inhalation 1:100 sol.; subcutaneous and I.M. injection 0.2 to 1 mg of 1:1000 sol.	excessive rise in blood pressure: check frequently; palpitations, rapid pulse, anxiety and headache
Isoproterenol (Aludrine) (Isonorin) (Isuprel) (Norisodrine)	adrenergic drug related to epinephrine; shrinks swollen mucous membranes and reduces mucus secretion	sublingual tablets 10, 15 mg; powder inhalant 10%-25%; solution for inhalation 1:100, 1:200, 1:400	may cause tachycardia accompanied by precordial distress; used with caution in cardiac cases
Ephedrine (Racephedrine)	reduces swelling of mucous membrane; long duration	p.o. 25 mg t.i.d.; parenteral 25 mg; nose drops 1%	excitation, tachycardia
Acetylcysteine (Mucomyst)	reduces thickness and stickiness of bronchial secretions for easier removal.	nebulization	stomatitis, nausea; can cause bronchospasm in asthmatic patients

Fig. 27-4 Bronchodilators

SUGGESTED ACTIVITIES

- Observe the cough medicines which are most frequently used. What is the desired action of the active ingredient of each one?
- Investigate the treatment of tuberculosis. Prepare a report on the effects of chemotherapy (treatment with synthesized chemicals), surgery, and streptomycin (an antibiotic) on tuberculosis.
- Observe and compare four patients suffering from respiratory ailments, one of which is emphysema. Prepare a report identifying one of the respiratory diseases, symptoms, drugs administered, their effects, and nursing care (focusing on the medication).

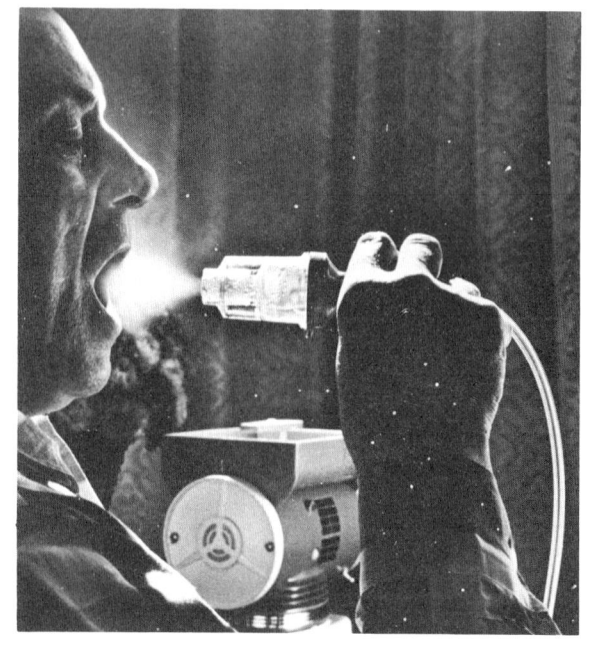

Fig. 27-5 Administration by Nebulizer

Unit 27 Medications that Affect the Respiratory System

- There is a rule in some hospitals which requires that stimulants be kept in a specific area in the medicine cupboard. Where are they kept in your hospital? What is this rule? Which stimulant is most frequently used? Explain why.

REVIEW

A. From Column II select the term which best fits each description in Column I. Place the appropriate letter in the blank provided.

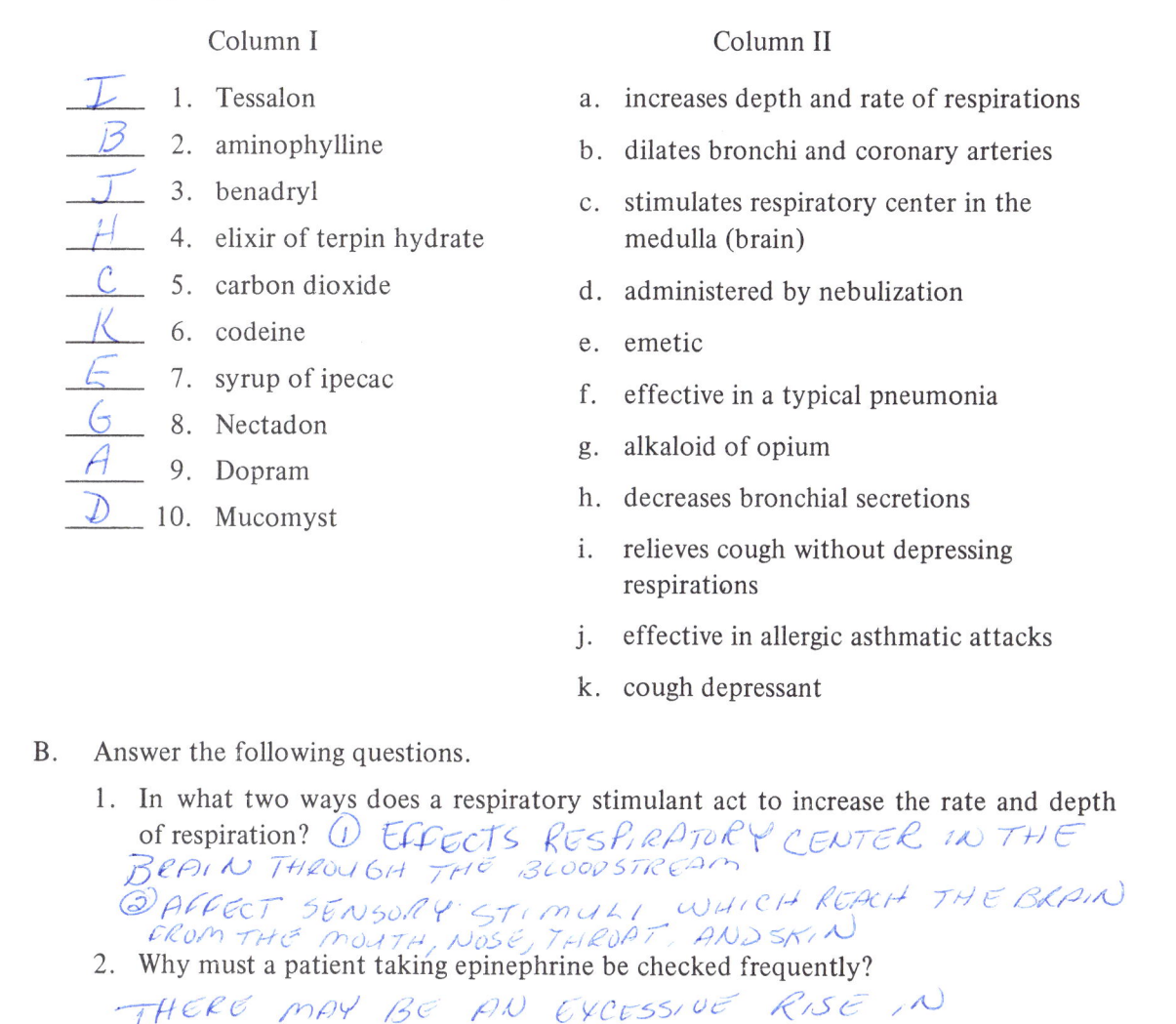

Column I

_I_ 1. Tessalon
_B_ 2. aminophylline
_J_ 3. benadryl
_H_ 4. elixir of terpin hydrate
_C_ 5. carbon dioxide
_K_ 6. codeine
_E_ 7. syrup of ipecac
_G_ 8. Nectadon
_A_ 9. Dopram
_D_ 10. Mucomyst

Column II

a. increases depth and rate of respirations
b. dilates bronchi and coronary arteries
c. stimulates respiratory center in the medulla (brain)
d. administered by nebulization
e. emetic
f. effective in a typical pneumonia
g. alkaloid of opium
h. decreases bronchial secretions
i. relieves cough without depressing respirations
j. effective in allergic asthmatic attacks
k. cough depressant

B. Answer the following questions.

1. In what two ways does a respiratory stimulant act to increase the rate and depth of respiration? ① EFFECTS RESPIRATORY CENTER IN THE BRAIN THROUGH THE BLOODSTREAM ② AFFECT SENSORY STIMULI WHICH REACH THE BRAIN FROM THE MOUTH, NOSE, THROAT, AND SKIN

2. Why must a patient taking epinephrine be checked frequently?
THERE MAY BE AN EXCESSIVE RISE IN BLOOD PREASSURE

3. Explain how a stimulating expectorant differs from the action of a cough depressant.
STIMULATING EXPECTORANTS TENDS TO INDUCE HEALING TO THE BRONCHIAL MUCOSA BY DECREASING THE AMOUNT OF MUCOUS SECRETIONS WHICH ARE IN THE RESPIRATORY TRACT

4. Of the following drug substances, which one is the chief respiratory stimulant?
   a. Tessalon
   b. (Carbon dioxide)
   c. Adrenalin
   d. Aminophyllin

THE DEPRESSANT INCREASES THE AMOUNT OF MUCOUS THUS REDUCING THE COUGHING.

Section 5 Effects of Medications on Body Systems

    5. Which one of the following statements is NOT correct.
       a. Respiratory stimulants increase the carbon dioxide in the blood
       b. Respiratory stimulants help the patient to expectorate and loosen secretions
       c. Respiratory stimulants act on the respiratory center in the brain
       d. Respiratory stimulants increase the rate of inspiration

EXTENDED STUDY

    Learn the meaning and proper use of the following terms:

achlorhydria	demulcent
acidity	digestant
absorbent	emetic
adsorbent	emollient
alkalinity	flatus
antacid	hyperacidity
anthelmintic	hypochlorhydria
antidiarrheic	laxative
antiemetic	purgative
carminative	systemic alkalosis
cathartic	opium alkaloid
colloidal	

Unit 28 Medications Used for Gastrointestinal System Disorders

OBJECTIVES

After studying this unit, the student should be able to:

- State the effects of the various types of antacids on the gastric secretions.
- Name the commonly used digestants.
- Define carminatives, emetics, antiemetics, cathartics, and anthelmintics.
- Explain the action of the different types of cathartics.

Digestion is the process by which the body changes solid food into energy and building material for the body cells. The sales of medications for disorders of the gastrointestinal system are probably promoted to the general public more than any other types of drugs. Through television and other means of commercial advertisement, drugs and the "wonders" they perform are brought to the attention of the public just as any of our common everyday products. The effect of this is to cause their widespread misuse by individuals who make a self-determined diagnosis of their ailment, or who know nothing about the drug except its advertised claims. The implication for the nurse is that the administering or taking of drugs is not a decision to be made on the basis of hearsay but only upon a doctor's recommendation.

Study figure 28-1; it is suggested that the illustration be referred to frequently when reading this unit.

The gastrointestinal tract has many curves and turns between the mouth and the anus. It is really one long tube through which food enters at the mouth and from which waste products are excreted at the anus. Between these two points many complicated processes take place which break down, liquefy, and transport the digested foods until they are ready for absorption in the small intestine. Food is considered to have actually entered the body only after it has been absorbed through the villi in the small intestine to enter the circulation for transportation throughout the body. The chemical processes of

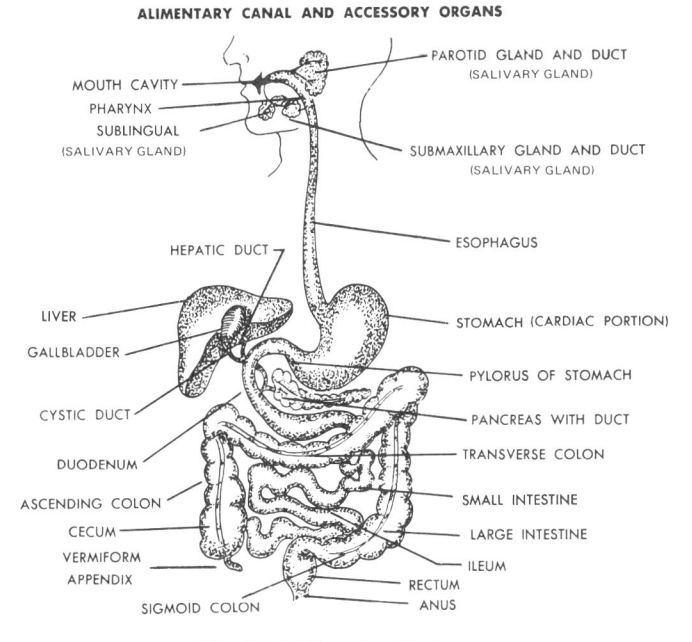

Fig. 28-1 Digestive System

digestion involve the use of many juices and enzymes which convert the food into liquid and its component parts for use in the tissues. There are also mechanical processes which break up and move forward the food in order that each part of the digestive system can perform its particular function. The medications discussed in this unit also aid in the functioning of the digestive glands and muscles.

DRUGS WHICH AFFECT THE MOUTH

Medications used for the gastrointestinal system include those which act specifically in the mouth. Oral hygiene can do a great deal toward promoting a healthy appetite and good mechanical breaking up of foods, both of which may lead to improved digestion. Among the medications or drugs used specifically in the mouth are flavoring substances which disguise the taste of medicines, (flavor is a mixed sensation in which taste and smell are both involved) astringents which contract tissues, medications which stimulate the taste buds, and medications which increase the flow of saliva. They also include mouthwashes and gargles.

Flavoring and Coloring Agents

Flavoring and coloring agents are added when the medication must be taken in liquid or powder form. These include cherry, raspberry, peppermint, vanilla, cinnamon, chocolate, and licorice. Medicines are made more attractive by the addition of vegetable colors such as red, green, and brown.

Mouthwashes and Gargles

Mouthwashes are, at best, temporary in effect. Good prophylactic care by the dentist and personal oral hygiene measures will go a long way toward preventing "bad breath" and dental caries. Mouthwashes may contain antiseptics, astringents, flavoring agents, and oxidizing agents. Hospital formularies (HF) usually make up their own mouthwashes and gargles. Proper dilutions are either on the stock bottle label or printed in the formulary.

Sodium bicarbonate is used in weak solution (1/2 tsp. to a glass of water). It removes mucus from the mouth and nasopharynx.

Salt (sodium chloride) in weak (1/2 tsp. to a glass of water) solution is a pleasant and a very inexpensive mouthwash.

Sodium perborate is an unpleasant, salty-tasting mouthwash which bubbles in the mouth as it frees its oxygen content. It is an effective mouthwash and gargle. It may be obtained with flavoring which disguises its unpleasant taste. It is effective in cases of Vincent's disease and in pyorrhea (gum disease) because it kills the anerobic bacteria which cause the condition. These bacteria cannot live in the presence of oxygen.

Weak solutions of hydrogen peroxide (1:4) and potassium permanganate (0.1% solution), both oxidizing agents, are good oral anti-infective agents.

Dentifrices usually contain the following components: a flavoring agent, an abrasive agent, and a foaming agent. In addition, some dentifrices contain fluorides, hard soap, and calcium carbonate. Toothpaste or powders must be effective as cleansing agents but must not injure the gums or teeth. Stannous fluoride added to the dentifrice has been recognized as being of use in reducing dental decay. Sodium fluoride is effective in reducing dental caries when added to the water supply. Acceptance of fluoridation of the water supply is still under discussion in some areas of our country.

DRUGS THAT AFFECT THE STOMACH

Drugs affecting the stomach are used chiefly for their effects upon the acidity or alkalinity of the gastric juice. They include such groups as antacids, digestants, carminatives, emetics, antiemetics and drugs used in diagnostic procedures.

The aim in treatment of peptic ulcers is to give the ulcer a chance to heal. The relief from hyperacidity and hyperactivity of the stomach muscles helps the healing process. In addition to a required diet, the drugs used for patients with peptic ulcers include antacids, antispasmodics, sedatives and/or tranquilizers.

Antacids

The aim of antacids is to lower the gastric acidity to pH 3 or 4. This helps to reduce the irritating effect upon the ulcer. Antacids are effective only when in the stomach. When the stomach becomes empty, the effect of the antacid is lost and the stomach begins to secrete more acid. The antacid should be effective enough so that a small dosage will control a good amount of gastric acid. It should not change the electrolyte balance and should not cause a general systemic alkalosis. It should have a long-lasting effect rather than a short one, after which there should not be a secondary increase in gastric acidity.

The nurse must remember that fluids should be taken after the antacid is administered, especially if the dose is a small amount, or the medication would only coat the esophagus. Also, an adverse symptom to watch for is systemic or general alkalinity.

Aluminum hydroxide gel is a nonsystemic antacid. It is an insoluble, colloidal substance which does not interfere with the acid-base balance in the blood. Its neutralization reaction is slower than sodium bicarbonate. There is no acid rebound, no abdominal distention, and no carbon dioxide produced. The hydrochloric acid in the stomach clings to the colloidal particles to cause chemical neutralization. This medication is a mild astringent which soothes the ulcer. Constipation may follow its use. Amphojel, Creamalin, Al-U-Creme, Alkagel are brand names for this antacid.

It is important to take fluid after small amounts of this medication or it will only coat the esophagus and have no effect on the ulcer.

> Dosage: p.o. 4 to 8 ml four to six times a day. Can have dosage of 15 to 30 ml hourly also. It is also available in tablets of 300 and 600 mg which should be chewed slowly and thoroughly.

Magnesium trisilicate. This nonsystemic antacid powder develops a gelatinous consistency in the stomach. Thus it forms a coating over the ulcer, soothing it. It has a prolonged effect. Because of its tendency to cause diarrhea, it is often prepared with aluminum hydroxide gel. Gelusil and Trisogel are two examples of this combination.

> Dosage: Acute phase: p.o. 2-4 Gm every 1-2 hours.
> Maintenance dose: p.o. 1 Gm q.i.d.

Aluminum Phosphate Gel is a nonsystemic antacid which has properties similar to those of aluminum hydroxide gel. This medication is used for those ulcer patients unable to be kept on a high-phosphate diet or who suffer from diarrhea. Phosphagel is an example of this antacid.

> Dosage: 4% suspension
> Acute phase: p.o. 15-30 ml with milk every 2 hours.
> Maintenance: p.o. 15 ml after meals and at bedtime.

Section 5 Effects of Medications on Body Systems

Calcium carbonate is an insoluble white powder which neutralizes the gastric acid. It is broken down by acids. It is used as a nonsystemic antacid for patients with hyperacidity, gastritis, and peptic ulcer.

    Dosage: Acute phase: p.o. 1-2 Gm every 1-2 hours
        Maintenance: p.o. 1 Gm after meals four times a day.

Magnesium oxide, a nonsystemic antacid, is a white powder insoluble in water. Its neutralizing ability is outstanding among antacids. It has a saline cathartic effect instead of the constipating effects of other antacids. It may alkalinize the urine. This preparation appears as light or heavy magnesia. Oxabid capsules contain magnesium oxide.

    Dosage: p.o. 250 mg

Other magnesium compounds are:

- Magnesium carbonate. Action is similar to that of magnesium oxide except that it frees carbon dioxide when neutralizing hydrochloric acid in stomach. It is a white powder.

      Dosage: p.o. 0.6 Gm

- Magnesium Magna (Milk of Magnesia). Mixture of magnesium hydroxide. It has same action as other magnesium salts.

- Maalox contains aluminum hydroxide gel and magnesium hydroxide.

      Dosage: p.o. 8 ml followed by milk or water

- Sippy powders developed by Dr. Sippy many years ago, are mixtures of nonsystemic acids. They were once widely used in conjunction with a milk and cream diet. Sippy powder #1 is a combination of magnesium oxide and sodium bicarbonate; Sippy powder #2 is made up of bismuth subcarbonate and sodium bicarbonate. The two powders were alternately given with the milk and cream.

Sodium bicarbonate (Baking Soda) is a systemic antacid, meaning that it is capable of altering the electrolyte balance. Sodium bicarbonate is used indiscriminately in many households. The alkaline reaction in the stomach slows down the action of pepsin because acid activates this digestive enzyme. The "belching" which frequently occurs following its use is nature's effort to rid itself of the accumulated carbon dioxide. Sodium bicarbonate passes out of the stomach rapidly, leaving an "acid rebound" or increased secretion of acid in the stomach.

    Dosage: 1-2 Gm once or twice a day.

ANTISPASMODICS, ANTIHISTAMINES AND SEDATIVES

The antispasmodics decrease gastric acidity, decrease gastric motility, and relieve spasms. Examples of them are:

    Methscopolamine bromide (Pamine bromide)
            Dosage: 2.5 mg a.c. and h.s.
            Side effects: dry mouth, constipation, blurred vision.

Methantheline bromide (Banthine bromide)
>Dosage: usually 100 mg t.i.d., a.c. and h.s.
>Side Effects: dry mouth, dilated pupils, inability to read fine print, urinary retention in patients with prostatic hypertrophy.

Tagamet (Cimetidine)
>Use: short-term treatment of duodenal ulcers
>Dosage: 300 mg
>Side Effects: diarrhea, muscle pain, dizziness, rash

The sedatives used in the treatment of patients with ulcer include Phenobarbital and Donnatol which is a mixture of atropine, scopolamine and phenobarbital.

DIGESTANTS

Digestants, as one might suspect, are medications which aid in the digestive process. They are usually prescribed to make up for deficiencies in the gastrointestinal tract. The nurse must be aware that overdose may cause a burning sensation and/or vomiting.

Hydrochloric Acid

Hydrochloric acid has important functions in the digestive process. It is needed to activate the pepsin needed for protein digestion. It has a germicidal effect upon many bacteria which enter the stomach. It stimulates absorption in the small intestines, and it helps to keep the electrolyte balance. It is ordered to relieve the symptoms of gastric hypochlorhydria, a decreased secretion of hydrochloric acid in the stomach and achlorhydria, the absence of hydrochloric acid.

Dilute hydrochloric acid 10% (4 milliliters diluted in glass of water) is taken through a drinking tube to prevent tooth decay. It may be taken during the meal or just after the meal. The mouth should be rinsed with an alkaline solution following administration.

Glutamic Acid Hydrochloride (Aciduline)

The hydrochloric acid is released when the preparation comes in contact with water.
>Dosage: Capsules: p.o. 0.3 Gm (equal to 0.6 ml of dilute hydrochloric acid) a.c. (before meals)

Pepsin

Pepsin is a gastric enzyme. It is secreted by the stomach. It is a proteolytic enzyme which helps in the digestion of proteins. It is used infrequently as a medication now. The source of the drug is the glandular part of a hog's stomach.
>Dosage: p.o. 0.5 to 1 Gm p.c. (after meals)

Pancreatin

The pancreas of hogs is the source of pancreatin. It may be ordered in cases of pancreatitis or insufficient pancreatic secretion. It contains three enzymes from the pancreas: amylase, trypsin, and pancreatic lipase. When ordered, it is given in enteric-coated pills, so that the stomach secretions will not destroy it.
>Dosage: p.o. 500 mg, usually a.c.

Section 5 *Effects of Medications on Body Systems*

Bile and Bile Salts

The chief function of bile is the digestion and absorption of fats and fat-soluble vitamins. Bile provides a mild laxative action in the intestines. The bile acids stimulate the liver to produce more bile. Bile is used to treat liver disorders, to stimulate biliary drainage, and to aid in the digestion of fats.

Preparations and Dosage:
- Dehydrocholic acid (Decholin) p.o. 250-500 mg; 2-3 times daily. (Increases volume of bile and biliary drainage.)
- Florantyrone (Zanchol) p.o. 750 mg to 1 Gm daily. This is a synthetic product which increase the flow of bile.

CARMINATIVES

Carminatives are drugs given to increase the expulsion of gas from the stomach and intestines (flatus). The active substances in carminatives are usually aromatic volatile oils; these give a feeling of warmth in the stomach, and help to expel gas from the intestines. A few drops of oil of peppermint or spirits of peppermint in hot water or brandy in hot water are frequently used in the home. Rhubarb and soda mixture, 4 ml, is used for the same purposes. Simethecone (Mylicon) is also used to relieve flatus.

EMETICS

Emetics induce vomiting either by stimulating the vomiting center in the brain or by local stomach action as in drinking large quantities of lukewarm water. They are used chiefly in cases of poisoning. Gastric lavages are being used more frequently than emetics. Adverse effects to emetics may be salivation, lacrimation, weakness and dizziness.

Apomorphine Hydrochloride

A narcotic which directly stimulates the vomiting center in the medulla, is apomorphine hydrochloride. Vomiting occurs shortly after injection. Large doses may increase depression if this is already present. The Controlled Substances Act must be observed.

Dosage: 5 mg (2-8 mg) s.c. or I.V.

Ipecac

Ipecac is used as an expectorant (Sorbutuss) as well as an emetic (Ipecac Syrup). Warning: Ipecac Syrup can exert a cardiotoxic effect if it is not vomited.

Usual dosage: 15 ml (1 tablespoonful) in persons over one year of age. The dosage may be repeated in twenty minutes if vomiting does not occur. Then, if the patient does not vomit, the dosage should be recovered by lavage if necessary.

ANTIEMETICS

Antiemetics relieve nausea and vomiting. They have, as the name implies, an effect opposite to that of emetics. Vomiting may be caused by irritation of the gastric mucosa or by stimuli affecting the vomiting center in the brain. Plain hot tea or carbonated drinks may relieve the vomiting.

Antiemetics are often given intramuscularly for acute nausea and vomiting, and orally to control nausea. The following drugs have been proven effective as antiemetics:

- Chlorpromazine (Thorazine)
    Dosage: p.o. 10-15 mg q. 4-6 h.; I.M. 25 mg q. 3-4 h.; rectal 25 and 100 mg suppositories q. 6-8 h.

- Dimenhydrinate (Dramamine)
    Dosage: p.o. 50 mg t.i.d.; rectal suppositories 50-100 mg; I.M. 50 mg

- Meclizine (Bonine)
    Dosage: p.o. 25 mg t.i.d.

- Prochlorperazine (Compazine) (tranquilizer)
    Dosage: p.o. 5 mg q.i.d.

The nurse should observe the patient for signs of drowsiness and report this fact to the charge nurse and/or physician.

CATHARTICS

Cathartics act to empty the colon by increasing the bulk or by irritating the mucosa. Constipation resulting in the need for carthartics may be due to inadequate diet, insufficient fluid intake, nervous tension, lack of exercise, insufficient bulk in the diet or poor routinized training. A daily bowel evacuation is not essential unless the person feels very uncomfortable. We should remember that cathartics should never be taken when there is abdominal pain, nausea, or vomiting unless ordered by the physician.

Bulk-increasing Cathartics

These drugs stimulate peristalsis because, taken by mouth, with water, they increase in volume. At least one full glass of water should be taken with the drug.

Agar. Obtained from seaweed, agar swells in the presence of water and forms a soothing mass. Agarol is a cathartic containing agar. The dosage is 4 Gm.

Psyllium seed. This product also swells in the presence of water. It produces a soft, moist stool. An example of a cathartic containing psyllium seed is Metamucil. The dosage is 4-7 Gm.

Methylcellulose. A synthetic product, methycellulose swells in the presense of water. Cathartics which contain methylcellulose are Hydrolose, Cellothyl and Cologel. The dosage is 1 Gm.

Saline Cathartics

Saline cathartics are soluble salts which are only slightly absorbed from the gastrointestinal tract. They draw water into the intestines because of their osmotic effect and increase the fluid content of the feces. Peristalisis is increased, and many liquid and semi-liquid stools may be evacuated. Saline cathartics are especially helpful in food or drug poisoning and in the relief of cardiac and cerebral edema when given with some anthelmintics.

Section 5 *Effects of Medications on Body Systems*

Preparations include:

- Sodium sulfate (Glauber's Salt).
    Dosage: p.o. 15 Gm
- Magnesium sulfate (Epsom Salt). A potent cathartic.
    Dosage: p.o. 15 Gm dissolved in water.
- Magnesium citrate. Contains sugar; therefore not given to a diabetic.
    Dosage: p.o. 6-12 ounces
- Milk of Magnesia. An effective antacid as well as a saline cathartic.
    Dosage: p.o. 15 ml

Emollient Cathartics

Mineral oil is an example of an emollient cathartic. It is not digested or absorbed to any degree. The result is that it softens the fecal mass and thus prevents too much absorption of water. Many physicians object to the use of mineral oil because it dissolves some of the bile salts and fat-soluble vitamins, thereby preventing their absorption. Other emollients which become cathartics when taken in large doses are olive oil and cottonseed oil. In ordinary amounts these oils are absorbed.

Irritant Cathartics

These drugs irritate the mucosa of the colon, causing contraction of the smooth muscles followed by expulsion. Aloe, rhubarb and senna fall in this group. Other preparations are:

- Castor oil (Oleum Ricini). The fatty acid is an irritant to the mucosa of the small intestine; it empties the bowel completely because of the rapid propulsion of the feces.
    Dosage: p.o. 15 ml
- Cascara Sagrada (Hinkle Pills, Cascara tablets, Fluidextract of Cascara). A mild action results.
    Dosage: p.o. 1 to 4 ml of fluidextract
- Phenolphthalein (Exlax, Feenamint). This medication is part of several candy laxatives.
- Bisacodyl (Dulcolax). This reflexly stimulates peristalsis upon contact with the mucosa of the colon.
    Dosage: 5 to 10 mg in 5 mg tablets. Do not chew tablets and they should not be taken within 1 hour after an antacid. Dulcolax acts in 6-12 hours. Rectal suppositories 10 mg (may cause a burning sensation and proctitis) act in 15 to 60 minutes.

Fecal Softeners

Fecal softeners are new surface agents which mix with the fecal material, softening it and reducing surface tension. They are the choice for cardiac patients because they are nonirritating and do not form bulk; stools are produced in 8-12 hours.

Preparations include:

Plain type: Colace and Doxinate

Combined type: Dialose, Dialose Plus, and Pericolace

ANTIDIARRHEICS

Antidiarrheics are used to treat diarrhea. This condition may be due to intestinal infection, nervous disorders, contaminated foods, or inflamed visceral organs. The types of antidiarrheics are:

- Demulcents which soothe the irritated membrane of the gastrointestinal system. For example, boiled milk, Bismuth Subcarbonate and Calcium Carbonate.

- Adsorbents which remove the irritating material. Examples are Kaolin, and Kaolin mixed with pectin (Kaopectate).

Antispasmodics, Sedatives, and Opium Alkaloids

Drugs which have another primary effect are also used at times for antidiarrhetic action. Some antispasmodics, sedatives, and opium alkaloids are often prescribed in the treatment of diarrhea.

Tincture of Belladonna is an antispasmodic drug which decreases tone and peristalsis in the intestines. The dosage is 10 minims in a small amount of water (20-30 ml).

Phenobarbital has a sedative action. The usual dosage is 15 milligrams every four hours by mouth.

Donnagel is a combination of Kaolin, pectin, atropine and belladonna. It is used for its adsorbent, demulcent, and antispasmodic effects. The usual dosage is 15 to 30 milliliters every 3 hours. In household measures, Donnagel is often taken as 1 or 2 tablespoons every 3 hours.

Papaverine relaxes the smooth muscles of the intestines. The dosage is 100 milligrams by mouth or 30-60 milligrams by intramuscular injection.

Laudanum (tincture of opium) decreases propulsive peristalsis. Its dosage is 0.3 to 1 milliliter by mouth; it is diluted in a small amount of water.

Paregoric is camphorated tincture of opium. It, too, decreases propulsive peristalsis. The dosage is 5 to 10 milliliters by mouth, diluted.

Lomotil is a trade name for Diphenoxylate. It is a synthetic narcotic which decreases gastrointestinal motility. The dosage is 15 to 30 milliliters every 3 hours.

ANTHELMINTICS AND AMEBICIDAL DRUGS

Anthelmintics are drugs used to eliminate parasitic organisms such as worms. The action of these drugs is to paralyze the muscles of the worms so that they cannot remain attached to the intestinal wall and can, therefore, be eliminated from the body. The most

Section 5 Effects of Medications on Body Systems

common types of intestinal parasites are hookworms, tapeworms, flat worms and round worms, figure 28-2.

Amebicidal drugs are used to kill amebae in the bowel. These drugs are sometimes referred to as *amebicides.* Infections of the bowel, caused by the ameba microorganisms, can be found in many parts of the world. It can be caused by poor sanitation. Amebiasis can be caused by poor sanitation; it may be transmitted through food and water which has been contaminated by feces. The nurse must be careful to wash the hands thoroughly and to be sure that patients and other persons follow the same precautions to prevent transmission of this disease. People who travel often become afflicted with amebic dysentery. Some of the drugs used to treat diseases of this kind are explained in figure 28-3.

Medication	Action	Administration and Dosage	Side Effects and/or Toxic Effects
Hexylresorcinol	paralyzes hookworms, pinworms, whipworms, dwarf tapeworms	p.o. 1 Gm for adults. A saline purgative is given the evening before and 2 to 4 hours after the administration of the drug. Food is withheld during treatment.	irritation of gastrointestinal tract
Piperazine (Antepar) (Perin)	induces paralysis in roundworms and pinworms	tablets 250-500 mg; syrup 100 mg per cc dose based on body weight; pinworms: 7 day course roundworms: 5-7 day course	vomiting, also urticaria, muscular weakness
Pyrvinium (Povan)	dye for treatment of pinworms; prevents uptake of oxygen by the worms	oral suspension 50 mg in 5 ml or in 50 mg tablets; dose is based on body weight; treatment is periodic over 2-3 weeks because of recurrence	nausea, vomiting and cramping. It colors the stools bright red. Vomitus may stain clothing or furniture
Quinacrine hydrochloride (Atabrine)	treatment of beef and pork tapeworms.	0.5 to 1 Gm with 1 Gm of sodium bicarbonate in the A.M. No food is given before the medication. A saline purgative is given the evening before and 2 hours after administration of the drug. It may be given through a duodenal tube	gastric irritation and vomiting

Fig. 28-2 Anthelmintics

Medications	Action	Administration and Dosage	Side Effects and/or Toxic Effects
Carbasone	an arsenic preparation for treatment of amebic dysentery; kills amebae in bowel	**p.o.** 250 mg 2 or 3 times daily for 7 to 10 days rectally is a cleansing enema followed by a retention enema of 2 Gm dissolved in 200 ml of warm 2% sodium bicarbonate solution repeated every other night for 5 times	rash, loss of weight, abdominal distress
Diiodohydroxyquin (Diodoquin)	iodine preparation which kills amebae in the bowel	650 mg to 1 Gm t.i.d. between meals	itching, dermatitis, diarrhea, headache
Paromomycin (Humatin)	antibiotic with direct amebicidal action	available in capsules 250 mg; syrup 125 mg per ml; dosage: 35 to 60 mg per kilogram of body weight. Given in divided doses with meals for 1 to 2 weeks	diarrhea, nausea, vomiting, headache

Fig. 28-3 Amebicides

DIAGNOSTIC AIDS

Indicators of Gastric Acidity

Histamine is a strong stimulant of gastric glands. It is used in gastric function tests to diagnose *achlorhydria*, a condition in which the stomach is unable to produce hydrochloric acid.

Dosage for diagnosis: s.c. or I.M. 0.3 to 0.5 mg

Some preparations are:

- Histamine Phosphate.
    Dosage: s.c. 0.04 mg/kg of body weight

- Betazole hydrochloride (Histalog) is used more frequently than histamine phosphate
    Dosage: s.c. 0.5 mg/kg of body weight

- Azuresin is used to diagnose achlorhydria.
    Dosage: p.o. 2 Gm (Urine will be blue-green for several days.)

Roentgenographic Studies

Barium sulfate is a powder, insoluble in water. It is used for X rays of the gastrointestinal tract. For colon X rays the barium must be given as an enema; after this diagnostic series is completed, a cleansing enema is given to rid the bowel of the barium.

Dosage: 300 Gm powder suspended in liquid is taken orally.

Section 5 Effects of Medications on Body Systems

Organic Iodine Compounds are used in x-ray examinations as they outline certain areas: liver, gallbladder, and bile ducts. The compounds are excreted by the liver into the bile which empties into the gallbladder. Iodine compounds must be used cautiously where there is kidney disease.

- Iodoalphionic Acid (Priodax) is used for cholecystography; it is entirely secreted by the kidney. There may be dysuria, nausea, vomiting, and diarrhea.
  > Dosage: p.o. 0.5 Gm as prepared. Adult dosage is 3 Gm taken with several glasses of water followed by a fat-free supper with no further food until the next morning.

- Iopanoic Acid (Telepaque) is used for cholecystography. It usually has no side effects. Nausea, diarrhea and dysuria sometimes develop.
  > Dosage: 3 Gm orally 10 hours before every X ray. (Drug is available in 500 mg tablets, and envelopes of 6 tablets (3 Gm, adult dose). A fat-free supper is served, and then food is withheld until after X rays.

SUGGESTED ACTIVITIES

- Study the charts of two patients hospitalized for peptic ulcer. Report to the class on the method of diagnosis, the medications ordered and diet therapy.
- Select one antacid and one cathartic for closer study. Investigate the active ingredients, dosage, adverse reactions, and recommended uses. Report your findings to the class.

REVIEW

A. The doctor's order reads: Give 25 mg of dramamine q.2h. until nausea is relieved. The tablets of dramamine are labeled 50 mg. What will be administered to the patient? How often?

B. Complete the following statements:
  1. Flavor is a mixed sensation in which_____ and _____ are both concerned.
  2. Soluble salts which are only slightly absorbed from the gastrointestinal tract are called _____.
  3. Flavoring agents used to cover up or disguise the unpleasant taste of medicines are _____.
  4. A dentifrice contains _____.
  5. Mouthwashes usually contain _____.
  6. Hypochlorhydria and hyperacidity are conditions concerned with the secretion of _____ in the stomach.
  7. Relief from hyperacidity is necessary for (a, an) _____ to heal.

8. An "acid rebound" may result from the administration of _____.
9. A systemic antacid alters the _____ of the body.
10. _____ is a nonsystemic antacid which coats the stomach.
11. Gelusil contains _____ to avoid the side effect of diarrhea.
12. Belching relieves excess _____ in the stomach.
13. Three commonly used digestants are _____ , _____ , and _____ .
14. _____ are drugs used to help the stomach and intestines expel flatus.
15. An emetic is used to _____.
16. Three commonly used antiemetics are _____ , _____ and _____ .
17. Methylcellulose acts as a cathartic by _____ .
18. Two cathartics which act by colon irritation are _____ and _____ .
19. Fecal softeners are used for cardiac patients because _____ .
20. Betazole hydrochloride is used in the diagnosis of _____ .

EXTENDED STUDY

Learn the meaning and proper use of the following terms:

acidosis	glomerular filtrate
dehydrate	nephrosis
diuresis	osmosis
diuretic	tubular reabsorption
electrolyte	urinary antiseptic

209

Unit 29 Medications Used for Urinary System Disorders

OBJECTIVES

After studying this unit, the student should be able to:

- Explain two functions of the kidney.
- State the action of the following kinds of diuretics: osmotic, mercurial, carbonic anhydrase inhibitors, hormone antagonists, and thiazide compounds.
- Identify examples of drugs used as diuretics, urinary antiseptics, alkalizers, and acidifiers.

The kidneys have two important, interrelated functions: (1) to purify the blood by removing the waste products of metabolism and (2) to regulate the loss of water and electrolytes in order to keep the body fluids stable in composition. In some patholgical conditions the kidneys are not able to maintain the water balance, and fluids begin to build up in the tissues. Sometimes the accumulation of body fluids is primarily due to a disorder within the kidney itself, as in nephrosis. *Nephrosis* is a degenerative condition of the kidneys characterized by marked edema, and albumin in the urine. However, the accumulation of body fluids is more frequently due to a primary disorder in the heart itself. In congestive heart failure, for example, the amount of blood pumped to the kidneys is upset and water accumulates in the body. Edema occurs in the lungs, preventing the proper amount of oxygen from getting to the lungs.

A current misuse of diuretics is for weight loss. The diuretics dehydrate the patient, and show a loss in weight. However, this is only a water loss which will be regained in a few days.

Each kidney is composed of a million or more functional units called nephrons, figure 29-1. Each nephron has a Bowman's capsule which encloses many capillaries. Waste products brought by the renal artery filter through the capillaries into the Bowman's capsule. Waste then goes through the collecting tubules to the renal pelvis and,

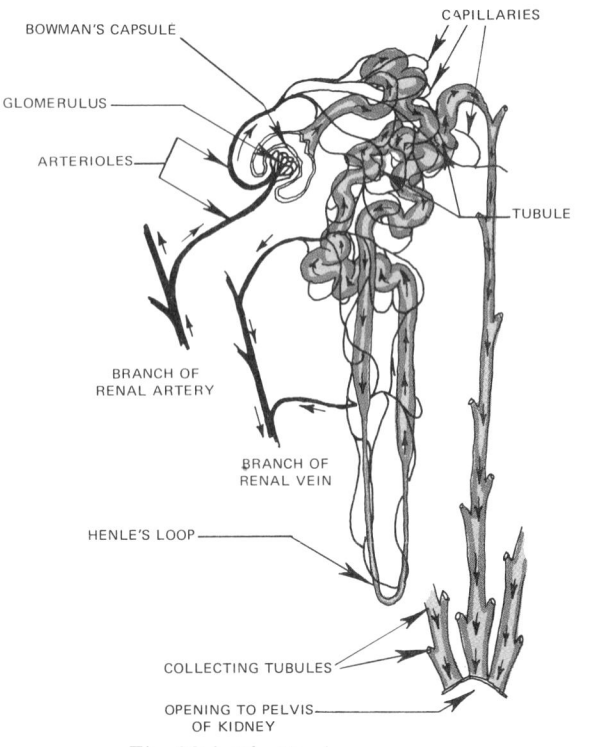

Fig. 29-1 The Nephron

in turn, down to the ureter, to the bladder, and is eliminated. Most of the filtered fluid, however, returns to the blood circulation.

DIURETICS

Urinary diuretics are medications which increase the amount of urine and sodium excreted, thus reducing the amount of fluid retained in the body and avoiding edema. The currently used diuretics fall into the following classifications:

- Osmotic diuretics
- Acid-forming diuretics
- Xanthine diuretics
- Mercurial diuretics
- Carbonic anhydrase inhibitors
- Hormone or steroid antagonists
- Thiazide compounds

Osmotic Diuretics

When two solutions of different concentrations are separated by a membrane, the solvent flow from the less concentrated solution to the more highly concentrated solution to equalize the percentage of solute in both solutions. This equalization process is called osmosis. In the kidney, the renal threshold determines how much of a certain substance can be reabsorbed by the tubules. When this threshold is exceeded, the body tries to equalize the concentration on both sides of the membranes. To balance the concentration, a greater amount of water must be excreted and diuresis results.

Glucose. Generally, the large amount of glucose in the Bowman's capsule is reabsorbed into the circulation. When the renal threshold is reached, glucose is excreted into the urine and large amounts of water are also excreted.

Urea. Urea is found normally in the body tissues. Carbamide is an example. To be effective, urea must be given in large doses. Much of it remains in the glomerular filtrate, thus increasing the urinary output.

Acid-forming Diuretics

Ammonium chloride and ammonium nitrate are acid-forming diuretics. They contain the NH_4 ion (ammonium) which, after the drug has been absorbed, is converted to urea in the liver. The large amount of urea promotes diuresis. Acidosis results from the presence of an excess of chloride ions, an effect of the conversion to urea.

Xanthine Diuretics

Xanthine diuretics are found in coffee, tea, and cocoa. Caffeine and aminophylline are the two most important xanthine diuretics.

Caffeine. Caffeine dimishes tubular reabsorption. It is seldom used as a medical diuretic because more effective drugs are available and because it has a short period of duration.

Section 5 Effects of Medications on Body Systems

Aminophylline. Aminophylline is a mild diuretic which increases the flow of urine moderately. It is also used in the treatment of severe bronchial asthma to relax the smooth muscles of the bronchioles. It is readily absorbed by all modes of administration: oral, intramusclar, intravenous, and rectal suppositories.

Mercurial Diuretics

The mercurial diuretics are the most reliable and effective of all the diuretics. They inhibit the work of the kidney tubule by inhibiting the reabsorption of fluid filtered through the glomeruli. As a result, the urinary output is practically doubled. The fact that most mercurial diuretics are required to be given by injection is difficult in many cases. The most widely used mercurials are: meralluride (Mercuhydrin), mersalyl and theophylline (Salyrgan-Theophylline), and mercaptomerin (Thiomerin).

Carbonic Anhydrase Inhibitors

These drugs prevent the action of an enzyme in the cells of the kidney tubules, resulting in the excretion of more water and sodium. Their mode of action is similar to the mercurials. Acetazolamide (Diamox) is an example of this type of drug.

Hormone Antagonists

An example of one of the hormone antagonists is spironolactone (Aldactone A). This medication antagonizes the function of the hormone aldosterone which increases sodium retention by the kidney. As a result, spironolactone decreases sodium retention. This drug has proved beneficial in overcoming edema caused by cirrhosis. In short, aldosterone increases sodium retention; spironolactone decreases sodium retention by the kidney.

Thiazide Compounds

Thiazide compounds were the first significantly effective oral diuretics. They act on the kidney tubules by supressing the reabsorption of sodium, potassium, and chloride ions resulting in increased urinary output. An example is chlorothiazide.

Because they also have antihypertensive effects, thiazide compounds are used in treating high blood pressure. They may also be used selectively for premenstrual tension and other emotional problems. With most thiazide diuretics, potassium is excreted and foods rich in potassium such as orange juice and bananas must be included in the diet. However, Dyazide is an exception. Dyazide is a potassium-sparing drug.

URINARY ANTISEPTICS

Urinary antiseptics are drugs used to treat minor infections of the urinary tract. Major infections are now treated with antibiotics and other chemotherapeutic drugs. Urinary antiseptics act best in an acid medium. Therefore, the nurse should provide cranberry juice in the diet.

Unit 29 Medications Used for Urinary System Disorders

Medication	Action	Administration and Dosage	Side Effects and/or Toxic Effects
Osmotic	produces diuresis by osmosis; urine output increases when renal threshold exceeded		
Urea (Carbamide)	diuretic	**p.o.**, based on wgt. 0.1 to 1 Gm per kg of body weight	gastric distress, vomiting
Glucose	diuretic	50 ml of 50% solution	thirst, headache, chills
Acid-Forming	is converted to urea in the liver		
Ammonium chloride	acidifier	**p.o.**, 8-12 Gm daily, divided doses	gastric distress
Xanthines	reduces tubular reabsorption		
Aminophylline	increases rate of urine formation	**p.o.**, 100-200 mg tablets I.M., 250-500 mg rectal, 125-500 mg	gastric discomfort, nausea, CNS symptoms: headache, anxiety, delirium, restlessness, convulsions, pain at injection site
Mercurials	inhibits reabsorption in kidney tubules		
Meralluride (Mercuhydrin)	diuretic	I.M., I.V. 1-2 ml, slowly 1 or 2 times a week	
Mercaptomerin (Thiomerin)	diuretic	s.c. or I.M. 0.5 to 2 ml rectal: 500 mg sup.	local tenderness after injection; personal sensitivity to mercurials
Chlormerodrin (Neohydrin)	diuretic	**p.o.**, 10 mg tablets 1-4 times daily	gastrointestinal upset
Carbonic Anhydrase Inhibitors	prevents action of enzyme in tubules		
Acetazolamide (Diamox)	diuretic; onset 1/2 hr. peaks in 2 hr., lasts 12 hr.	**p.o.**, I.V., 250-500 mg daily	drowsiness
Hormone Antagonists	antagonizes function of aldosterone to increase sodium retention		
Spironolactone (Aldactone A)	produces diuresis but minimizes potassium loss	**p.o.**, 25 mg q.i.d.	abdominal cramps, mental fogginess, skin rash

Fig. 29-2 Diuretics (continued on page 214)

Medication	Action	Administration and Dosage	Side Effects and/or Toxic Effects
Thiazides	suppresses reabsorption of sodium		
Chlorothiazide (Diuril)	diuretic; antihypertensive	p.o. I.V., 0.5 to 1 Gm daily	blood dyscrasias
Hydrochlorothiazide (Hydrodiuril) (Esidrix)	as above	p.o. 25-100 mg once or twice daily	as above
Methyclothiazide (Enduron)	as above	p.o., 2.5-10 mg per day	as above
Polythiazide (Renese)	as above	p.o., 1-4 mg per day	as above
Bendroflumethiazide (Naturetin)	diuretic	p.o., 2.5-10 mg per day	as above
Trichlormethiazide (Naqua) (Metahydrin)	diuretic	p.o., 2-4 mg per day	as above
Furosemide (Lasix)	rapidly absorbed; short duration, but potent; used in congestive heart failure, cirrhosis, nephrosis	p.o., 1-2 tablets of 40 mg daily in A.M.	dehydration, vascular collapse, thrombosis, embolism, hepatic coma; observe patient closely
Ethacrynic acid (Edecrin)	short duration but potent; used in acute pulmonary edema, renal edema, cirrhosis	p.o., 50-100 mg; in 50 mg tablets; I.V., 50 mg in 50 mg vials	severe diarrhea, severe loss of water; hepatic coma, weakness, dizziness, skin rash; observe patient closely
Others			
Chlorthalidone (Hygroton)	similar to chlorothiazide but has longer action	p.o., 100 to 200 mg per day	dizziness, nausea, blood dyscrasias
Quinethazone (Hydromox)	diuretic	p.o., 50-100 mg per day	as above
Dyazide	antihypertensive, diuretic, reduces reabsorption of sodium, chlorides, and water, spares potassium elimination	p.o., 1-4 capsules per day after meals	Dry mouth; headache, muscle cramps, dizziness, weakness, nausea, vomiting, G.I. disturbances

Fig. 29-2 Diuretics (continued from page 213)

Medication	Action	Administration and Dosage	Side Effects and/or Toxic Effects
Methenamine mandelate (Mandelamine)	antiseptic (urine must be acid)	**p.o.** 1-1.5 Gm q.i.d.	not ordered in hepatitis or renal insufficiency
Sulfisoxazole (Gantrisin)	sulfa product used in urinary infections	**p.o.** 2-4 Gm, then maintenance dose of 0.5-1 Gm q. 4-6h	nausea, vomiting, rash
Nitrofurantoin (Furadantin)	antibiotic	**p.o.** 100 mg q.i.d.	nausea, vomiting
Phenylazopyridine (Pyridium)	urinary analgesic and was formerly used as urinary antiseptic	**p.o.** 200 mg t.i.d. 100-200 mg t.i.d. a.c.	changes color of urine (red-orange)
Nalidixic acid (NegGram)	urinary antiseptic	**p.o.** 250-500 mg q.i.d. .5 to 1 Gm q.i.d.	rash and pruritus, convulsions occasionally (don't give to epileptics)

Fig. 29-3 Urinary Antiseptics

Acidifiers

Some drugs are used to increase the acidity of the urine because, when administering urinary antiseptics, an acid medium should be created. Ammonium chloride (p.o. 3-9 Gm or 8-12 Gm in divided doses daily) and sodium biphosphate (p.o. 0.6 Gm 1 to 6 times daily) may be used.

Alkalizers

Other drugs act to decrease the acidity of the urine. These are chiefly alkaline salts. They are usually dilutions of sodium and potassium. Sodium bicarbonate is often given routinely with sulfonamide drugs to make the urine alkaline.

SUGGESTED ACTIVITIES

- There are several mercurial diuretics. Investigate the action upon the kidneys which brings about diuresis.
- Investigate the diagnosis of three patients to whom diuretics were administered. How did these patients respond to the drug? Were these patients given a special diet? Did the patients' weight change during the administration of the drug? Were they permitted to drink all the fluids they wished?
- Kidney stones are fairly common. Find out why these develop in some people and not in others.
    a. Why are urinary antiseptics used in these cases?
    b. Why is morphine sulfate necessary in some of these cases?

Section 5 Effects of Medications on Body Systems

- The body builds up a resistance to antibiotics. Furadantin is a chemical which has not had this response. Investigate the drug and report your findings to the class.
- Select a urinary antiseptic and submit a written report describing the uses, dose, actions and nursing care.

REVIEW

A. Match the columns by placing the letter of the medication listed in Column II by its description in Column I.

	Column I		Column II
_G_	1. mercurial diuretic	a.	potassium carbonate
_I_	2. acidifier	b.	Furadantin
_E_	3. chemotherapy	c.	sodium biphosphate
_F_	4. urinary analgesic and antiseptic	d.	morphine sulfate
_J_	5. alkalizer	e.	Gantrisin
_B_	6. antibiotic	f.	Pyridium
_A_	7. oral alkalizer used especially during sulfonamide therapy	g.	Mercuhydrin
		h.	Diamox
_H_	8. oral medication which acts on kidneys to eliminate fluid from body	i.	ammonium chloride
		j.	sodium bicarbonate
_C_	9. oral acidifier and diuretic	k.	salyrgan

B. Answer the following questions.

1. What are the two functions of the kidney? (1) To purify the blood by removing the waste products of metabolism (2) To regulate the loss of water and electrolytes in order to keep the body fluids stable in composition.

2. Describe the action of the following diuretics:

   a. Osmotic - it equalizes the pressure in the kidney

   b. Acid-forming - converts urea in the liver in the cells of the kidney tubules re

   c. Carbon anhydrase inhibitors - prevents the action of enzymes in the cells of the kidney tubules, resulting in the excretion of more water and sodium

   d. Hormone antagonists - it antagonizes the function of the hormone aldosterone which increases sodium retention by the kidney

   e. Thiazide compounds - they suppress the reabsorption of sodium, potassium, and chloride ions resulting in increased urinary output.

3. Why are diuretics ordered for congestive heart failure? *To alleviate the water pressure of (on) the heart.*

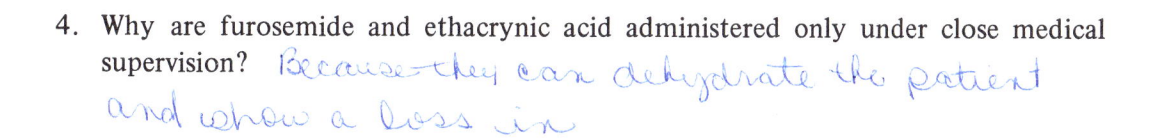

4. Why are furosemide and ethacrynic acid administered only under close medical supervision? *Because they can dehydrate the patient and show a loss in*

5. Is an alkaline or acid urine desirable when administering urinary antiseptics? *Acid*

C. Select the correct response.

1. Xanthine diuretics are found in all but one of the following
    a. coffee
    b. *milk*
    c. cocoa
    d. tea

2. Diuril is a/an
    a. thiazide compound diuretic
    b. mercurial diuretic
    c. Xanthine diuretic
    d. osmotic diuretic

3. Minor infections of the urinary tract are treated with
    a. urinary antiseptics
    b. chemotherapeutic drugs
    c. antibiotics
    d. forcing of fluids

EXTENDED STUDY

Learn the meaning and proper use of the following terms:

Addison's disease
acromegaly
basal metabolism rate
cortex
cretinism
diabetes mellitus
endocrine
glycosuria

hormone
hypoglycemia
hyperthyroidism
hypophysis
hypothyroidism
medulla
metabolism
myxedema

Unit 30 Medications Used in Treatment of Endocrine Conditions

OBJECTIVES

After studying this unit, the student should be able to:
- Identify the hormones secreted by the endocrine glands and state their functions.
- List important toxic and side effects of hormone therapy.
- Associate hormone deficiencies with the conditions they cause.

The endocrine system is composed of a number of ductless glands which secrete chemical compounds called hormones. Hormones are secreted into and carried by the bloodstream to specific organs which they stimulate or inhibit.

The most important endocrine glands include the pituitary gland in the skull, the thyroid gland in the throat, the parathyroid glands located on the thyroid glands, the pancreas located in back of the stomach, the adrenal glands over the kidneys, and the sex glands, or gonads, figure 30-1. All these glands work together to help the organism to grow and develop normally and to carry on the normal functions of the healthy person. If this coordination of body function is upset, serious conditions arise that require medical treatment.

THE PITUITARY GLAND

The *pituitary* gland (hypophysis) is called the master gland because it exerts control over the other endocrine glands. This gland is located at the base of the brain within the *sella turcica*, a small bony cavity at the base of the skull. The pituitary gland is composed of three parts, the anterior lobe, the posterior lobe, and the pars intermedia. The latter is a group of secreting cells about which little is known. We have evidence that the anterior lobe discharges at least six hormones which, in turn, regulate other endocrine glands, figure 30-2.

The improper functioning of the pituitary gland can cause marked clinical conditions.
- Hypofunction: if previous to puberty, underactivity of the gland

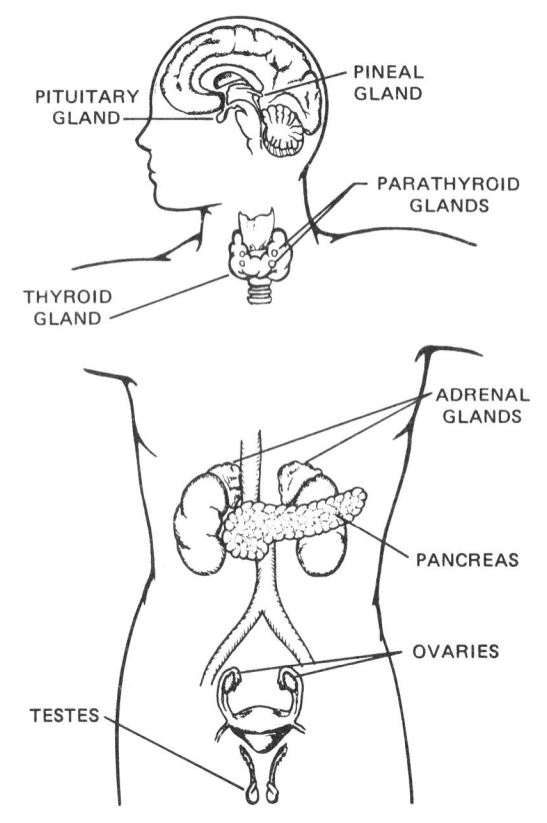

Fig. 30-1 Location of the Endocrine Glands

ANTERIOR LOBE

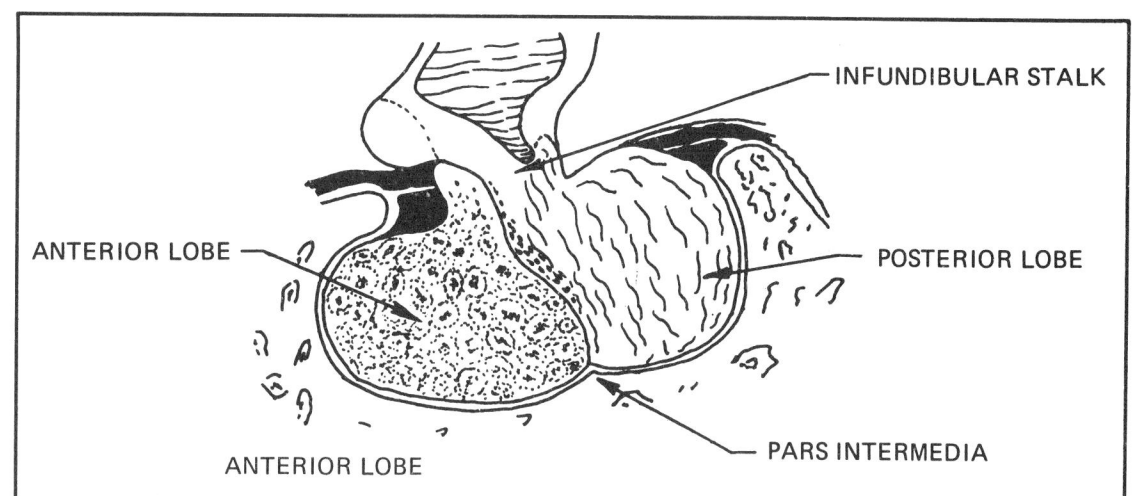

LTH (Lactogenic Hormone): stimulates mammary glands and production of progesterone.

TSH (Thyrotropic Hormone): stimulates thyroid gland.

LH (Luteinizine Hormone): stimulates maturity of Graafian follicle and ovulation in female; testosterone in male.

ACTH (Adrenocorticotropic Hormone, Corticotropin): stimulates cortex of adrenal gland to secrete glucocorticoids, mineralcorticoids and androgens.

STH (Growth Hormone, Somatrotrophic Hormone): stimulates growth of bones and organs.

FSH (Follicular-Stimulating Hormone): stimulates secretion of estrogen in female and production of sperm in male.

MSH (Melanocyte-Stimulating Hormone): influences deposition of melanin in skin; absence cause albinism.

POSTERIOR LOBE

Oxytocin: stimulates uterine muscles to contract.

ADH (Antidiuretic Hormone, Vasopressin): stimulates intestinal muscles and superficial blood vessels to contract; maintains water balance by reducing urinary output.

Fig. 30-2 The Pituitary Gland

can cause dwarfism and poor growth and functioning of the thyroid gland, sex glands, and adrenal cortex.

- Hyperfunction: if occuring before puberty, overactivity of the gland can cause gigantism. If occuring after puberty, when the epiphyses of the long bones have become complete, the feet, hands, and face will show overgrowth. This condition is known as acromegaly.

Due to the dominance of the pituitary gland and its interrelation with other endocrine glands, the many effects of endocrine therapy are carefully weighed by the physician before he prescribes hormones. ACTH (corticotropin) is used extensively. ACTH stimulates the adrenal cortex to produce cortisone and hydrocortisone. Adrenocorticotropic Hormone, ACTH and Corticotropin are terms used for the same hormone.

THYROID GLAND

The thyrotropic hormone (TSH) from the anterior lobe of the pituitary gland regulates the activity of the thyroid gland. There are two closely related hormones produced

Section 5 Effects of Medications on Body Systems

Medication	Action	Administration and Dosage	Side Effects and/or Toxic Effects
Anterior Lobe			
TSH (Thyrotropin) (Thytropar)	stimulates thyroid gland to release thryoid hormone	I.M. or s.c. 10 units diluted in 2 ml sodium chloride	headache, irritability, restlessness, rapid pulse, bowel hypermotility, sweating, menstrual irregularities. Contraindicated: coronary thrombosis or untreated Addison's disease.
ACTH (Adrenocorticotropic hormone) (Acthar) (Acthar gel) (Corticotropin) (Depo-ACTH)	stimulates adrenal cortex to secrete cortisone; normal adrenal glands are essential to its success	I.M. ampules 10-40 I.V. units 10-25 units q.6h. average adult dose: I.M. 20U q. 6h. I.V. 5-20U q. 8h.	may induce diabetes; cautious use with cardiac failure; interferes with healing of wounds, rounded face, striae of skin, edema
Sterile corticotropin (Zinc hydroxide suspension)	as above; prolonged action	I.M. 40 units initially then 20U 2 or 3 times a week	as above
Posterior Lobe			
Vasopressin (Pitressin)	antidiuretic; used in diabetes insipidus therapy	20 units/ml dose is 20U s.c. or I.M.	coronary artery constriction, general cramps
Oxytocin (Pitocin)	improves uterine contractions in obstetrics; stops post partum bleeding	10-20 units 5-10U I.M.-post partum, 10U in 1000 ml 5% glucose in water I.V. to induce labor	rupture of uterus
Posterior pituitary extract	same uses as vasopressin and oxytocin	10U/ml dose .3 to 1 ml	as above

Fig. 30-3 Pituitary hormonal drugs

by the gland: thyroxin and triiodothyronine (T3). Both hormones have essentially the same action in their effect on *metabolism* (the rate at which foods are burned in the tissues). Iodine is necessary for the production of these hormones, and it is stored in the thyroid gland. When the thyroid hormones are produced in excessive amounts, the patient suffers from hyperthyroidism and has a high basal metabolism rate. Too small a secretion causes the opposite effect and the patient has hypothyroidism with a low basal metabolism rate. In a child, hypothyroidism results in cretinism; in an adult, myxedema. Hyperthyroidism results in exophthalmic goiter (Graves' disease).

Hyperthyroidism

Hyperthyroidism (oversecretion of the thyroid hormones) is usually medically treated by the following:

- Radioactive iodine I^{131} is used to treat certain cases of hyperthyroidism and selected cases of cancer of the thyroid.
    Dosage: Oral capsules: 1-100 microcuries

- Propylthiouracil: Interferes with the making of thyroid hormones by the thyroid gland. It is used to control the symptoms in Graves' disease and in toxic goiter as well as to prepare the patient for thyroid surgery by reducing basal metabolism.
    Dosage: p.o. 50 mg q.8h., usually is increased for severe hyperthyroidism

- Methylthiouracil (Methiacil, Muracil, Thimecil)
    Dosage: p.o. 200 mg daily in divided doses

- Methimazole (Tapazole)
    Dosage: p.o. 5-10 mg q.8h. initially

Hypothyroidism

Myxedema and cretinism (undersecretion of thyroid hormone) may be treated medically with:

- Sodium Liothyronine (Cytomel)
    Dosage: 5-200 micrograms daily

- Levothyroxine sodium (Synthroid)
    Dosage: p.o. 0.1 mg to 0.6 mg daily, preferably before breakfast

Cretinism often occurs in the "Goiter Belt" of the midwestern United States. (People living in this area may have diets deficient in iodine.) If the child is started on a thyroid product early in life, he will develop normally. If not, he may remain dull mentally and show various growth deficiencies, such as dry skin, thick tongue, coarse hair, etc.

Patients on thyroid must be watched for toxicity — rapid pulse, headache, gastric upsets, insomnia and nervousness. The nurse should take the patient's pulse before each dose and if the pulse is 100 or over, withhold the drug and notify the physician. Surgical removal of the thyroid gland and radiation therapy for cancer of the thyroid results in the need for replacement therapy.

PARATHYROID GLANDS

The parathyroid glands, located on top of each thyroid lobe, secrete parathormone. This hormone regulates calcium and phosphorus metabolism and affects the irritability of nerves and muscles. It has a considerable influence on bone formation.

The nurse should observe the patient for muscle spasms and convulsions. Parathyroid deficiency may be treated with:

- Parathyroid extract
    Dosage: I.M. 40 units q.12h.

Section 5 Effects of Medications on Body Systems

ADRENAL GLANDS

There are two adrenal glands; one is located on top of each kidney. Each gland consists of two distinct parts, the outer cortex and the inner medulla, each of which secretes different hormones. Its hormones are secreted when the gland is stimulated by ACTH from the anterior lobe of the pituitary gland. Its chief functions are to regulate fat, salt, and water metabolism and to produce anti-inflammatory effects on the body. It secretes three important hormones:

- Cortisone and hydrocortisone which are secreted by the cortex of the adrenal.
- Epinephrine and norepinephrine, secreted by the medulla of the adrenal. They are powerful stimulants which stimulate the heart, constrict the blood vessels, increase the rate of carbohydrate metabolism, and stimulate the central nervous system.

Addison's disease is a progressive condition of adrenal insufficiency. The patient's skin becomes a copper color with mottled marks. Nausea and vomiting become increasingly severe, and there is danger of dehydration and circulatory collapse. Adrenal cortex hormones (corticosteroids) are used to treat this condition.

Cortisone and hydrocortisone are good anti-inflammatory medications. These hormones are administered in cases of bursitis, rheumatoid arthritis, and topically in certain skin diseases. They offer only temporary relief from any condition. When the hormone is stopped, the symptoms of the disease reappear. Dosage varies widely, depending on the severity of the disease. Continued use may cause hirsutism (hairy face), "moon face," and muscular weakness, as well as retention of salt and water in the body. These hormones are dangerous in that they suppress pain and discomfort from gastric ulcers, tuberculosis, and severe infections. Newer synthetic products, called corticoids, have fewer side effects and have greater relative potency than cortisone.

The corticosteroids should be given with meals or milk since peptic ulcers may result from therapy. Refer to the charts in the unit on musculoskeletal disorders (next unit, figures 31-3 and 31-4) for more details regarding corticosteroid and corticoid preparations.

THE PANCREAS

Insulin is the hormone secreted by the islets of Langerhans which are embedded throughout the pancreas. Like all hormones, the secretion is poured directly into the bloodstream. Acting as a catalyst, insulin metabolizes sugar rapidly; it is essential to carbohydrate (starch and sugars) metabolism. An undersecretion of insulin will produce symptoms of diabetes mellitus; an oversecretion will produce *insulin shock*.

Hypoglycemic reactions of the diabetic patient are due to low blood sugar because of the administration of an overdose of insulin or because the patient has not eaten his entire prescribed diet. A simple sugar as is found in orange juice will usually build the blood sugar to the desired level. However, the patient taking PZI insulin will need more substantial nourishment following the use of orange juice. Crackers and milk will provide adequate and more lasting calories to balance the insulin taken.

Medication	Absorption and Peak Times	Administration and Duration	Side and/or Toxic Effects
Insulin	acts as catalyst in cell metabolism to replace deficient glandular secretion of insulin	subcutaneous; units prescribed; always check expiration date on vial	weakness, sweating, nervousness, fall in blood pressure, pallor, anxiety
Regular (crystalline)	as above: rapid action within hour or less; peak 2-4 hrs.	subcutaneous; administered 30 min. before meals; Duration 5-8 hours.	as above
Globin zinc insulin	as above; intermediate action 2-4 hrs.; peak effect 6-10 hours	s.c. given once daily, 1 hr. before breakfast Duration 18-24 hours	as above
Isophane insulin (NPH)	as above; intermediate action 2-4 hrs.; peak effect 8-12 hours	s.c. given once daily 1 hr. before breakfast; thoroughly mix by rotating vial gently Duration 28-30 hours	as above
Lente insulin	as above; intermediate action 2-4 hrs.; peak effect 8-12 hours	s.c. given once daily 1 hr. before breakfast; thoroughly mix; Duration 28-32 hours	as above
Protamine zinc (PZI)	as above; slow action 4-6 hrs.; peak effect 16-24 hours	s.c.; administered 1/2 to 1 hr. before breakfast or supper once a day; thoroughly mix solution by rotating gently between palms Duration 24-36 hours	as above
Ultra lente insulin	as above; slow action 8 hrs.; peak effect 16-24 hours	s.c. 1 hr. before breakfast; Duration 36 or more hrs. thoroughly mix	as above

Fig. 30-4 Types of insulin

Types of insulin are described in figure 30-4. Before using any insulin, the nurse should always check the expiration date on the vial of insulin. She should also thoroughly mix NPH, PZI, Lente and Ultra-Lente insulins by gently rotating the vial between the palms before withdrawing the dose. The insulin must be measured accurately and the right syringe used; insulin syringe with U40 markings should be used when U40 insulin (vial) is administered, U80 syringe for U80 insulin, etc.

Oral medications used in the treatment of certain types of diabetes are available. They are not used in complicated cases or

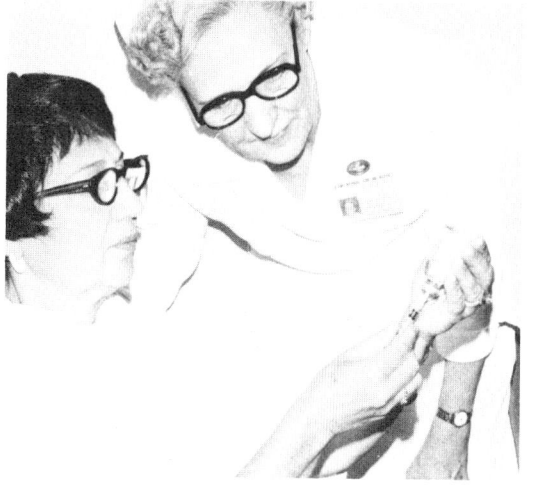

Fig. 30-5 Insulin must be measured accurately and the right syringe used.

223

Insulin Overdose (Insulin Reaction)	Diabetic Coma (Deficiency of Insulin)
Rapid development of symptoms	Slow development of symptoms, more rapid in the child
Skin cold and clammy	Skin hot and dry
Trembling, twitching of lips, mental confusion	Fruity odor to breath
Double vision	Extreme thirst, nausea, vomiting
Shallow breathing	Deep heavy breathing
Hunger	Loss of consciousness
Loss of consciousness	
Convulsions occasionally	
NPH insulin overdose has a slow reaction occurring late in day	
Treatment: Insulin Overdose	**Treatment: Diabetic Coma**
Give orange juice with or without sugar.	Check urine; it will have a heavy sugar content.
Check urine; it will probably be sugar-free.	Call physician for order of regular insulin and further direction.
Call physician for further direction.	

Fig. 30-6 Symptoms and treatment of insulin reactions

for young diabetics. The patient is required to continue on a diabetic diet and to remain under close medical supervision during their administration. These drugs are not substitutes for insulin but are synthetic compounds. Those listed are scored tablets given in divided dosages.

Gastrointestinal symptoms such as nausea and loss of appetite may follow long-continued administration of these drugs. The oral antidiabetic drugs are readily absorbed. They are excreted by the kidneys in 12-24 hours. The most frequent difficulty is excessive lowering of the blood sugar accompanied by its toxic reaction. They are contraindicated in pregnancy because of possible harm to the fetus. The following are the commonly used oral antidiabetic drugs.

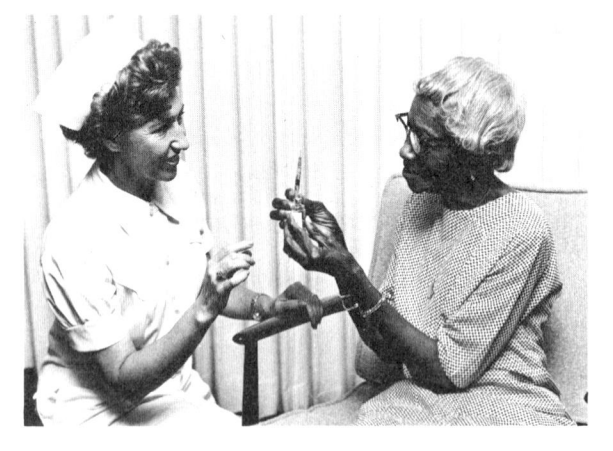

Fig. 30-7 Patients are taught how to measure and administer their own insulin.

- Tolbutamide (Orinase) Side effects are common.
    Dosage: 500 mg tablets available

- Chlorpropamide (Diabinese) Reactions more common than with Orinase. Drug rash, liver damage, nervous symptoms.
    Dosage: 100-250 mg tablets available

- Acetohexamide (Dymelor)
    Dosage: 250-500 mg tablets available

- Phenformin (DBI)
    Dosage: 25 mg and 50 mg tablets available

THE GONADS

The gonads are the sex organs. In the female they are the ovaries; in the male, the testes. The functions of the gonads and the hormones they secrete are directed by the pituitary gland. A discussion of medications used will be covered in Unit 33 which deals with drugs that affect the reproductive system.

SUGGESTED ACTIVITIES

- The nurse must have the proper measuring syringe to match the strength of the insulin to be administered. Investigate the official unit measuring scale of syringes being currently manufactured. Discuss your findings in class.

- Review urine testing for the presence of sugar. Tes-Tape, and Clinitest tablets are the most popular to the layperson. Since urine testing is part of diabetic detection, control, and instruction regarding insulin intake, each student should be able to test urine for the presence or absence of glucose and acetone.

- Select a patient with a glandular disorder. Study the chart and prepare a report for class discussion. In the report include the causes, signs and symptoms, treatment, and nursing care of the patient.

REVIEW

A. Complete the following chart.

Kind of Insulin	Absorption Time	Peak Effect	Duration
Regular insulin	1 HR OR LESS	2-4 HRS	5-8 HRS
Globin zinc insulin	18-24 HRS	2-4 HRS	6-10 HRS
Protamine zinc insulin	24-36 HRS	4-6 HRS	16-24 HRS
NPH insulin	28-30 HRS	2-4 HRS	8-12 HRS
Lente insulin	28-32 HRS	2-4 HRS	8-12 HRS
Ultra-lente insulin	36 OR MORE	8 HRS	16-24 HRS

Section 5 Effects of Medications on Body Systems

B. Match the items in Column I with their description in Column II.

Column I

H 1. ACTH
J 2. cortisone
A 3. epinephrine and norepinephrine
L 4. insulin
G 5. thyroxin
___ 6. Orinase
C 7. sella turcica
D 8. lactogenic hormone
F 9. ADH factor
E 10. cretinism

Column II

a. secreted by the medulla of the adrenal glands
b. an oral tablet used by an older diabetic to lower the blood sugar
c. a bony cavity in which the pituitary gland is housed
d. stimulates mammary glands to secrete milk
e. hypothyroidism in childhood due to lack of secretion of thyroid hormones
f. maintains water balance; reduces output of urine
g. secreted by the thyroid gland
h. stimulates the cortex of the adrenal gland to secrete cortisone
i. Graafian follicle
j. secreted by the cortex of the adrenal gland
k. growth hormone
l. secreted by islets of Langerhans in pancreas

C. Answer the following questions.

1. Name the two hormones secreted by the posterior lobe of the pituitary gland. Describe their functions. (1) Oxytocin - Stimulates uterine muscles to contract. (2) ADH (Antidiuretic Hormone) - Stimulates intestinal muscle and superficial blood vessels to contract; maintain water balance by reducing urinary output

2. State the relationship between iodine and the thyroid hormones.
(A) Iodine - is necessary for production of hormones
(B) Thyroid -

3. What side effects may occur in patients on thyroid therapy?
Toxicity - rapid pulse, headache, gastric upsets, insomnia, and nervousness

Unit 30 Medications Used in Treatment of Endocrine Conditions

4. What are the functions of epinephrine and norepinephrine?

    They stimulate the heart, constrict the blood vessels, increase the rate of carbohydrates metabolism, and stimulates the central nervous system

5. Differentiate between insulin overdose and diabetic coma by stating three symptoms which are opposites.

Insulin Overdose	Diabetic Coma
rapid development of symptoms	slow development of symptoms (more in child)
skin cold & clammy	skin, hot and dry
Trembling, twitching of lips, mental confusion	Fruity odor to breath

EXTENDED STUDY

Learn the meaning and proper use of the following terms:

> analgesic
>
> anticoagulant
>
> corticosteroid
>
> corticoid
>
> curariform
>
> cyanosis
>
> edema

227

Unit 31 Medications Used for Musculoskeletal System Disorders

OBJECTIVES

After studying this unit, the student should be able to:

- State the purpose of analgesics.
- List important desirable and adverse reactions to specific drugs used to relieve conditions of the musculoskeletal system.

The skeleton gives the body its shape, protects the internal organs, and forms a place for attachment of the muscles. The movement of the body is dependent upon the muscles. Bones are unable to contract because of the hard layers of calcium of which they are made; therefore, we must depend upon the four hundred or more different muscles which make up nearly one-half of our body weight to move these bones. The musculoskeletal system is made up of muscles and bones and the ligaments and tendons which support them. Because it is made up of living tissue, the musculoskeletal system is subject to as many ailments as other systems. For treatment of these ailments, drugs and hormones are very often prescribed.

The medications shown in figures 31-1 through 31-4 are used for treatment of disorders of the musculoskeletal system. An explanation of their functions, methods of administration, average dosage, and symptoms to report to the doctor or charge nurse are included.

The student should review the anatomy and physiology of the musculoskeletal system in order to understand the action of drugs included in this unit.

ANALGESICS

Analgesics are drugs used to relieve pain. Two of the most commonly used of these are aspirin (acetylsalicylic acid) and salicylates which are salt forms of salicylic acid. While these drugs are seldom dangerous when taken in their prescribed dosages, some people are sensitive to them. Aspirin, for example, may cause stomach upsets, severe hives, and swelling of the skin and mucous membranes in hypersensitive persons. Aspirin is not usually prescribed when the patient is taking anticoagulants because of interactions affecting coagulation time. Figure 31-1 gives analgesics specifically ordered to relieve pain affecting the musculoskeletal system. Other kinds of analgesics are described in Unit 32.

Unit 31 Medications Used for Musculoskeletal System Disorders

Medication	Action	Administration and Dosage	Side Effects and/or Toxic Effects
Acetylsalicylic acid (aspirin)	relieves pain of arthritic conditions	p.o. 0.6 Gm q. 3-4h.	ringing in ears, rash, dizziness, sweating, nausea, heartburn, bleeding
Sodium salicylate	relieves pain of arthritic conditions, rheumatic fever	p.o., I.V., I.M. 0.6 Gm q. 2-4h.	as above
Ibuprofen (Motrin)	relieves pain and stiffness of arthritis. Reduces swelling, improves grip strength and joint flexion	p.o. 300 mg white, 400 mg orange tabs q.i.d.	nausea, vomiting, blurred vision, itching of skin
APC Capsules (Aspirin compound) (Empirin compound)	relieves pain	combination of acetylsalicylic acid, acetophenetidin, caffeine; p.o. .3 to .6 Gm q.4h.	habituation
(Anacin)	relieves pain	combination of aspirin and caffeine	habituation
Acetanilid	relieves pain	p.o. 0.2 Gm q.4h.	difficult breathing, cold sweat, irregular pulse, cyanosis, subnormal temperature
Acetaminophen (Tylenol) (Apamide)	relieves pain, non-addictive	p.o. 0.3 Gm tablets	none
Phenylbutazone (Butazolidin)	relieves pain, inflammation of arthritic conditions	p.o. 300-600 mg initial dose; then 100-200 mg daily	edema; agranulocytosis
Propoxyphene (Darvon)	relieves pain; used when aspirin is contraindicated as in bleeding	p.o. 32 and 65 mg capsules 4 times daily	none
Indomethacin (Indocin)	relieves pain, inflammation	p.o. 25 mg tablets 2-3 times daily	peptic ulceration, gastric irritation, headache, dizziness, bone marrow depression, skin rashes

Fig. 31-1 Analgesics

Section 5 Effects of Medications on Body Systems

Medication	Action	Administration and Dosage	Side Effects and/or Toxic Effects
Tubocurarine (Curare)	skeletal muscle relaxant; aids in anesthesia	I.V. 0.5-3.0 mg	respiratory depressant; cardiac accelerator; paralysis of muscles may indicate overdose or toxic reaction
Gallamine triethiodide (Flaxedil)	as above	I.V. 50-60 mg (average dose)	as above
Decamethonium bromide (Syncurine)	as above	I.V. 0.5-3.0 mg	as above
Carisoprodol (Rela) (Soma)	skeletal muscle relaxant; closely related to meprobamate	250, 300 and 350 mg tablets; usually q.i.d.	value to be proven
Methocarbamol (Robaxin)	skeletal muscle relaxant	0.5 and 0.75 Gm tablets usually q.i.d.	value to be proven
Succinylcholine (Anectine) (Sucostrin)	brief action; like curariform drugs; used in anesthesia and shock therapy	I.V. by slow drip single-injection; vials 10 cc with 20 mg per cc	respiratory depressant; cautious use in malnutrition cases; liver disease and anemia

Fig. 31-2 Muscle Relaxants

Medication	Action	Administration and Dosage	Side Effects and/or Toxic Effects
Cortisone (Cortone)	relieves pain of arthritis rheumatic fever; anti-inflammatory agent	**p.o.** 25-100 mg, I.M. 300 mg 1st day, then 100 mg daily thereafter	hypertension, hairiness and moonlike contour of face, change in glucose tolerance, edema
Hydrocortisone (Cortef) (Hydrocortone)	used in treating some types of arthritis; anti-inflammatory agent	**p.o.** 20 mg 2-3 times a day; I.V., I.M.: 10-100 mg; Topical: 1% lotion	same as above
ACTH (Adrenocorticotropic hormone) (Acthar Gel) (Cortrophin)	stimulates adrenal cortex to produce cortisone and hydrocortisone; anti-inflammatory agent	I.M., I.V. 10-40 units (ampule pulv., Acthar Gel)	hypertension, hairiness and moonlike contour of face, edema, elevated blood sugar

Fig. 31-3 Corticosteroids

Medication	Action	Administration and Dosage	Side Effects and/or Toxic Effects
Prednisolone (Meticortelone) (Delta-Cortef)	synthetic; less risk of side effects than hormones; relieves severe joint pain	injected into joint space, 25-30 mg; tablets and ointments also available	hypertension, hairiness and moonlike contour of face, edema, elevated blood sugar
Methylprednisolone (Medrol)	synthetic; anti-inflammatory	p.o., 2, 4 and 16 mg tablets	as above
Clinoril (Sulindac)	anti-inflammatory agent: osteoarthritis, gouty arthritis	200-400 mg b.i.d. with food	gastrointestinal upset, nausea, anorexia
Dexamethasone (Decadron) (Deronil) (Gammacorten)	synthetic; similar to hydrocortisone; very potent; does not retain salt and water	p.o. 0.75 mg tablets I.M. 4 mg per cc	osteoporosis, other effects as above

Fig. 31-4 Corticoids

MUSCLE RELAXANTS

The drug most commonly used as a muscle relaxant is curare. It is a highly toxic drug obtained from a tropical plant family and functions so as to paralyze motor nerve endings. It was first used by South American Indians for poisoning the tips of their arrows. Early Spanish explorers who encountered these arrows very appropriately named the poison "curare", meaning "he to whom it comes, falls." Drugs used to relax muscles are called curariform after the drug. Curare and curariform drugs are given by the anesthesiologist before surgery to increase the effectiveness of anesthesia. The medication enables less potent anesthesia to be given in smaller amounts. Chlorpromazine and meprobamate, commonly used as tranquilizers, are sometimes ordered for muscle relaxation.

CORTICOSTEROIDS AND CORTICOIDS

Drugs such as cortisone and hydrocortisone are hormones which are produced by the cortex of the adrenal gland. Adrenocorticotropic hormone or ACTH as it is commonly called, is produced by the anterior pituitary gland. They are called corticosteroids and affect the musculoskeletal system. They are prescribed when the patient's body is deficient in its production of these hormones.

While corticosteroids cannot cure disease, they provide relief from such conditions as Addison's disease, rheumatic fever, arthritis and certain allergies. They also have an antiinflammatory effect that is very important. Corticosteroids may have important effects on the mineral and water balance in the body. Synthetic drugs, called corticoids, are more potent and less toxic.

Section 5 Effects of Medications on Body Systems

LOCAL APPLICATION

Of the local medications used for diseases of the musculoskeletal system, the most commonly used is oil of wintergreen, also known as methyl salicylate. Applied to the skin, it acts as a counterirritant, relieving pain by producing a superficial irritation which is intended to relieve an already present irritation. If the oil is rubbed in too vigorously, it may cause extreme and undesirable effects due to rapid absorption.

SUGGESTED ACTIVITIES

- Study the charts of four patients receiving hydrocortisone for various conditions. From your study determine:

    a. The patient's diagnosis

    b. The length of time the patient has been taking the steroid

    c. Any signs of permanent improvement or symptoms of adverse reactions

    d. Appropriate nursing care to be taken

- Refer to an appropriate text and study the two recognized types of arthritis. Distinguish between the two types. Which type is relieved by steroid therapy? Be prepared to discuss your findings with the class.

- Investigate the reason why aspirin is not administered to patients taking anticoagulants.

REVIEW

A. Answer the following questions.

1. The nurse must realize that aspirin can be dangerous under the following two conditions.

2. If a surgical patient were given an injection of 0.4 mg of curare by the anesthesiologist, what effect would be produced?

3. Is cortisone manufactured by the body or is it synthetic? Explain your answer.

Unit 31 Medications Used for Musculoskeletal System Disorders

B. Complete the table by filling in the reactions associated with the drugs which are listed.

Drug	Desirable Reactions	Undesirable Reactions
Hydrocortisone		
ACTH		
Propoxyphene		
Ibuprofen (Motrin)		
Acetylsalicylic acid		
Sodium salicylate		
Prednisolone		

EXTENDED STUDY

Learn the meaning and proper use of the following terms:

adrenergic-stimulating agent	habituation
adrenergic-blocking agent	hypnotic
analeptic	intraocular
analgesic	interoceptor
anticonvulsant	local anesthetic
barbiturate	miotic
conjunctiva	mydriatic
exteroceptor	narcotic
glaucoma	sedative
general anesthetic	strabismus

233

Unit 32 Medications that Affect the Nervous System

OBJECTIVES

After studying this unit, the student should be able to:

- Identify the action of stimulants, depressants, narcotics, analgesics, barbiturates, anesthesias and anticonvulsants.
- State the toxic effects of narcotics, barbiturates and amphetamines.
- Compare the effects of adrenergic-stimulating and adrenergic-blocking agents.
- State the difference between miotics and mydriatics.
- Explain why silver nitrate eye drops are given to the newborn.
- Discuss the effect of certain eye medications on glaucoma.
- Name drugs used for specific eye infections.

The nervous system is composed of the central nervous system (the brain and spinal cord) and the peripheral nervous system. Working together, they coordinate many essential functions that keep us alive and constantly adjusting to life.

The central nervous system is concerned with coordination and control of all the functions of the body. It has the ability to receive and transmit stimuli to and from the higher center, the cortex of the cerebrum. The cortex of the brain is the center of highest mental process that controls thought, reason, judgment, memory, and learning. The central nervous system enables us to respond to stimuli from our environment.

The nurse must know how various drugs affect people in order to be able to observe patients, report observations intelligently, and take appropriate action. The brain can be either stimulated or depressed. We read a great deal about actions resulting from people taking amphetamine tablets such as Benzedrine. We read of others "taking trips" on L.S.D. We read of others committing acts beyond their control after becoming addicted to sedatives and narcotics. However, drugs can be used in many beneficial ways when properly controlled.

STIMULANTS

Drugs which stimulate the higher centers help us think and make judgments faster than would happen otherwise. Although there are many drugs used as central nervous systems stimulants, there are two groups which have medicinal value. These are the respiratory stimulants and stimulants used to overcome the effects of depression.

Respiratory stimulants were discussed in Unit 27. Stimulants tend to restore consciousness, raise the blood pressure, and make the patient mentally alert again. The chief central nervous system stimulants are: xanthines, amphetamines, and miscellaneous agents such as cerebrospinal stimulants.

Xanthines

Caffeine is an example of xanthine. It stimulates the cerebral cortex so the person is more alert, thinks faster and reacts faster.

Caffeine stimulates the heart muscle, increasing the heart rate and output. There is a slight but temporary rise in the blood pressure. It temporarily stimulates urinary secretion by increasing glomerular filtration. Caffeine is not usually given to patients with gastric ulcers because it stimulates the output of gastric pepsin and hydrochloric acid.

Amphetamines

The *amphetamines* are synthetic, habit-forming drugs which stimulate the cerebral cortex. They overcome fatigue, increase the desire to work, alertness, and talkativeness. Continued use causes sleeplessness, irritability, dizziness and loss of appetite. Large doses are frequently followed by depression.

Amphetamines may be used to treat mild cases of depression following childbirth and in old age, and to alleviate chronic fatigue. They are sometimes used to reduce the appetite of those trying to overcome obesity although other methods of weight reduction are preferred. The amphetamines are not given in cases of hypertension and cardiovascular disease. They are also contraindicated for anxious and excited patients. Side effects include dryness of mouth, headache, insomnia, irritability and constipation.

Cerebrospinal Stimulants

Cerebrospinal stimulants are drugs which increase the activity of the brain and spinal cord. They tend to markedly increase the blood pressure and stimulate alertness. They are frequently ordered as antidepressants for depressed patients, as indicated in Unit 25.

DEPRESSANTS

Depressants act to make us less concerned with our environment. They decrease our ability to concentrate. Of course, the individual's reaction to them has a great deal to do with his fundamental personality.

Depressants are classified in the following three ways: analgesics which relieve pain; sedatives and hypnotics which produce rest and sleep; and general anesthetics which produce loss of sensation and unconsciousness.

Analgesics

Analgesics should be strong enough to relieve pain for the required period. They should have minimum side effects such as nausea, vomiting, respiratory depression, and constipation, should act promptly, causing little sedation, and should be inexpensive.

Narcotics

Narcotics are addictive drugs, derived from cocaine and derivatives of opium, such as morphine and codeine. They provide relief from pain and induce sleep, depending on the dosage.

Section 5 Effects of Medications on Body Systems

Medication	Action	Administration and Dosage	Side Effects and/or Toxic Effects
Class: Xanthines			
Caffeine	mild CNS stimulant, increases heart rate, respiration, dilates most blood vessels, (constricts cerebral vessels)	p.o. 0.2 Gm	tachycardia, restlessness, insomnia, irritability
Caffeine and sodium benzoate	mild CNS stimulant; increases heart rate; respiration; dilates blood vessels (constricts cerebral vessels	I.M., I.V. 0.5 Gm - 1 Gm	tachycardia, restlessness, insomnia, irritability
Aminophylline	mild respiratory stimulant; antispasmodic; dilates coronary arteries; relaxes bronchioles in asthma attack	p.o. 100 and 200 mg tabs I.M., I.V. as ordered rectal: 0.2-0.5 Gm	fall in blood pressure
Class: Amphetamines			
Amphetamine (Benzedrine)	stimulates the central nervous system	p.o. 5, 10, 15 mg tabs 10-15 mg spansules I.M., I.V. 5-10 mg b.i.d. avoid giving drug after 4 p.m.	restlessness, dry mouth, insomnia, excitation, elevated blood pressure
Dextroamphetamine sulfate (Dexedrine)	same as above	p.o., tablets, elixir, spansules; 2.5 to 15 mg t.i.d., a.c.; last dose at least 6 hr. before hour of sleep	same as above but less toxic
Phenmetrazine hydrochloride (Preludin)	mild stimulant; depresses appetite when taken 1 hour before meals	p.o. 25 mg t.i.d. 1 hr. a.c.	restlessness, insomnia, excitation, elevated blood pressure
Methamphetamine (Amphedroxyn) (Dexoval) (Methedrine)	CNS simulant, more potent than amphetamine, and with less cardiovascular action; used in treatment of narcolepsy depression and alcoholism	p.o. initially 2.5 mg daily, increased to 2.5-5 mg t.i.d.; 10-15 mg I.V. as emergency drug	same as above
Class: Cerebrospinal Stimulants (Emergency Drugs)			
Picrotoxin injection	powerful CNS stimulant and convulsant; used in barbiturate poisoning	I.V., 3% solution; dosage depends on patient's condition	convulsions
Pentylenetetrazol (Metrazol)	stimulates respiratory system	I.V. 100-500 mg	convulsions in large doses

Fig. 32-1 Stimulants

Medication	Action	Administration and Dosage	Side and/or Toxic Effects
Morphine sulfate (Controlled Substances Law)	relieves deep-seated pain; narcotic action on cerebrum which results in analgesia and sleep; addictive; depresses respirations and heart action	**p.o.**, s.c. 8-30 mg as ordered	respirations at 10 or below per minute: discontinue and report; addiction, constipation, nausea, vomiting
Codeine sulfate (Controlled Substances Law)	narcotic; sedative; relieves pain; 1/6 as analgesic as morphine; cough depressant	**p.o.** and parenteral 30-60 mg as ordered	addiction, constipation
Paregoric (Controlled Substances Law)	checks intestinal peristalsis, diarrhea	**p.o.** 5-10 ml	as above
Pantopon (Pantopium) (Controlled Substances Law)	similar to morphine; sometimes tolerated by patients who are hypersensitive to morphine	I.M., s.c. 5-20 mg	as above
Papaverine hydrochloride (Controlled Substances Law)	less depressive action on brain than morphine; antispasmodic on smooth muscle	**p.o.** 100 mg; I.M. 30 mg; I.V. as ordered (slowly)	usually none, non-addicting
Dihydromorphinone hydrochloride (Dilaudid) (Controlled Substances Law)	less hypnotic action than morphine; depresses respirations; increases intracranial pressure; 10 times potency of morphine	**p.o.**, s.c. 2 mg suppository	nausea, vomiting, excitation

Fig. 32-2 Narcotic Analgesics

Narcotics may lead to systemic poisoning due to overdose as in an attempt to commit suicide or because of personal sensitivity to products of opium. The respirations continue to fall until they reach a rate below 10 per minute. The pupils of the eyes constrict until they are the size of pinpoints. Stupor and coma result. *Stop the drug immediately. Call the physican and/or the emergency squad.* Be ready with respiratory stimulants which will be administered immediately.

The Harrison Narcotic Act regulated the manufacture and sale of many opium and cocaine derivatives. It was amended many times. It has been replaced by the Controlled Substances Law of 1970.

Section 5 Effects of Medications on Body Systems

Synthetic Narcotic Analgesics. Analgesics which have fewer of the undesirable side effects of morphine and other opium derivations have been synthesized. A few of these are included in figure 32-3.

Narcotic Antagonists. Narcotic antagonists are also called analeptics. They are administered in narcotic poisoning cases, figure 32-4.

Sedatives and Hypnotics

A sedative quiets and relaxes the patient without producing sleep. It is not an analgesic. Many drugs may be either hypnotic or sedative, depending on the dosage. Hypnotics are drugs which induce sleep. They do not relieve pain by themselves although they may be combined with an analgesic. A good hypnotic should give as normal sleep as possible. It should act fairly rapidly and should not give the patient a delayed effect the following day.

Medication	Action	Administration and Dosage	Side and/or Toxic Effects
Meperidine hydrochloride (Demerol) (Controlled Substances Law)	depresses central nervous system; effective analgesic for visceral pain especially; increases intracranial pressure; helpful for asthmatic patients	p.o. 50-100 mg; severe pain up to 150 mg; I.M. 100 mg	addictive: promotes spasms of biliary tract, nausea, vomiting, sweating, postural hypotension
Methadone (Adanon) (Dolophine) (Methadon) (Controlled Substance Law)	potent analgesic; non-sedative; withdrawal drug in morphine addiction; suppresses cough	p.o. available in 2.5-10 mg, ampule 1 cc = 10 mg usual dose 7.5 mg q. 4h.	addictive; respiratory depression; nausea, vomiting, skin rash, itching, constipation
Oxycodone (Percodan) (Eucodol) (Controlled Substance Law)	derivative of morphine; 5-6 times as potent as codeine; analgesic for moderate pain; cough suppressant	p.o. 3-20 mg; s.c. 5 mg	drowsiness; psychic, physical dependence and tolerance may develop
Carbamazepine (Tegretol)	relieves pain of trigeminal neuralgia (tic douloureux)	p.o., 200 mg tablets increased as tolerated	intraocular pressure; given with caution in heart and liver disease

Fig. 32-3 Synthetic Narcotics

Medication	Action	Administration and Dosage	Side and/or Toxic Effects
Nalorphine hydrochloride (Nalline) (Controlled Substance)	antagonist to respiratory depression of morphine, meperidine, and methadone; not useful in addiction cases	I.V., I.M., s.c. ampules 5-10 mg.	not addictive
Levallorphan tartrate (Lorfan)	as above	vials of 1 mg. per ml available	as above

Fig. 32-4 Narcotic Antagonists

Medication	Action	Administration and Dosage	Side Effects and/or Toxic Effects
Propoxyphene hydrochloride (Darvon)	relieves mild to moderate pains; similar to action of codeine	p.o. capsules 32-65 mg q 4h	nonaddictive; few side effects with average doses
Ethoheptazine (Zactane)	similar to meperidine; effective for musculo-skeletal disorders; analgesic	p.o.: 75 mg tablets range 75-150 mg t.i.d. or q.i.d.	rarely present epigastric distress, dizziness, pruritis
Pentazocine (Talwin)	potent analgesic, relieves pain during labor, after surgery	I.V., I.M., s.c., 30 mg q 4h p.o. 50 mg tabs	nausea, vomiting, dizziness, euphoria

Fig. 32-5 Synthetic Analgesics (Non-narcotic)

Medication	Action	Administration and Dosage	Side Effects and/or Toxic Effects
Acetylsalicylic acid (Aspirin) (Ecotrin)	relieves elevated temperature, minor aches and pains; anti-inflammatory action; large doses suppress blood clotting	p.o. 0.3-0.6 Gm (leading cause of death among children. Never tell them it is candy)	gastrointestinal distress, ringing in ears, dizziness; acute poisoning: stupor and coma. Action: stop drug. Give plenty of fluids p.o. Gastric lavage may be necessary
Indomethacin (Indocin)	potent anti-inflammatory analgesic and antipyretic drug	p.o. 25 mg b.i.d., p.c.	peptic ulcerations and gastric irritation, headache, dizziness, skin rash, bone marrow depression
Phenylbutazone (Butazolidin)	as above; used for rheumatoid arthritis, acute attacks of gout	p.o. initial dose 300-600 mg; maintenance 100-200 mg	use restricted because of toxicity; edema, nausea, gastric distress; hepatitis, hypertension, temporary psychosis, leukopenia, agranulocytosis
Acetaminophen (Tylenol)	analgesic; antipyretic	p.o. 0.3 Gm q. 3-4 h.	none

Fig. 32-6 Analgesics which are also antipyretics

Section 5 Effects of Medications on Body Systems

Barbiturates

The barbiturates act at all levels of the central nervous system. They may provide a state ranging from mild sedation to deep sleep and anesthesia, depending upon the drug and dosage prescribed and the individual reaction of the patient, figure 32-8.

Medications	Action	Dosage	Side and/or Toxic Symptoms
Ethchlorvynol (Placidyl)	mild hypnotic; no addiction results; used for patients who are unable to take barbitals	p.o.: 100-500 mg	hypotension, mental confusion, nightmares, nausea
Glutethimide (Doriden)	depresses the central nervous system; is quickly effective; duration 4-8 hrs.	p.o.: .25 to 0.5 Gm	nausea and rash; suspected habituation
Methyprylon (Noludar)	depresses central nervous system; for simple and nervous insomnia, duration same as short-acting barbiturates	p.o.: 200-400 mg	morning drowsiness, dizziness, gastric upset. Physical and psychological dependence

Fig. 32-7 Sedatives and Hypnotics

Medication	Action	Administration and Dosage	Side and/or Toxic Effects
Phenobarbital (Luminal)	slow onset but long-acting; used to prevent seizures in epileptics; duration 12-24 hours	p.o. 100-200 mg sedative — 16 to 32 mg hypnotic — 100 to 320 mg	restlessness, skin rashes, facial edema, asthmatic attack
Sodium Phenobarbital (Sodium Luminal)	rapid onset; injectable preparation of above	I.M. 15 mg — 130 mg	as above
Secobarbital Sodium (Seconal)	a rapid-acting barbiturate; duration 3-8 hours, preanesthetic medication	p.o. 100 mg (sleep) 300 mg (preoperative) suppositories; ampules 0.25 to 0.5 Gm	same as above
Pentobarbital sodium (Nembutal)	short onset and length of action; action 3-8 hrs.	p.o.: 100-200 mg I.V.: 50 mg in 5 cc	same as above
Amobarbital (Amytal)	intermediate in action; 6-10 hrs. duration	p.o., I.V. and I.M. tablets 50, 100 mg ampule: 0.25-0.5 Gm sedatives: 65 mg b.i.d. hypnotic: 100-200 mg	same as above
Butabarbital (Butisol)	intermediate action, 5-6 hours	p.o. sedative 15-30 mg t.i.d.: hypnotic 50 to 100 mg	same as above

Fig. 32-8 Barbiturates

Large doses depress the respiratory and vasomotor centers. Death from these drugs is usually the result of overdose, either accidental or suicidal. Death results from respiratory paralysis. Therapeutic doses have no effect on the respiratory and vasomotor centers. Continued use of very large doses of barbiturates will cause habituation, and for this reason many states now have laws controlling their sale.

Barbiturates have several uses:

- To produce sleep and sedation.
- To serve as a preoperative medication.
- To produce sedation in obstetrical patients.
- To prevent convulsions.
- To calm hyperactive, psychiatric patients.
- To relieve pain in combination with an analgesic.

Barbiturates are readily absorbed when administered orally. They may also be given rectally, intramuscularly, subcutaneously, and intravenously. They undergo changes in the liver and are excreted by the kidney.

In selecting a barbiturate, the physican decides upon the length of time the drug will serve his patient. The onset of action of the barbiturates varies; they have been classified as ultrashort-acting, short-acting, intermediate, and long-acting. If the patient has trouble getting to sleep, a short-acting agent is indicated. However, if the patient goes to sleep readily but awakens during the night, a long-acting barbiturate may be indicated.

Side effects and toxic effects include bad dreams and restlessness, skin rashes, edema of the face, and sometimes asthmatic attacks. The longer acting agents may produce a "barbiturate hangover" upon awakening. The drinking of alcoholic beverages with the taking of barbiturates is contraindicated since alcohol intensifies the depressant effect of the drug.

OTHER HYPNOTICS

- Chloral hydrate: one of the oldest hypnotics. It depresses the central nervous system, acts promptly in from 10-15 minutes, and produces sleep for 5 or more hours. The sleep is very like normal sleep. There is little or no effect upon the heart or respiratory center when taken in average dosages. An overdose will cause cardiac depression. It is an effective hypnotic when patient has no pain. Its chief drawback is that it may cause gastric irritation. The patient should not take chloral hydrate with alcohlic beverages, as alcohol enhances the depressant effect.

    Dosage: Gelatin capsules: 250 mg (sedative), 500 mg (hypnotic) t.i.d. If liquid is used, it should be given in milk or syrup to cover its taste.

- Petrichloral: derived from chloral. Its action as a hypnotic and sedative is similar to chloral hydrate. It is well tolerated because it is odorless and tasteless. It does not irritate the gastric mucosa and is a safe drug.

    Dosage: p.o. 300 mg (sedative), 600 mg (hypnotic)

- Paraldehyde: a clear liquid with a strong odor and an unpleasant taste. Its hypnotic effect occurs in about 20 minutes and the effect lasts for 4-8 hours. Ordinary doses do not depress the heart, respiratory center, or the medullary centers. Some of the drug is excreted through the lungs, giving a characteristic odor to the breath. The drug is frequently used to quiet noisy alcoholics. The liquid should be administered cold and well-diluted in wine, syrup, or fruit juice because of its odor and taste. Some addiction may develop. Never give by subcutaneous injection. When given by I.M., it should be given deeply into a large muscle because of its irritating effect (an abscess or tissue sloughing could occur).

    Dosage: p.o. 8 ml

    rectal: 4-8 ml in oil, as retention enema

    I.M.: 2-4 ml, deep in large muscle. Use Z-track technique

ANESTHETICS

Anesthetics are drugs which make patients insensitive to pain. A general anesthetic is one which extends to the entire body and results in a state of unconsciousness. Some general anesthetics are inhaled; others are administered intravenously. The patient's general response to the anesthetic is caused by the functioning of his nervous system instead of the nature of the anesthetic. In other words, two patients may react very differently to the administration of the same anesthetic and, therefore, dosages vary according to age, weight, sex and idiosyncrasies. Refer to the preceding unit for information about caution in the administration of muscle relaxants, especially before anesthesia.

Medication	Action	Administration and Dosage	Toxic Symptoms
Ether	produces loss of sensation for prolonged periods	inhalation (dosage varies)	drop in blood pressure, weak, irregular pulse, clammy skin, nausea, dilated pupils, shallow respirations, vomiting during recovery period
Cyclopropane	prolonged anesthetic	inhalation (dosage varies)	cardiac irregularity
Nitrous oxide (Laughing gas)	low anesthetic potency; used with oxygen as analgesic; used after preanesthetic medication with oxygen and muscle relaxant as anesthetic	inhalation (dosage varies)	breathing difficulty (anoxia)
Halothane (Fluothane)	potent general anesthetic; four times more potent than ether; used with oxygen or oxygen and nitrous oxide	inhalation (dosage varies)	respiratory depression, hypotension

Fig. 32-9 General Anesthetics

The effect of a local anesthetic is confined to one area of the body. The anesthetic makes that area insensitive to pain but the patient remains conscious. Local anesthetics are nerve block anesthetics and sprayed-on anesthetics. They may include: cocaine, procaine, tetracaine and dibucaine for injections and local application, and ethyl chloride which is sprayed on.

ANTICONVULSANTS

Anticonvulsant drugs are depressants. There are various types of convulsive seizures. Epilepsy is considered to be a symptom of brain disorder. The *electroencephalogram* shows many changes in the activity of the cerebral cortex. Epileptic seizures are grouped as: grand mal seizures, petit mal seizures, Jacksonian epilepsy, and psychomotor attacks. Some people have mixed seizures.

Medication	Action	Administration and Dosage	Toxic Symptoms to Report
Cocaine	Ophthalmic use, penetrates mucous membrane, blocks nerve conduction	ophthalmic solution, 0.5-4.0% topical, 2-5%	dizziness, palpitation, fainting
Dibucaine hydrochloride (Nupercaine)	more potent and more toxic; absorbed from skin and mucosa, relieves burns and hemorrhoid discomfort	topical and injection 0.05 to 0.1% solution topical – ointment	dizziness, palpitation, fainting (more toxic than cocaine)
Procaine (Novocain)	blocks nerve conduction	regional anesthetic 0.5-2.0%; spinal anesthetic 1.5%	dizziness, palpitation, fainting, overdose; convulsions, respiratory failure, reduced B/P
Lidocaine (Xylocaine)	twice potency of procaine	infiltration 0.5%; nerve block 1 or 2%; peridural .5 to 2%; spinal anesthesia 5%; topical – ointment	same as procaine in 0.5% 50% greater at 2%
Ethyl chloride	anesthetizes skin before incising boils, or removing superficial foreign bodies; freezes tissue for 30-60 sec.	volatile liquid in special spray containers, used as topical spray	local pain and swelling following freezing
Tetracaine (Pontocaine)	ophthalmic use, also for spinal and nerve block anesthesia	ophthalmic sol. 0.5-1% ung. 1%	pain following use

Fig. 32-10 Local Anesthetics

Section 5 Effects of Medications on Body Systems

All drugs useful in epilepsy stop the spread of the seizure, but we do not know how this is accomplished. Anticonvulsive drugs should be effective against mixed seizures as well as against specific types. They should have a lengthy but nontoxic action. They should be tolerated well by the patient and should be inexpensive. Some of the anticonvulsives are given in figure 32-11.

AUTONOMIC NERVOUS SYSTEM

The autonomic nervous system is a self-governing system. The autonomic nervous system has two parts: the parasympathetic and the sympathetic systems. One stimulates and the other inhibits actions.

This system has control over the nerves and ganglia which regulate the heart, blood vessels, glands, and the smooth internal muscles of the body. The circulation, metabolism, respiration and digestion of the body are regulated by the autonomic nervous system. Its ganglia are usually found close to the thoracic and lumbar vertebrae. The *hypothalamus* in the brain coordinates and regulates activities such as water balance, blood pressure, body temperature, and emotions as well as carbohydrate and fat metabolism. This structure influences the autonomic system and the central nervous system. To repeat, the central nervous system is made up of the brain and spinal cord. The autonomic system is made up of the sympathetic and parasympathetic systems.

Medication	Action	Administration and Dosage	Side Effects and/or Toxic Effects
Diphenylhy-dantoin (Dilantin)	controls grand mal and psychomotor seizures in epilepsy	p.o. 100 mg t.i.d. I.M. 100-200 mg	nausea, vomiting, skin eruptions, soreness of gums; CNS complications: ataxia, dizziness, tremors, psychosis
(Phelantin)	Dilantin combined with phenobarbital		
(Hydantal)	combined with phenobarbital		
(Mebroin)	combined with methobarbital		
Mephenytoin (Mesantoin)	same action as Dilantin	p.o. children 100-400 mg; adults 400-600 mg	destruction of blood cells; aplastic anemia, jaundice
Trimethadione (Tridione)	anticonvulsive; effective against petit mal epilepsy	p.o. 900-1200 mg in divided doses for adults and 300-900 mg for children	blood dyscrasias, gastric irritation, vision disturbances
Paramethadione (Paradione)	action same as Tridione	p.o. initial 900 mg in divided doses for adults, 300 to 600 mg for children	photophobia, skin rashes

Fig. 32-11 Anticonvulsants

Examples of the effects produced by the autonomic nervous system are shown below.

Sympathetic	Parasympathetic
Dilated pupils of eye to adjust to light (dark)	Constricted pupils to adjust to light (bright)
Increase heart rate	Decreased heart rate
Dilated coronary arteries	Constricted coronary arteries
Relaxed smooth muscle of bronchial tubes	Constricted blood vessels of bronchial tubes
Decreased smooth muscle action in gastrointestinal tract	Increased gastrointestinal action (peristalsis)
Decreased uterine muscle activity	Increased uterine muscle activity
Constriction of sphincter muscles	Relaxation of sphincter muscles

Sympathomimetic Agents

Adrenergic-stimulating agents mimic and produce the effect of stimulation of the sympathetic nervous system. They are our bodily defense in case of emergencies. Many, but not all, have about the same chemical structure. Some of these drugs were discussed in relation to the endocrine glands; epinephrine and norepinephrine, which have a typical adrenergic-stimulating action, will be considered here.

Epinephrine and Norepinephrine. These chemical substances are produced in the medulla of the adrenal gland. In emergencies the adrenal gland secretes an overabundance of these hormones. They are the best heart stimulants in cases of acute heart failure and are used often as emergency drugs. Under ordinary conditions, these drugs are used to treat acute bronchial asthma. Overdoses may cause overstimulation of the heart muscle, the myocardium.

Other drugs used include: levarterenol bitartrate (Levophed, Arterenol, Nor-Epinephrine), ephedrine (Racephedrine), phenylephrine (Neo-synephrine), and the amphetamines.

Sympatholytic Agents

Adrenergic-blocking agents neutralize or oppose the effect of the stimulation of the sympathetic nervous system. Generally, they are effective vasodilators; they lower the blood pressure and increase the action of the smooth muscles of the gastrointestinal tract. There are both natural and synthetic products in this group. One drug in this group, Dibenzyline, will be discussed briefly and others named for your consideration and further research.

Phenoxybenzamine hydrochloride (Dibenzyline). It dilates the blood vessels of the extremities and is useful in the treatment of Raynaud's disease. It blocks adrenergic stimuli, lowers peripheral resistance and increases the size of the vascular space. It lowers the blood pressure of some patients. The maintenance dose is 20 to 60 mg daily.

Others in this group include: ergot alkaloids (used extensively in obstetrics), dihydroergotamine (D.H.E. 45) used chiefly to treat migraine headaches, and methysergide maleate (Sansert), also used in the treatment of migraine headaches.

Section 5 *Effects of Medications on Body Systems*

SENSE ORGANS

Observation and knowledge of the world comes through the sense organs: the eye for vision, the ear for hearing, the nose for smell, the tongue for taste, and the skin for touch. Each of the sense organs is made so that it responds to one type of stimulation. The *exteroceptors* (sensory nerve endings in the skin) are stimulated by the outside environment. The *interoceptors,* sensory nerve endings located in the respiratory and gastrointestinal tract, are stimulated by the internal environment, for example, gas distention causes pain.

Sensation or impression really takes place in the brain, but the sensation seems to be in the area of the body from which the message came. Our sense organs are very important to us because they are really our connection with our environment. Life would be meaningless if we could not see, hear, smell, taste and feel. In this unit, we will consider medications which affect the eye, one of the most important organs of sense perception, figure 32-12.

MIOTICS

The miotics are used to lower the eyeball pressure in cases of glaucoma and in the treatment of some types of strabismus. Care must be taken in the instillation of miotics (and mydriatics). Figure 32-13 illustrates the method. Examples of miotics are given and described in figure 32-14.

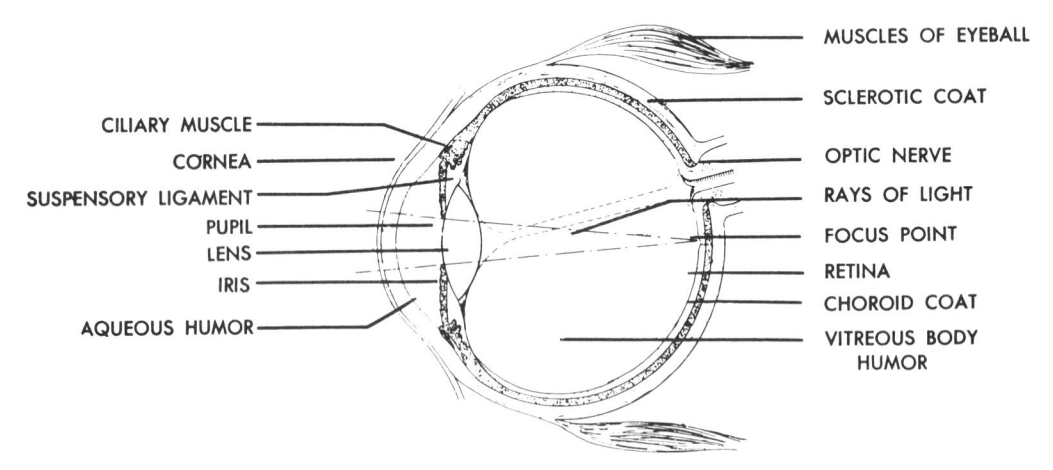

Fig. 32-12(A) Internal view of the eye

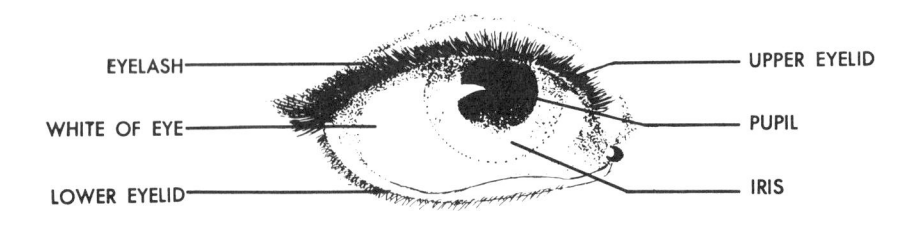

Fig. 32-12(B) External view of the eye

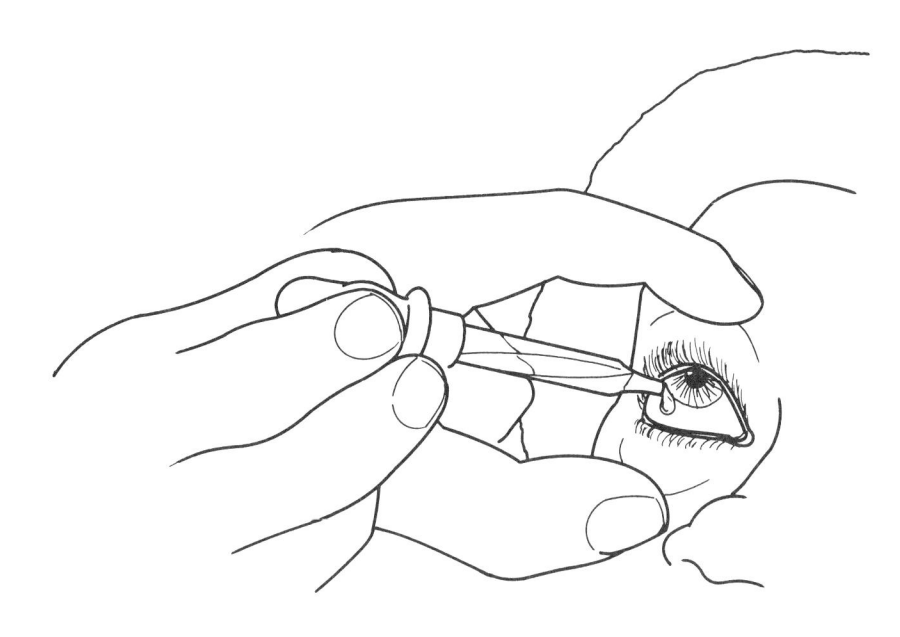

Fig. 32-13 Instillation of eye drops

Medication	Action	Administration and Dosage	Side Effects and/or Toxic Effects
Pilocarpine nitrate (Pilocarpine hydrochloride)	causes miosis (contraction of pupil) in 15 minutes; lasts several hours	eye drops: 0.5 to 4% solution	overdose or sensitivity to drug will cause headache, sweating, salivation
Carbachol (Doryl) (Carcholin)	miotic, as above	eye drops: 0.75 to 3.0%	as above
Physostigmine salicylate (Eserine salicylate)	miotic, longer acting	eye drops: .5% - 1%	as above
Demecarium bromide (Humorsol)	powerful miotic; lasts 5-10 days	eye drops: 0.25% solution	avoid systemic absorption
Isoflurophate DFP (Floropryl)	same as physostigmine but more powerful; longer acting	eyedrops in peanut oil 0.1% solution	take care to prevent tears from contaminating the solution.

Fig. 32-14 Miotics

Section 5 Effects of Medications on Body Systems

MYDRIATICS

Mydriatics are used to dilate the pupil of the eye, thus aiding the oculist in making his examination of the retina and eye grounds (back of eye). If mydriatics are absorbed into the system, some serious side effects may develop, such as dryness of the mouth, flushing, tachycardia, delirium, and coma. *Care must be used in administering these drugs either locally or systemically because of individual sensitivity to the drugs.* Great care should be used with patients for whom an increase in intraocular pressure may be hazardous. For example, atropine sulfate would be contraindicated in patients with glaucoma.

Medication	Action	Administration and Dosage	Side Effects and/or Toxic Effects
Atropine sulfate	dilates pupil of eye	aqueous solution of 0.5 to 4% for eye drops; lasts 7 to 12 days	difficulty in focusing eyes
Scopolamine hydrobromide (Hyoscine hydrobromide)	as above	aqueous solution for eye drops 0.2 to 0.5% lasts 7 to 12 days	as above
Homatropine hydrobromide (Mesopin) (Novatrin)	see atropine sulfate	eye drops of 1% to 5% solution; lasts 24 hours	as with atropine but for shorter period
Eucatropine hydrochloride (Euphthalmine hydrochloride)	as above	2% solution eye drops; lasts only a few hours	as with atropine but for short time
Cyclopentolate hydrochloride (Cyclogyl hydrochloride)	as above	eye drops 0.5 to 2%; rapid; brief dilation	as with atropine but for only a brief time
Epinephrine hydrochloride (Adrenalin)	treats local allergies in ophthalmology; also superficial hyperemia; mixed with other drugs to lower intraocular pressure in glaucoma	2% Epitrate®	avoid use in cardiac patients
Phenylephrine hydrochloride (Neo-Synephrine)	Dilates pupils for ocular exam	2.5 to 10% solution	rise in blood and intraocular pressure; avoid systemic absorption

Fig. 32-15 Mydriatics

IRRIGATIONS

Eye washes or irrigations are used to flush the conjunctiva (delicate membrane which covers the eyeballs) to cleanse and aid in removing foreign bodies, and to relieve inflammation and pain. Hands are thoroughly washed before proceeding with any eye treatments. All equipment and solutions should be sterile. Always wipe away from the nose toward the temple. Some examples of medications used in eye irrigations are normal saline and weak preparations of boric acid.

- Normal Saline

    Isotonic sodium chloride 0.9%

    No adverse effects

- Boric Acid Solution

    3-5% solution (weak acid)

    Adverse effects: excessive burning sensation

    Action: Flush freely with water

ANTIBIOTICS

Many antibiotics are available for ophthalmic use. The tetracyclines, chloramphenicol, erythromycin, and streptomycin are prepared as solutions, ointments, and suspensions in strengths varying from 0.5 to 1 percent. These drugs are administered systemically as well as topically for eye infections. Chloramphenicol has particular merit in the treatment of intraocular infections (infections within the eye) because the eye absorbs the medication easily. Bacitracin is especially useful as an ophthalmic anti-infective because it is non-irritating to the eye and produces no side effects. Many microorganisms do not develop resistance to it. It is available for topical application in an ophthalmic ointment of 500-1000 units. Amphotericin B is ordered for fungus infections of the eye as a 0.5 percent ointment. Isoniazid 10% is used for tuberculous infection of the eye. Idoxuridine in 0.1% solution is effective against the herpes simplex virus.

Steroids are sometimes used in the treatment of eye conditions. Dexamethasone, Prednisolone and Hydrocortisone are examples of those used to treat allergic reactions, severe injury and some inflammations.

MISCELLANEOUS AGENTS

Miscellaneous and unclassified drugs are drugs used for various purposes which do not fall under any special classification. These include: antiseptics against gonococcus (silver nitrate 1%), against staphylococcus (Metaphen), against fungus (Merthiolate) and antiseptics and stimulants (yellow oxide of mercury).

Section 5 Effects of Medications on Body Systems

Medication	Action	Administration and Dosage	Side Effects and/or Toxic Effects
Silver nitrate	to prevent gonorrheal eye infections (Law requires it put in eyes of newborn.)	eye drops 1% or 2%	low toxicity, therefore few symptoms, discoloration of skin, gastritis if swallowed
Nitromersol (Metaphen)	to treat gonorrhea and other infections	ointment 1:3000 eyewash 1:1000 to 1:10,000	discoloration of skin due to chemical action
Thimerosal (Merthiolate)	especially effective against fungus infections	ointment 1:5000	few symptoms if used as directed, skin discoloration results from color of chemical
Yellow oxide of mercury	to treat eye infections	ointment 1 and 2% (poison if taken by mouth)	none

Fig. 32-16 Miscellaneous ophthalmic drugs

SUGGESTED ACTIVITIES

- Study the charts of three patients who have undergone surgery. What preoperative medications were ordered? For what purpose were these medications ordered? What medications were ordered postoperatively? What were their effects?
- Locate a patient for whom narcotic drugs have been prescribed. What is the patient's diagnosis? List the narcotic, dosage, and specific purpose for which the narcotic is being given. What is the patient's response to the drug?
- Explain the care of narcotics in the clinical area to which you have been assigned. Describe the records which must be kept relative to the use of narcotics.
- Investigate the symptoms and treatment of glaucoma. How is early diagnosis of the condition made? Why is early diagnosis important?
- Boric acid solution can be toxic when swallowed in any amount. Investigate the symptoms of this type of poisoning. What emergency treatment should be administered in such cases?

REVIEW

A. Complete the following sentences.

1. a. Amphetamines are classified as _____ .
      (stimulants, depressants)

   b. They _____ habit-forming.
      (are, are not)

2. Narcotics are addictive drugs derived from _____ and _____ .

3. Two signs of an overdose of narcotics are a reduction in _____ and constriction of the _____ .

4. a. Demerol _____ a narcotic.
         (is, is not)

   b. It _____ addictive.
         (is, is not)

5. Barbiturates may be _____ or _____ in effect, depending on the dosage.

6. Alcoholic beverages are contraindicated when the patient is taking chloral hydrate because _____ .

7. The general anesthetic _____ is combined with oxygen as an analgesic.

8. Anticonvulsant drugs are _____ (stimulants, depressants).

9. Epinephrine and norepinephrine are used as emergency drugs in _____ .

10. The autonomic nervous system has two parts, _____ and _____ .

B. Match the drugs listed in Column I with their description in Column II.

   Column I
   _____ 1. amphetamines
   _____ 2. topical anesthesias
   _____ 3. hypnotics
   _____ 4. analgesias
   _____ 5. general anesthetics
   _____ 6. synthetic analgesias
   _____ 7. narcotic antagonists
   _____ 8. antipyretics
   _____ 9. adrenergic agents
   _____ 10. Dilantin

   Column II
   a. drugs which relieve pain
   b. man-made or chemically made drugs which relieve pain
   c. drugs which reduce fever
   d. drugs which stimulate the sympathetic nervous system
   e. drug used to prevent epileptic seizures
   f. drugs which anesthetize the skin for surgery
   g. synthetic, habit-forming drugs which stimulate the cerebral cortex
   h. drugs which produce loss of sensation and unconsciousness
   i. drugs which produce a block anesthesia
   j. drugs which are administered in narcotic poisoning cases
   k. drugs used to overcome the effects of depressant drugs
   l. drugs which produce sleep

C. Answer the following questions.

   1. What are the contraindications and side effects of the amphetamines?

   2. Name three narcotic analgesics and three non-narcotic analgesics.

Section 5 Effects of Medications on Body Systems

3. Upon what basis does the physician select a barbiturate?

4. How do the sympathetic *and* parasympathetic nervous systems affect each of the following?
    a. heart rate

    b. coronary arteries

    c. peristalisis

    d. muscles of bronchi

D. In each of the following all but one answer is correct. Select the *incorrect* item.
   1. Drugs which stimulate the nervous system include
      a. caffeine and sodium benzoate
      b. benzedrine
      c. pantopon
      d. dexedrine
   2. Some synthetic non-narcotics which relieve pain but do not have the undesirable side effects of morphine and opium, include
      a. Demerol
      b. Darvon
      c. Zactane
      d. Talwin
   3. Some nonbarbituate sedatives and hypnotics include
      a. Doriden
      b. Placidyl
      c. Noludar
      d. Amytal
   4. Some general anesthetics include
      a. Cocaine
      b. Cyclopropane
      c. Fluothane
      d. Halothane

E. Answer the following questions.

1. Why does state law require silver nitrate to be put in the eyes of the newborn?

2. Why is a mydriatic given before an eye examination?

3. What side effects may result from the systemic absorption of mydriatics?

4. For what purposes are miotics ordered?

5. For what purposes are eye irrigations ordered?

EXTENDED STUDY

Learn the meaning and use of the following words.

amenorrhea	lactation
androgen	luteal hormone
climacteric	menopause
contraceptive	menstruation
estrogen	ovulation
follicular hormone	oxytocic
gonadotropic	progesterone
hirsutism	spermatogenesis

Unit 33 Medications that Affect the Reproductive System

OBJECTIVES

After studying this unit, the student should be able to:

- Explain the relationship between the gonadotropic hormones, the processes of ovulation and menstruation, and estrogen and progesterone.
- Identify the uses of the estrogens, progesterone, and the androgens.
- Explain the cycle of administration for the oral contraceptive agents.

The sex glands are the ovaries in the female and the testes in the male. They release their hormones when stimulated by the gonadrotropic hormones from the pituitary gland. These hormones are the follicle-stimulating hormone (FSH), the luteinizing hormone (LH), and the luteotropic hormone (LTH). The sex organs and sex characteristics develop as a result of the activity of the follicle-stimulating hormone. This hormone is responsible for maintaining these characteristics throughout life. It stimulates the growth of the ovarian follicle in the female and spermatogenesis in the male. The luteinizing hormone also contributes to ovulation, spermatogenesis, and the secretion of male and female sex hormones. The luteotropic hormone stimulates the secretion of progesterone and also stimulates the secretion of milk by the mammary glands.

FEMALE HORMONES

In order to understand the functions of the female hormones, it is necessary to study the processes of ovulation and menstruation. These two processes are interrelated. Ovulation is the process by which a mature ovum is developed, and the uterus is made ready to receive the fertilized ovum. Menstruation is the process of casting off the unnecessary uterine lining when conception does not occur after ovulation.

During menstruation, a graafin follicle develops in the ovary. The ovum grows to maturity in this follicle. About 12 to 16 days after the beginning of the menstrual period, the ovum reaches maturity and it is expelled from the follicle. When the ovum appears on the surface of the ovary, it is drawn into the fallopian tube.

As the follicle and its ovum grow, it produces the hormone, estrogen, which stimulates the glands of the uterine lining (endometrium) to thicken. Because of its origin, estrogen is called the follicular hormone. When ovulation occurs, the follicle, now termed the corpus luteum, secretes another hormone, progesterone, which increases the blood vessels in the endometrium and causes uterine secretions. Progesterone is called the luteal hormone. These changes prepare the uterus to receive the fertilized ovum. At this point, the uterine lining is engorged with blood, and it is thick and spongy. If conception does not occur, the secretion of hormones falls off, and a portion of the endometrium is discharged through the vagina. The menstrual flow consists of mucus secretions, tissue fragments, and blood. After menstruation, the endometrium of the uterus is very thin.

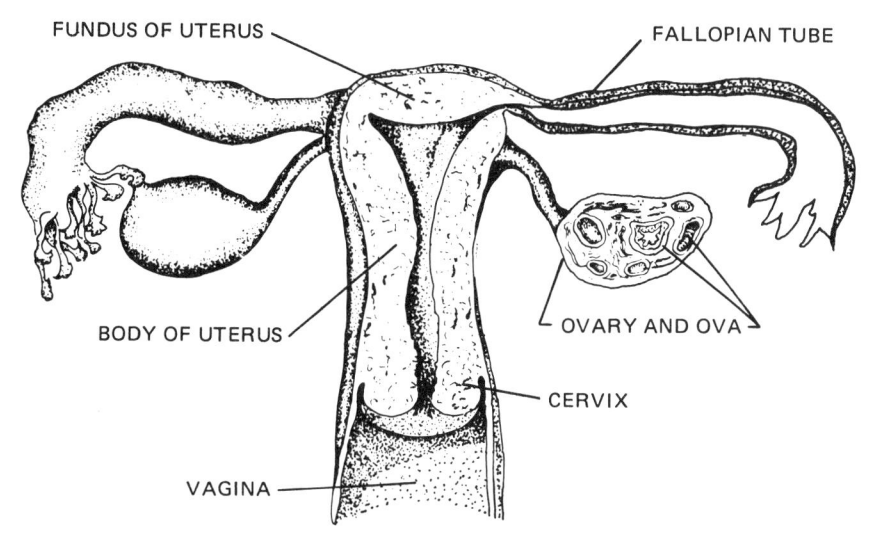

Fig. 33-1 Uterus, tubes, and ovaries

The hormones estrogen and progesterone and their synthetic preparations are used to treat many conditions. In general, these medications have a low toxicity. Some gastrointestinal symptoms may occur as well as headaches, dizziness, and allergic symptoms.

During pregnancy chorionic gonadotropin is produced by the placenta. Large amounts of gonadotropic substances are excreted in the urine. This is the basis of the A-Z test for pregnancy.

Estrogens

Estrogens are ordered for a wide variety of medical purposes. They relieve uncomfortable symptoms of menopause. During post menopause they are used in the treatment of senile vaginitis and urinary infections associated with post menopause. They suppress lactation in the postpartum period. Estrogens are used in palliative therapy for breast cancer in women and prostatic cancer in men. Both natural and synthetic estrogens are available.

Natural Estrogens. The nurse should be familiar with the following natural estrogens.

- Estrone (Theelin)
    Dosage: I.M., 0.2-1 mg twice weekly

- Estradiol (Progynon)
    Preparations: topical, tablets, suppositories
    Dosage: I.M., parenteral solution, 0.25-1 mg

- Estradiol Benzoate (Diogyne B, Dimenformon Benzoate): a form of estradiol more suitable for intramuscular injection than estradiol
    Dosage: I.M. 0.1-5 mg

- Estradiol Dipropionate (Ovocylin Dipropionate): slow absorption and excretion.
    Dosage: I.M. (in oil), 0.1-5 mg weekly

- Ethinyl Estradiol (Estinyl): a potent estrogen.
    Dosage: p.o., tablets and elixir, 0.02-0.05 mg t.i.d.

Conjugated Estrogens. Estrogenic substances, conjugated (Premarin). This drug is made up of mixed estrogens from the urine of pregnant mares. It is used in menopausal conditions, breast engorgement, senile vaginitis, and pruritis vulvae.

    Dosage: p.o., 1.25-3.75 mg

Synthetic Estrogens. The following synthetic estrogens are available.

- Diethylstilbestrol (Stilboestrol, Stilphostrol): this drug duplicates inexpensively all the known actions of natural estrogens. Headache, nausea, and vomiting are common side effects. It is used for menopausal symptoms,—for discomfort in mammary cancer, and for prostatic cancer. It suppresses lactation when administered after childbirth.

    Preparations: plain tablets, enteric-coated tablets, capsules, suppositories, and vials for injection

    Dosage: menopausal symptoms, p.o. 0.5-1 mg daily suppression of lactation, p.o. 5 mg b.i.d. for 2-4 days

    prostatic cancer: I.M., 3 mg daily, then 1 mg daily

    breast cancer: p.o. 15 mg daily

- Diethylstilbestrol Dipropionate: has fewer side effects than free stilbestrol. Has a prolonged effect when given intramuscularly in oil.

    Dosage: p.o., 0.5-2 mg, 2-3 times weekly

- Hexestrol: less potent and less toxic than diethylstilbestrol.

    Dosage: p.o., 1-3 mg available

    menopausal symptoms, 2-3 mg daily

- Dienestrol (Restrol, Synestrol): has few side effects.

    Dosage: p.o., 0.1-1.5 mg daily

    solutions for I.M. and s.c. injections

- Chlorotrianisene (Tace): this has the same actions and uses as other estrogens. It is stored only in body fat and is released slowly.

    Preparation: 12 and 25 mg capsules

    Dosage: menopause, p.o. 12-24 mg daily

    mammary engorgement, p.o. 48 mg daily for 1 week

Progesterone

The LTH, or luteotropic hormone, from the anterior lobe of the pituitary gland, is responsible for the secretion of progesterone. This hormone prepares the uterus for the implantation of the fertilized ovum. It suppresses ovulation during pregnancy. After delivery of the newborn, LTH stimulates the breasts to secrete milk.

Progesterone is also made synthetically. It is used to prevent uterine bleeding, and it is combined with estrogen in the treatment of amenorrhea. It is also ordered in cases of infertility and habitual abortion. Some forms of progesterone are combined with other medications in the oral contraceptive agents.

- Progesterone (Lipo-lutin, Proluton): ineffective when given orally. It is prepared in oil and in aqueous suspension.
    Dosage: I.M., 25 mg
    sublingual, 10-25 mg 3-4 times daily

- Ethisterone (Pranone)
    Dosage: p.o., 5, 10, or 25 mg q.i.d.

- Norethindrone (Norlutin): semisynthetic. It is used in amenorrhea, irregularity, and infertility.
    Dosage: p.o. 10-20 mg

- Medroxyprogesterone acetate (Provera): synthetic. It is active when given orally.
    Preparations: tablets: 2.5 and 10 mg
    Dosage: individualized, range 2.5 to 30 mg daily

Oral Contraceptive Agents

The oral contraceptive pills are ordered for persons who wish to limit the size of their families. A modified progesterone and small amounts of estrogens form the basis of these pills. They prevent the occurrence of pregnancy by preventing ovulation. The woman takes a total of 20 pills and then stops. The first pill is taken on the fifth day of her menstrual cycle and then each day until the 20 pills have been taken. Menstrual bleeding begins upon cessation of the medication. The procedure is repeated.

Side effects include nausea, vomiting, headache, fatigue, pain in the breasts, and phlebitis. Weight gain and fluid retention are common occurrences.

Some of the brand names are: Ovulen, Provest, Norlestrin, Norinyl, and Enovid.

Another type of oral contraceptive schedule requires two kinds of pills. For 15 days the woman takes estrogen. For the next 5 days she takes a pill containing both estrogen and progesterone. No pills are taken during the menstrual period. Fewer side effects have been reported from this method.

ANDROGENS

Male sex characteristics depend upon an adequate supply of androgens. They are chemical compounds called steroids and as such are chemically similar to progesterone. Androgens function in the development of the sex organs. Given therapeutically, they replace missing hormones. The androgens produce marked changes in the sex organs, body build, and voice, provided that the secretion of male hormones has not been deficient for too long a period. They are used for replacement therapy in cases of castration and in the treatment of undescended testicles. Good results have also been noted from their administration during the male climacteric and in menopausal symptoms in women. They are used to relieve pain in inoperable breast cancer.

Section 5 Effects of Medications on Body Systems

Side effects may include fluid retention, jaundice, nausea, and gastrointestinal upsets. When used in the female, they may cause deepening of the voice, hirsutism, flushing, and regression of the breasts. Their use is contraindicated in cases of prostatic cancer.

- Testosterone propionate (Oreton)
    Dosage: buccal tablets (held in space between teeth and cheek, 5-10 mg)
    intramuscular: 10-60 mg 2-6 times weekly
    breast cancer: 150-300 mg weekly in divided doses

- Testosterone (Delatestryl)
    Dosage: I.M. in oil lasts up to 3 weeks, 200 mg given every 2-4 weeks

- Deladumone: a combination of estradiol and testosterone in oil; it is used to suppress lactation. Given intramuscularly once immediately following delivery

- Methyltestosterone (Oreton M, Metandren)
    Dosage: oral, buccol, and sublingual tablets, 10 mg t.i.d.

- Fluoxymesterone (Halotestin): synthetic.
    Dosage: 4-10 mg

DRUGS USED DURING LABOR AND DELIVERY

Two kinds of drugs, uterine sedatives and uterine stimulants, deserve mention for their specific action in hastening or delaying birth. Narcotics, such as morphine, methadone, and meperidine, are ordered to relieve pain, delay or control uterine contractions, and to allay anxiety. Promethazine hydrochloride, an antihistamine, is also used for obstetric sedation in combination with lesser doses of Demerol or morphine.

Oxytocic drugs are uterine stimulants. They cause contractions of the uterus and, therefore, are used during birth. They may be used to induce labor or to hasten it in the later stages. They are frequently used at the end of labor because the prolonged contraction helps to prevent postpartum bleeding.

Oxytocic drugs also have a vasoconstricting effect in addition to increasing the force and length of contractions in the third stage of labor. The action of oxytocics is similar to the action of the hormone oxytocin secreted by the posterior lobe of the pituitary gland. They must be administered with care to those patients who have had previous cesarean deliveries, in heart cases, and when there is an abnormal presentation of the fetus. Some of these drugs are given in figure 33-2.

SUGGESTED ACTIVITIES

- Investigate the use of the sex hormones in cancer therapy. Be able to report on the conditions for which they are used, their action, dosage, and side effects.

- Study the medications ordered for three patients on the obstetrics service. What drugs were given during labor, delivery and the postpartum period? What was the purpose of each?

Medication	Action	Dosage	Side Effects and/or Toxic Effects
Ergonovine maleate (Ergotrate-maleate)	used in third stage of labor to prevent postpartum bleeding	I.V.: 0.2-0.4 mg p.o.: 0.2-0.4 mg postpartum	increase in blood pressure
Oxytocin injection extract (Pitocin)	prevents postpartum bleeding, also increases force of uterine contractions	s.c. or I.M.: 3 to 10 units; or I.V.: drip, diluted	may produce uterine rupture
Oxytocin injection synthetic (Syntocinon)	prevents postpartum bleeding	I.M.: 3-10 units I.V.: drip, diluted	same as extract
Methylergonovine (Methergine)	used in third stage of labor to prevent postpartum bleeding	I.M. or I.V.: 0.2-0.4 mg p.o.: 0.2 mg postpartum	increase in blood pressure
Sparteine sulfate (Spartocin) (Tocosamine)	speeds up slow labor in first and second stage	I.M.: 75 mg	not given in cardiac cases; may produce uterine rupture

Fig. 33-2 Oxytocics

REVIEW

A. Match the drug in Column I with its use in Column II

Column I
_____ 1. estrogen
_____ 2. oxytocic
_____ 3. Ovulen
_____ 4. testosterone
_____ 5. progesterone

Column II
a. relieves pain of breast cancer
b. stimulates uterine contractions
c. uterine sedative
d. prevents uterine bleeding
e. suppresses lactation
f. oral contraceptive

B. Answer the following questions.

1. List three gonadotropic hormones and give one function of each.

2. a. What is the function of estrogen during the menstrual cycle?

    b. What is the function of progesterone during the menstrual cycle?

Section 5 *Effects of Medications on Body Systems*

3. When is the use of the oxytocics contraindicated?

4. Explain the schedule for taking oral contraceptive pills which have estrogen and progesterone in a combined form.

5. What side effects may result when a female patient takes one of the androgens?

Achievement Review 5

Section 5 Effects of Medication on Body Systems

A. Complete the following statements by filling in the blank spaces with the appropriate word or words.

1. Aspirin is classified as an analgesic because _____ and as an _____ because it reduces fever.
2. Hormone drugs are not given to cure disease but to provide _____ from _____.
3. Cortisone is administered by _____ means or by _____ injection.
4. A drug which produces a superficial irritation is often called a _____.
5. Retention of body fluid is a toxic symptom usually associated with the drug _____.
6. _____ is a cardiotonic which strengthens the cardiac muscle, increases the force of systolic contraction, and slows the heart.
7. The action of phenacetin is much the same as aspirin but care must be taken in its use to avoid its becoming _____.
8. An overdose of the drug _____ may cause paralysis of muscles.
9. Vasoconstrictor drugs raise the blood pressure by _____ the blood vessels.
10. Quinidine is a drug often used as a heart _____.
11. A lowering of the blood pressure is brought about by the use of drugs known as _____.
12. Nitroglycerin is a drug often administered by the _____ method.
13. Drugs used to increase urinary output are called _____.
14. A rapid fall in blood pressure is a toxic symptom often associated with the drug _____.
15. Emetics are used to induce _____.
16. Heart stimulants quicken the heart action whereas heart tonics _____ the heart action.
17. Digitalis medications frequently cause such toxic symptoms as _____, _____, and _____.
18. Carbon dioxide is administered by the _____ method.

Section 5 Effects of Medications on Body Systems

19. An antispasmodic is a type of drug which _____ muscle contractions and _____ spasms of the bronchi.

20. Antihistamines are valuable in the treatment of _____ conditions.

21. Spirits of ammonia causes the patient to gasp by _____ the mucous membrane.

22. The hormones which regulate the rate of metabolism are _____.

23. The chief function of tranquilizer drugs is to tone down _____ overactivity.

24. Mydriatics are drugs which _____ the pupil of the eye.

25. Librium is classified as a _____ drug.

B. List a drug that is classified as a

1. Cerebrospinal stimulant

2. Narcotic analgesic

3. Non-narcotic analgesic

4. Mercurial diuretic

5. Local anesthetic

6. Corticosteroid

7. Vasodilator

8. Anticoagulant

9. Saline cathartic

10. Synthetic estrogen

C. In the following table, list one drug after each classification and give a toxic symptom, if any, associated with each drug listed.

Classification	Drug	Adverse or Toxic Symptoms
1. Nonsystemic Antacid		
2. Digestant		
3. Carminative		
4. Emetic		
5. Antiemetic		

Achievement Review

D. In the space provided before each statement, mark (T) for those which are true, and (F) for those which are false.

_____ 1. Cortisone is a drug which affects the endocrine and musculoskeletal systems.

_____ 2. Analgesics are not considered to be narcotics.

_____ 3. An allergic reaction is a toxic symptom very often associated with the drug Equanil®.

_____ 4. Drugs used in the treatment of cardiac cases are seldom potent.

_____ 5. The use of aminophylline may sometimes cause a fall in blood pressure.

_____ 6. Chemotherapeutics are drugs used in the treatment of bacterial and virus infections.

_____ 7. Astringents are used to stimulate the taste buds.

_____ 8. Histamine is used to cause vomiting.

_____ 9. Uremia is a toxic symptom defined as excessive urination.

_____ 10. Conditioned avitaminosis is due to inadequate vitamin absorption.

_____ 11. Mucomyst reduces consistency of bronchial secretions for easier removal.

_____ 12. When giving urinary antiseptics it is best to provide an alkali medium.

_____ 13. Estrone may sometimes cause uterine bleeding.

_____ 14. Miotics are drugs used to desensitize the eye.

_____ 15. Ethyl chloride is a local anesthetic administered by injection.

_____ 16. Fainting is a toxic symptom to look for following the administration of Novocain®.

_____ 17. Cyanosis is a toxic symptom in which the patient's skin turns blue.

_____ 18. Hypnotics are used to relieve pain.

_____ 19. Ovulen® is classified as an androgen.

_____ 20. Digitalis leaf is given for congestive heart failure.

E. Select the drug in Column II which applies to the appropriate item in Column I. Enter the letter in the blank provided.

Column I	Column II
1. _____ Androgen	a. Theelin
2. _____ Natural estrogen	b. Proluton
3. _____ Synthetic estrogen	c. Oreton
4. _____ Oxytocic	d. Enovid
5. _____ Oral contraceptive agent	e. Paregoric
6. _____ Progesterone	f. Diethylstilbestrol
	g. Pitocin
	h. Codeine sulfate

Section 5 Effects of Medications on Body Systems

F. The items in Column I and Column II pertain to the treatment of eye disorders. Select the appropriate letter and place it in the blank provided.

Column I		Column II
_____ 1. chloramphenicol	a.	miotic
_____ 2. 1% silver nitrate drops	b.	solution for eyewash:
_____ 3. amphotericin B	c.	eye anesthetic
_____ 4. inner coat of eye with nerve endings	d.	optic nerve
	e.	mydriatic
_____ 5. nerve endings which receive the stimulus	f.	prevents gonorrheal eye infections in the newborn
_____ 6. cocaine hydrochloride	g.	receptors
_____ 7. normal saline	h.	bacteriostatic
_____ 8. causes pupil to contract	i.	retina
_____ 9. causes pupil to dilate	j.	fungicide
_____ 10. nerve from eye to brain	k.	synthetic

G. Identify the adverse toxic symptom or symptoms associated with the following drugs by placing the letters of the symptoms which apply, in the spaces provided.

Drugs	
_____ Ibuprofen	_____ Lasix
_____ Pitocin	_____ Diodoquin
_____ Cortisone	_____ Protamine zinc insulin

Adverse/Toxic Symptoms		
a. diarrhea	m.	rise in blood pressure
b. dehydration	n.	hairiness
c. edema	o.	nausea and vomiting
d. tachycardia	p.	excessive secretion of saliva
e. vascular collapse	q.	loss of weight
f. insomnia	r.	itching of skin
g. slow pulse rate	s.	moonlike face
h. hypertension	t.	change in glucose tolerance
i. hypotension	u.	gastrointestinal
j. perspiration	v.	blurred vision
k. nervousness	w.	headaches
l. rupture of uterus	x.	hepatic coma

Appendix

	Page
GLOSSARY	266
LOOK-ALIKE AND SOUND-ALIKE DRUGS	269
POSSIBLE PHARMACOLOGICAL DRUG INTERACTIONS	270
METRIC DOSES AND APOTHECARY EQUIVALENTS	271
TEMPERATURE CONVERSION CHART	272

GLOSSARY

abatement: lessened pain or symptoms of a condition.
abortion: expulsion of fetus before it is viable.
abnormal: contrary to the usual condition.
absorbent: a medication which incorporates secretions or liquids into its substance.
acidosis: depletion of the alkaline reserve in the body.
acne: inflammatory condition of the sebaceous glands.
acromegaly: a pathological condition due to a pituitary tumor resulting in abnormal enlargement of bones of hands, feet and face.
actinomyces: a moldlike type of bacteria parasitic on man and animals.
addiction: compulsion to use drugs constantly.
adrenergic: pertaining to the sympathetic nervous system.
adsorbent: a medication which attracts other materials or particles to its surface.
aedes aegypti: mosquito which transmits yellow fever.
aerobe: a microorganism which can grow in the presence of oxygen.
aerosol: an inhalant medication mixed with air and prepared in spray.
agar agar: a gelatin made of various seaweeds; used as culture media.
agglutination: a clumping together of bacteria.
albolene: an oil made from petroleum.
alcohol: a liquid distilled from various ferments. Ethyl alcohol is an ordinary alcohol; methyl alcohol is a wood spirit alcohol poisonous to drink.
alkalosis: increased alkali reserve in blood and body tissues.
allergen: any substance capable of inducing a hypersensitivity, i.e., pollens, dust, etc.
allergy: an abnormal hypersensitivity to some protein found in certain foods, cosmetics, medications, etc.
alleviate: to make easier.
amnesia: loss of memory.
ampule: a small sealed glass vial usually containing a medication.
analgesic: a pain-relieving medication.
anaphylaxis: exaggerated reaction to increased susceptibility to a drug protein or toxin following its administration.
androgen: male hormone.
anaerobe: an organism which cannot live and grow in the presence of oxygen.
anesthetic: a drug which causes insensibility to pain.
anodyne: a medication which relieves pain.
anthelmintic: medication used to destroy worms.
antiemetic: medication given to overcome nausea and vomiting.
antibody: a protein substance produced by the body as a result of action of an antigen.
antidote: medication which counteracts poisons.
antigen: a substance which induces the body to produce antibodies.
antipyretic: medication used to reduce fever.
antiseptic: a substance used to slow down the growth of bacteria.
antispasmodic: medication used to relieve muscle spasms.
antitoxin: a particular kind of antibody produced in the body as a result of the stimulation of a toxin.
apprehension: fear or anxiety.
aromatic: a substance having a spicy odor, sometimes used in compounding medications. Ex: anise.
Aschheim-Zondek hormone: secreted by the placenta and appearing in the urine.
aseptic: freedom from infection of contamination.

astringent: medication which causes contraction of tissues and stops discharges.
ataractic: a tranquilizing drug.
ataxia: irregularity in muscle coordination.
atonic: lack of normal tone. Ex: muscle tone.
atrophy: wasting of body tissue.
aura: a sensation felt by a person before an epileptic seizure.
bactericidal: a chemical agent which destroys bacteria.
biliary: referring to gall bladder, liver, bile or bile ducts.
bradycardia: slow heart rate.
calculus: a stone formed in any part of the body.
capsule: gelatinous encasing for medications.
carcinomatous: pertaining to cancer.
cardiac: pertaining to the heart.
carminative: medication which helps to relieve gas in the stomach and intestines.
chemotherapy: a chemical agent used to treat disease.
colic: acute abdominal pain.
condiment: food flavoring which enhances the flavor.
contraindication: any symptom which makes the administration of a medication undesirable.
corrosive: chemical which can destroy tissue.
debility: lack of strength and energy.
demulcent: a soothing local medication application.
digestant: medicine which helps the digestive process.
dilute: to weaken by adding more fluid to the mixture.
disinfectant: substance which destroys microorganisms. Also called a germicide.
diuretic: medication used to increase the amount of urine excreted.
dyspnea: labored breathing.
emetic: a substance which produces vomiting.
emollient: a soothing and softening medicine.
emulsifier: a substance used to make an emulsion.
enzyme: an organic substance formed in the body and which alters the speed of chemical process.
estrogen: a preparation of estrin, female sex hormone.
exophthalmic: protruding eyeballs as seen in hyperthyroidism.
expectorant: medicine which aids in expectorating or coughing up of sputum.
flaccid: soft and flabby musculature.
fungicide: any substance which can destroy a fungus.
germicide: a chemical substance which destroys germs.
glycemia: presence of glucose in the blood.
griping: cramp-like pain in the abdomen usually associated with bowel activity.
hematocrit: the percent by volume of red blood cells in whole blood.
hirsutism: abnormal hairiness such as facial hair in women.
hormone: chemical substance secreted by an endocrine gland, carried by the bloodstream and stimulating other organs to activity.
hydrogen ion concentration: forms acids which affect all our life processes.
hypochondriac: person having extreme concern about his health.
icterus or jaundice: a yellowness of skin or eyes caused by excess bile pigment. One reason is rapid destruction of red blood cells.
infarct: damage caused by occlusion of the arterial blood supply. Ex: in a small artery in the heart.
inunction: rubbing of an ointment into the skin.
kilogram: a unit of weight; 2.2 pounds or 1000 grams.
lanolin: wool fat.
lethargy: drowsiness or lack of mental alertness.

Glossary

leukopenia: leukocyte deficiency.
lotion: a liquid used on the skin to soothe and heal the area.
millicurie: unit of radiation; one thousandth of a curie.
miotic: medication used to contract the pupil of the eye.
mydriatic: medication used to dilate the pupil of the eye.
nostrum: medicine with little value.
oxytocic: medication which stimulates contractions of the uterine muscle.
parenteral: medication administered by needle.
pathology: science which studies the results caused by a disease.
peripheral: outer part of the body.
placebo: a nonmedicinal substitute for a medication given to a patient to satisfy him but without therapeutic value.
prophylactic: treatment or medication which will prevent a disease.
pruritus: intense itching.
psychosomatic: refers to the mind and body relationship.
respiratory depressant: medication which slows down the respiratory rate by its action on the respiratory center.
respiratory stimulant: medication which stimulates the respiratory center thus increasing the rate of respiration.
roentgen rays: X-rays; discovered by Dr. Roentgen.
rubefacient: an agent used locally to dilate the blood vessels and thus redden the skin.
saline cathartic: increases the water in the intestines causing bowel evacuation.
soporific: drug which produces deep sleep.
steroid: a chemical compound such as sex hormones, cortical hormones, etc.
syndrome: the symptoms associated with a disease forming a complete clinical picture of that disease.
synthetic: man-made in the laboratory.
toxic: referring to a poison.
urticaria: "hives;" a skin condition showing skin wheals with burning and itching.
vesicant: a local irritant which causes blisters.
volatile: a substance which vaporizes rapidly.

Nurses often have to decipher physicians' handwriting. Look-alike and sound-alike drugs can be responsible for the administration of a drug not intended by the prescriber. Diuril may look like Darcil and Phenaphen may look like Phenergan when written in a hurry. Loridine sounds like Doriden and Tedral sounds like Teldrin. The nurse can reduce the possibility of such misunderstandings by being aware of such look-alike and sound-alike pairs. Listed below are a number of examples.

	Thyrar	**Tryptar**
Brand Name	Thyrar, Armour	Tryptar, Armour
Generic Name	Thyroid	Trypsin
Category	Hypothyroid	Enzyme
Recommended Dose	30 mg daily (initially)	Topically as indicated
Preparations	Tablets, 32 mg, 65 mg 130 mg	250,000 units per 30 ml vial

	Mestinon	**Mesantoin**
Brand Name	Mestinon, Roche	Mesantoin, Sandoz
Generic Name	Pyridostigmine Bromide	Mephentoin
Category	Myasthenia Gravis	Anticonvulsant
Recommended Dose	60 mg initially (must be individualized)	50-100 mg per day initially
Preparations	Syrup, 60 mg/5 ml Tablets, 60 mg Tablets (timed release) 180 mg injection, 5 mg/ml	Tablets, 100 mg

	Ethionamide	**Ethinamate**
Brand Name	Trecator-SC, Ives	Valmid, Lilly
Generic Name	Ethionamide	Ethinamate
Category	Anti-tubercular	Nonbarbiturate sedative
Recommended Dose	500 mg to 1 gram daily	500 mg to 1 gram
Preparations	Tablets, 250 mg	Tablets, 500 mg

It is strongly urged that personnel involved in the administration of medications check with the physician at the slightest doubt regarding drug nomenclature. Also, since dissemination of drug information is a very important function of the pharmacy, nurses should not hesitate to contact pharmacists for data on dosages, adverse reactions, precautions, warnings and other drug-related problems.

Look-Alike and Sound-Alike Drugs
(Courtesy of Benjamin Teplitsky, R.Ph. and the American Journal of Nursing)

POSSIBLE PHARMACOLOGICAL DRUG INTERACTIONS

	aminophylline	ampicillin	atropine	calcium	Coumadin	Demerol	digoxin and other cardiac glycosides	Dilantin	glucagon	Heparin	Inderal	Isuprel	Lasix	Levophed	morphine	nitroglycerin	potassium	Pronestyl	Prostaphlin	quinidine	Tensilon	Valium	Xylocaine
aminophylline					X																		
ampicillin					X																		
atropine					X						X		X	X	X			X		X	X		
calcium						X																	
Coumadin	X	X			X	X	X	X	X		X		X					X	X			X	
Demerol			X	X										X						X	X		
digoxin and other cardiac glycosides			X	X				X		X	X	X	X				X	X		X			
Dilantin				X		X				X	X								X		X		
glucagon					X																		
Heparin					X		X											X					
Inderal					X	X					X	X	X	X	X		X	X					
Isuprel		X			X					X			X										
Lasix			X		X	X		X			X										X		
Levophed		X						X		X	X												
morphine		X	X					X											X	X			
nitroglycerin		X		X			X	X	X														
potassium					X																		
Pronestyl		X			X			X										X	X	X			
Prostaphlin		X			X																		
quinidine		X	X		X	X		X									X		X		X		
Tensilon		X		X							X		X	X									
Valium			X	X			X				X	X											
Xylocaine																	X	X					

"X" indicates an interaction between two drugs given concurrently or within the span of action of either.
(Courtesy of Arthur F. Shinn, David N. Collins and Ellen J. Hoops with permission of American Journal of Nursing)

METRIC DOSES AND APOTHECARY EQUIVALENTS

VOLUME (liquids)			WEIGHT				
METRIC		APPROXIMATE APOTHECARY EQUIVALENTS	METRIC		APPROXIMATE APOTHECARY EQUIVALENTS	METRIC	APPROXIMATE APOTHECARY EQUIVALENTS
4000	ml	1 gallon (4 quarts)	360	Gm	1 pound (12 ounces)	30 mg	1/2 grain
1000	ml	1 quart (32 fluid ounces)	30	Gm	1 ounce (480 grains)	25 mg	3/8 grain
750	ml	1 1/2 pints	15	Gm	4 drams	20 mg	1/3 grain
500	ml	1 pint (16 fluid ounces)	10	Gm	2 1/2 drams	15 mg	1/4 grain
250	ml	8 fluid ounces	7.5	Gm	2 drams	12 mg	1/5 grain
200	ml	7 fluid ounces	6	Gm	90 grains	10 mg	1/6 grain
100	ml	3 1/2 fluid ounces	5	Gm	75 grains	8 mg	1/8 grain
50	ml	1 3/4 fluid ounces	4	Gm	60 grains (1 dram)	6 mg	1/10 grain
30	ml	1 fluid ounce (8 fluid drams)	3	Gm	45 grains	5 mg	1/12 grain
15	ml	4 fluid drams	2	Gm	30 grains (1/2 dram)	4 mg	1/15 grain
10	ml	2 1/2 fluid drams	1.5	Gm	22 grains	3 mg	1/20 grain
8	ml	2 fluid drams	1	Gm	15 grains	2 mg	1/30 grain
5	ml	1 1/4 fluid drams	0.6	Gm	10 grains	1.5 mg	1/40 grain
4	ml	1 fluid dram (60 minims)	0.5	Gm	7 1/2 grains	1.2 mg	1/50 grain
3	ml	45 minims	0.3	Gm	5 grains	1 mg	1/60 grain
2	ml	30 minims	0.25	Gm	4 grains	0.5 mg	1/120 grain
1	ml	15 minims	0.2	Gm	3 grains	0.4 mg	1/150 grain
0.75	ml	12 minims	0.15	Gm	2 1/2 grains	0.3 mg	1/200 grain
0.6	ml	10 minims	0.12	Gm	2 grains	0.25 mg	1/250 grain
0.5	ml	8 minims	0.1	Gm	1 1/2 grains	0.2 mg	1/300 grain
0.3	ml	5 minims	75	mg	1 1/4 grains	0.15 mg	1/400 grain
0.25	ml	4 minims	60	mg	1 grain	0.1 mg	1/600 grain
0.2	ml	3 minims	50	mg	3/4 grain		
0.1	ml	1 1/2 minims	40	mg	2/3 grain		
0.06	ml	1 minim					

271

TEMPERATURE CONVERSION CHART

\multicolumn{10}{c}{Celsius to Fahrenheit}
C°	F°	C°	F°	C°	F°	C°	F°	C°	F°
0	32	13.9	57	27.8	82	41.1	106	55	131
0.6	33	14	57.2	28	82.4	41.7	107	55.6	132
1	33.8	14.4	58	28.3	83	42	107.6	56	132.8
1.1	34	15	59	28.9	84	42.2	108	56.1	133
1.7	35	15.6	60	29	84.2	42.8	109	56.7	134
2.1	35.6	16	60.8	29.4	85	43	109.4	57	134.6
2.2	36	16.1	61	30	86	43.3	110	57.2	135
2.8	37	16.7	62	30.6	87	43.9	111	57.8	136
3	37.4	17	62.2	31	87.8	44	111.2	58	136.4
3.3	38	17.2	63	31.1	88	44.4	112	58.3	137
3.9	39	17.8	64	31.7	89	45	113	58.9	138
4	39.2	18	64.4	32	89.6	45.6	114	59	138.2
4.4	40	18.3	65	32.2	90	46	114.8	59.4	139
5	41	18.9	66	32.8	91	46.1	115	60	140
5.6	42	19	66.2	33	91.4	46.7	116	60.6	141
6	42.8	19.4	67	33.3	92	47	116.6	61	141.8
6.1	43	20	68	33.9	93	47.2	117	61.1	142
6.7	44	20.6	69	34	93.2	47.8	118	61.7	143
7	44.6	21	69.8	34.4	94	48	118.4	62	143.6
7.2	45	21.1	70	35	95	48.3	119	62.2	144
7.8	46	21.7	71	35.6	96	48.9	120	62.8	145
8	46.4	22	71.6	36	96.8	49	120.2	63	145.4
8.3	47	22.2	72	36.1	97	49.4	121	63.3	146
8.9	48	22.8	73	36.7	98	50	122	63.9	147
9	48.2	23	73.4	37	98.6	50.6	123	64	147.2
9.4	49	23.3	74	37.2	99	51	123.8	64.4	148
10	50	23.9	75	37.5	99.6	51.1	124	65	149
10.6	51	24	75.2	37.8	100	51.7	125	65.6	150
11	51.8	24.4	76	38	100.4	52	125.6	66	150.8
11.1	52	25	77	38.3	101	52.2	126	66.1	151
11.7	53	25.6	78	38.9	102	52.8	127	66.7	152
12	53.6	26	78.8	39	102.2	53	127.4	67	152.6
12.2	54	26.1	79	39.4	103	53.3	128	67.2	153
12.8	55	26.7	80	40	104	53.9	129	67.8	154
13	55.4	27	80.6	40.6	105	54	129.2	68	154.4
13.3	56	27.2	81	41	105.8	54.4	130	68.3	155

Temperature Conversion Chart

C°	F°	C°	F°	C°	F°	C°	F°	C°	F°
68.9	156	81.1	178	93.3	200	110	230	193.3	380
69	156.2	81.7	179	93.9	201	112.8	235	198.9	390
69.4	157	82	179.6	94	201.2	115	239	200	392
70	158	82.2	180	94.4	202	115.6	240	204.4	400
70.6	159	82.8	181	95	203	118.3	245	210	410
71	159.8	83	181.4	95.6	204	120	248	215.6	420
71.1	160	83.3	182	96	204.8	121.1	250	220	428
71.7	161	83.9	183	96.1	205	123.9	255	221.1	430
72	161.6	84	183.2	96.7	206	125	257	226.7	440
72.2	162	84.4	184	97	206.6	126.7	260	230	446
72.8	163	85	185	97.2	207	129.4	265	232.2	450
73	163.4	85.6	186	97.8	208	130	266	237.8	460
73.3	164	86	186.8	98	208.4	132.2	270	240	464
73.9	165	86.1	187	98.3	209	135	275	243.3	470
74	165.2	86.7	188	98.9	210	137.8	280	248.9	480
74.4	166	87	188.6	99	210.2	140	284	250	482
75	167	87.2	189	99.4	211	140.6	285	254.4	490
75.6	168	87.8	190	100	212	143.3	290	260	500
76	168.8	88	190.4	100.6	213	145	293	265.6	510
76.1	169	88.3	191	101	213.8	146.1	295	270	518
76.7	170	88.9	192	101.1	214	148.9	300		
77	170.6	89	192.2	107.7	215	150	302		
77.2	171	89.4	193	102	215.6	154.4	310		
77.8	172	90	194	102.2	216	160	320		
78	172.4	90.6	195	102.8	217	165.6	330		
78.3	173	91	195.8	103	217.4	170	338		
78.9	174	91.1	196	103.3	218	171.1	340		
79	174.2	91.7	197	103.9	219	176.7	350		
79.4	175	92	197.6	104	219.2	180	356		
80	176	92.2	198	104.4	220	182.2	360		
80.6	177	92.8	199	105	221	187.8	370		
81	177.8	93	199.4	107.2	225	190	374		

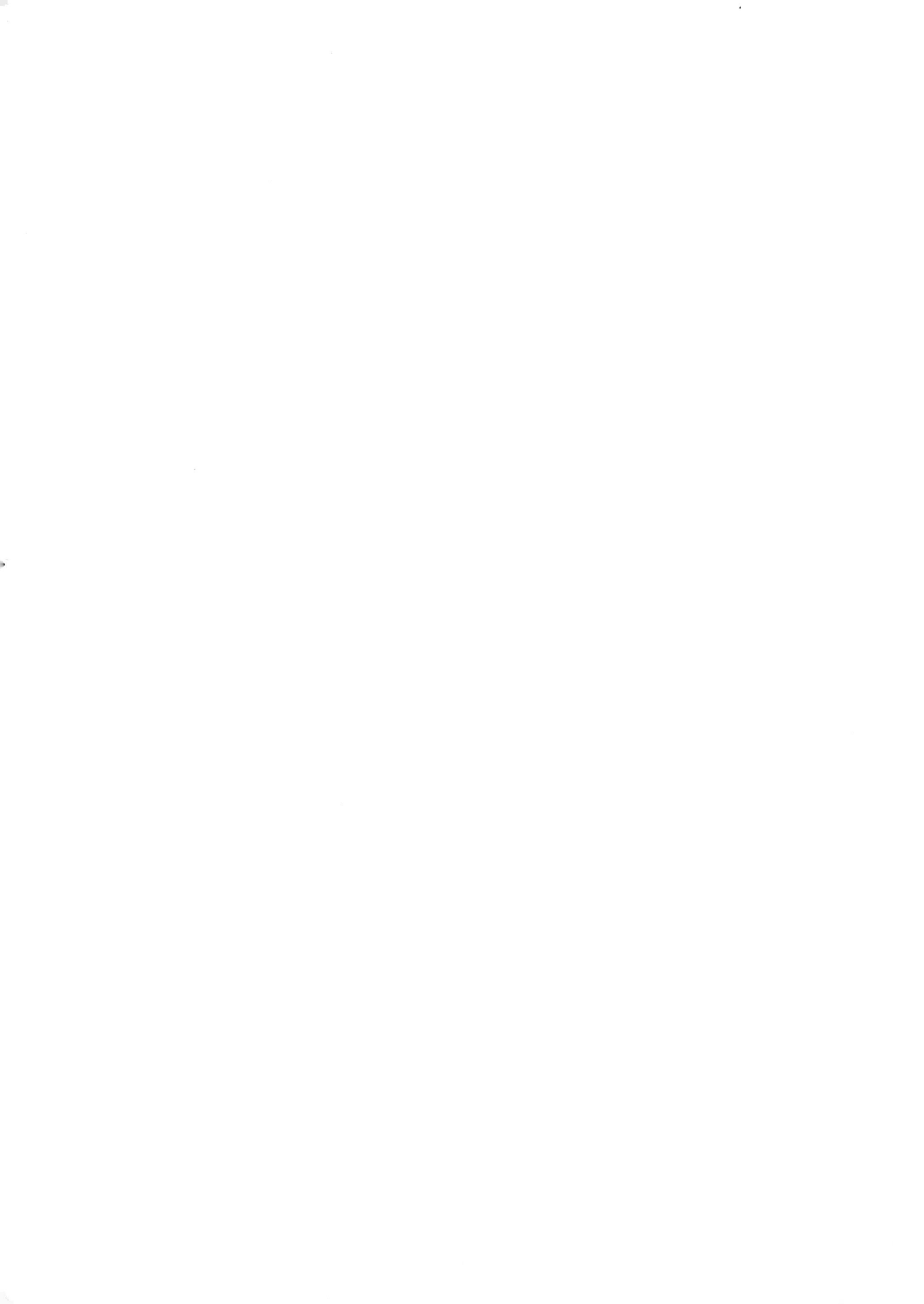

INDEX

A

Achlorhydria, 207
Acid-forming diuretics, 211
Acidifiers, 215
Aciduline. *See* Glutamic acid hydrochloride
ACTH, 231
Addiction, 73
Addison's disease, 222
Adrenal glands, 222
Adrenalin, 54. *See also* Epinephrine
Adrenocorticotropic hormone. *See* ACTH
Aerosols, 71
Agar, 203
Alcohol, 139
Alkalizers, 215
Allergic reaction, 154
Alpha rays, 128
Aluminum hydroxide gel, 199
Aluminum phosphate gel, 199
Alveolar sacs, 191
Amebiasis, 206
Ambicidal drugs, 205-206
Aminophylline, 212
Amphetamines, 235
Amphotericin B., 142, 249
Analeptics. *See* Narcotic antagonists
Analgesics, 228, 235
Anaphylactic shock, 154-55
Androgens, 257-58
Anesthetics, 242-43
Anions, 163-64
Antacids, 199-200
    aluminum hydroxide gel, 199
    aluminum phosphate gel, 199
    calcium carbonate, 200
    magnesium oxide, 200
    magnesium trisilicate, 199
    sodium bicarbonate, 200
Antibiosis, 139
Antibiotics, 139-44, 249
    antifungal, 142-43
    bacitracin, 141
    cephalosporins, 143-44
    chloramphenical, 141
    erythromycin, 142
    kanamycin, 142
    neomycin sulfate, 141
    novobiocin sodium, 142
    penicillin, 140
    streptomycin, 140-41
    tetracyclines, 141
    triacetyloeandomycin, 142
Antichlolesterol drugs, 185
Anticoagulants, 189
Anticonvulsants, 243-44
Antidepressants, 171-73
Antidiarrheics, 205
Antiemetics, 202-203

Antifungal antibiotics
    amphotericin B, 142
    Griseofulvin, 143
    Nystatin, 142-43
Antihelmintics, 205-206
Antihemorrhagic vitamin. *See* Vitamin K
Antihistamines, 154
Antiseptics
    alcohol, 139
    Iodine, 139
    organic formalin complexes, 139
    phenolics, 137
Antispasmodics, 194, 200-201, 205
Antitoxin serums, 168
Apomorphine hydrochloride, 202
Apothecaries' system, 4, 30-31
Arabic numerals, 5
Arrhythmias, 182-84
Ascorbic acid. *See* Vitamin C
Aspirin, 228
Ataractics. *See* Tranquilizers
Autonomic nervous system, 244-45

B

Bacitracin, 141, 249
Bactericidal, 137
Bacteriostatic action, 137
Baking Soda. *See* Sodium bicarbonate
Barbiturates, 240-41
Barium sulfate, 207
Beta rays, 128
Bile, 202
Bile salts, 202
Bioassay, 56
Blood, drugs affecting, 185-89
Blood vessels, drugs affecting, 185
Bromides, 163
Bronchodilators, 194
Buccal tablet, 89

C

Caffeine, 211-12, 235
Calciferol. *See* Vitamin D
Calcium carbonate, 200
Calcium ions, 163
Cancer, 149
Capsule, 72
Carbon anhydrase inhibitors, 212
Cardiotonics, 182
Carminatives, 202
Castor oil, 54
Catalyst, 160
Cathartics, 203-205
Cations, 163
Celsius scale, 22-24
Centigrade scale. *See* Celsius scale
Cephaloridine, 143
Cephalosporins, 143-44
Cephalothin, 143
Cerebrospinal stimulants, 235
Cevitamic acid. *See* Vitamin C

Children, drug preparation and administration, 94
Chloral hydrate, 241
Chloramphenical, 141, 249
Chlorides, 163
Chloromycetin, 55
Chlorotrianisene, 256
Cidex, 139
Circulatory system disorders, medications for, 181-84
Clark's rule, 46
Coagulants, 188
Coal tar, 54
Cobalt, 128
Common fractions, 6-11
    addition of, 8
    complex, 7
    compound, 7
    conversion to decimal, 13
    division of, 10
    equivalent, 7
    improper, 7
    mixed number, 7
    multiplication of, 10
    proper, 7
    relative values of, 11
    simple, 7
    subtraction of, 9-10
Conditioned Avitaminosis, 160
Congestive heart failure, 182
Conjugated estrogens, 256
Contact dermatitis, 154
Controlled Substance Act of 1970, 55-56
Corticoids, 231
Corticosteroids, 231
Cortisone, 54
Cough depressants, 192-93
Cresol, 137
Cretinism, 221
Curare, 231
Curariform drugs, 231
Cyanocobalamin. *See* Vitamin B12

D

Decimal fractions
    addition of, 14
    conversion to common fraction, 13
    defined, 12
    dividing by multiples of ten, 15-16
    division of, 15
    multiplication of, 14
    multiplying by multiples of ten, 15-16
    subtraction of, 14
Deladumone, 258
Delivery, drugs used in, 258
Denominator, 6
Dentifrices, 198
Depressants
    analgesics, 235
    Barbiturates, 240-41

279

Index

Depressants (cont'd)
  hypnotics, 238
  narcotics, 235
  sedatives, 238
Dibenzyline. See Phenoxybenzamine hydrochloride
Dienestrol, 256
Diethylstilbestrol, 256
Diethystilbestrol dipropionate, 256
Digestants
  glutamic acid hydrochloride, 201
  hydrochloric acid, 201
  pancreatin, 201
  pepsin, 201
Digitalis, 54, 182
Disinfectants, 137-39
Disposable syringe units, 98-101
Diuretics
  acid-forming, 211
  aminophylline, 212
  carbon anhydrase inhibitors, 212
  hormone antagonists, 212
  mercurial diuretics, 212
  osmotic, 211
  thiazide compounds, 212
  Xanthine diuretics, 211
Donnagel, 205
Dosages, calculation of
  hypodermic, 38-40
  insulin, 36-37
  methods of
    fixed forms, 35
    prescription bottles, 35
    stock bottles, 36
Dosages, children's, 45-46
Drug Abuse Control Amendments of 1965, 55
Drug administration
  inhalation, 119-24
  by local application, 124-26
Drug dosages, 57
Drug potency, loss of, 74
Drug legislation
  Controlled Substance Act of 1970, 55-56
  Federal Food, Drug, and Cosmetic Act, 55
  Social Security Amendments of 1965, 55
Drugs
  aerosols, 71
  anticholesterol, 185
  blood, affecting, 185-89
  blood vessels, affecting, 185
  capsules, 72
  classified action of, 73
  elixirs, 71
  emulsions, 70
  fluid extracts, 71
  labor and delivery, used during, 258
  liniments, 71

Drugs (cont'd)
  liquid preparations, 70
  lotions, 71
  malignant diseases, used in, 149-52
  mixtures, 70
  mouth, affecting, 198
  ointments, 72
  pills, 72
  preparing and administering to children, 94
  solutions, 70
  sources of, 53-55
  spirits, 71
  sprays, 71
  standardization of, 56-57
  stomach, affecting, 199-200
  suppositories, 72
  suspensions, 70
  syrups, 70
  tablets, 72
  tinctures, 71
  used to counteract infections, 137-45
Durham-Humphrey Amendment of 1951, 55

E

Electrolytes, 163
Elixirs, 71
Emetics
  apomorphine hydrochloride, 202
  ipecac, 202
Emollient cathartics, 204
Emulsions, 70
Endocrine conditions, medications used in treatment of, 218-25
Enteric coated, 72
Epilepsy, 243
Epinephrine, 155, 245
Erythromycin, 142
Estradiol, 255
Estradiol Benzoate, 255
Estradiol dipropionate, 255
Estrogens
  natural, 255
  synthetic, 256
Estrone, 255
Ethinyl estradiol, 255
Ethisterone, 257
Ethyl alcohol, 139
Expectorants, 192-93
Extremes, 20
Extrinsic factor, 162
Eye washes. See Irrigations

F

Fahrenheit scale, 22-24
Fat-soluble vitamins, 160-61
Fecal softeners, 204-205
Federal Food, Drug and Cosmetic Act, 55, 56
Female hormones, 254-57

Female hormones (cont'd)
  estrogens, 255-56
  oral contraceptive agents, 257
  progesterone, 256-57
Fixed forms, 35
Fluid extracts, 71
Fluoxymesterone, 258
Folic acid, 162
Follicle-stimulating hormone, 254
Formaldehyde, 139
Formalin, 139
Fractions. See also Common fractions
  reducing, 7
Fried's Rule, 45
FSH. See Follicle-stimulating hormone
Fungicides, 137

G

Gamma rays, 128
Gantrisin. See Sulfisoxazole
Gargles, 198
Gastric acidity, indicators of, 207
Gastrointestinal system disorders, medications for, 197-208
Germicides, 137
Glucose, 211
Glutamic acid hydrochloride, 201
Gonads, the, 225
Graduated cylinder, 90
Graduated medicine droppers, 90
Gram, 29
Griseofulvin, 143

H

Half-life, 128
Harrison Narcotic Act, 55
Heart action, drug affecting, 181-84
Heart failure, 182
Hematinics, 189
Hexestrol, 256
Homeostasis, 163
Hormone antagonists, 212
Hormones, 218. See also Female hormones
Household measurement system, 4, 32-33
Hydrochloric acid, 201
Hyperthyroidism, 221
Hypervitaminosis, 160
Hypnotics, 238
  chloral hydrate, 241
  paraldehyde, 242
  petrichloral, 241
Hypodermic needles, 101-103
Hypodermic solutions, 38-40
Hypodermic syringes, 98
Hypodermic tablets, 72
Hypotensives. See Vasodilators
Hypothalamus, 244
Hypothyroidism, 221
Hypovitaminosis, 160

I

Idoxuridine, 249
Immune serum, 167

Index

Immune serum globulin, 167-68
Immunity, types of, 167
Immunizations, 167-68
Immunization schedule, 168-69
Inderol. *See* Propranolol
Inhalation, administering drugs by, 119-24
Injections
   intradermal, 115-17
   intramuscular, 109-15
   intravenous, 116-17
   preparing an, 105-107
   subcutaneous method, 107-108
Insufflator, 125
Insulin, 54
Insulin dosages, 36-37
Insulin shock, 222
Insulin shock therapy, 174
Intradermal injections, 115-17
Intramuscular injections, 62, 109-15
Intravenous injection, 116-17
Inunction, 124
Iodine, 54, 139
Ipecac, 202
Irrigations, 249
Irritant cathartics, 204
Isoniazid 10%, 249
Isopropyl alcohol, 139

K
Kanamycin, 142
Kardex, 77
Kefauver-Harris Amendment of 1962, 55, 56
Keflex, 143
Keflin. *See* Cephalothin
Kilograms, 33

L
Labor, drugs used in, 258
Laudanum, 205
Leukemia, 149
LH. *See* Luteinizing
Lincomycin, 143
Liniments, 71, 124
Liter, 29
Local action, 73
Lomotil, 205
Loridine. *See* Cephaloridine
Lotions, 71, 124
Lozenges, 72
Luteinizing hormone, 254
Luteotropic hormone, 256
Lymphoma, 149

M
Magnesium ions, 163
Magnesium oxide, 200
Magnesium trisilicate, 199
Malignant diseases, drugs used in, 149-52
Means, 20
Measurement, systems of
   apothecaries' system, 4

Measurement, systems of (cont'd)
   household measurement system, 4
   metric system, 4
Medication, 62-65
   administration of, 53-130
      basic procedures in, 83-87
      ethics applied to, 67
      by injection, 105-17
      precautions in, 95
      responsibilities in the, 62-67
   charting of, 95
   equipment, aftercare of, 66
   in liquid form, 90-92
   not completely used, 66
   reaction to, 65
   respiratory system, affecting, 191-94
   rules for giving, 83-87
   in solid forms, 92-94
Medication order, 77-81
   abbreviations, 81
   Kardex, 77
   medicine card and, 79-81
   patient's chart, 77
   verbal order, 79
Medicine card, 79-81
Medicine glass, 90
Medicine ticket. *See* Medicine card
Medroxyprogesterone acetate, 257
Mercurial diuretics, 212
Metabolism, 220
Metastasis, 149
Meter, 28
Methylcellulose, 203
Methyl salicylate. *See* Oil of Wintergreen
Methyltestosterone, 258
Metric system, 4, 28-30
Milliliter, 29
Minerals, 163-64
Minim glass, 90
Minuend, 9
Miotics, 246
Mixed number, 7
   addition of, 9
   changing to improper fractions, 8
Mixtures, 70
Motion sickness drugs, 155-57
Mouthwashes, 198
Muscle relaxants, 231
Musculoskeletal system disorders, medications for, 228-32
Mydriatics, 248

N
Narcotic antagonists, 238
Narcotics, 235
Nasal catheter, 120-21
National Formulary, The, 56, 57
Needles, 101-103
Neomycin sulfate, 141
Nephrosis, 210
Nervous system, medications affecting, 234-50

New Drugs (pub.), 57
N.F. *See* National Formulary
Niacin, 162
Nicotinic acid. *See* Niacin
Nondisposable syringes, 98
Norepinephrine, 245
Norethindrone, 257
Norlutin. *See* Norethindrone
Novobiocin Sodium, 142
Numerals
   arabic, 5
   Roman, 5
Numerator, 6
Nystatin, 142-43

O
Oil of wintergreen, 232
Ointments, 72, 124
Opium Alkaloids, 205
Oral contraceptive agents, 257
Oral medications, administration of, 89-95
Order book, 78
Organic iodine compounds, 208
Oxygen
   administration of
      by tent method, 121-24
      nasal catheter, 120-21
Oxytocic drugs, 258

P
Pancreas, the, 222-25
Pancreatin, 201
Papaverine, 205
Paraldehyde, 242
Parathyroid glands, 221
Paregoric, 205
Patient's chart, 77
Penicillin, 140
Pepsin, 201
Percentage, 16-18
Petrichloral, 241
Phenobarbital, 205
Phenolics, 137
Phenoxybenzamine hydrochloride, 245
Phosphates, 163
Physicians' Desk Reference, 57
Pills, 72
Pituitary glands, 218-19
Polycythemia vera, 149
Potassium, 163
Pranone. *See* Ethisterone
Precipitate, 86
Prepackaged form, 35
Prescription, 62, 78-79
Prescription bottles, 35
Procainamide hydrochloride, 184
Pronestyl. *See* Procainamide hydrochloride
Prontosil, 144
Proportion, 20
Propranolol, 184
Provera. *See* Medroxyprogesterone

281

Index

Psychotropic drugs
    antidepressants, 171-73
    tranquilizers, 171
Psyllium seed, 203
Pyridoxin, 162

Q
Quinidine sulfate, 184

R
Radioactive substances, administration of, 128-30
Radium, 128
Ratios, 19-20
Registered pharmacist, 63
Remission, 149
Remote action, 73
Reproductive system, medications affecting, 254-58
Respiratory stimulants, 192
Respiratory system, medications affecting, 191-94
Restrol. *See* Dienestrol
Riboflavin, 162
Roentgenographic studies, 207-208
Roman numerals, 5
Rounding off numbers, 15

S
Salicylates, 228
Saline cathartics, 2-3, 204
Salk, Jonas, 168
Scored tablets, 72
Sedative expectorant, 193
Sedatives, 62, 200-201, 205, 238
Selective action, 73
Selective depressants. *See* Tranquilizers
Sense organs, 246
Shock therapy, 174
Side effects, 73
    of psychotropic drugs, 174
Social Security Amendments of 1965, 55
Sodium, 163
Sodium bicarbonate, 198
Sodium perborate, 198
Solute, 41, 43
Solutions, 70
    adding the solute, 43
    making dilute from stock solutions, 43
    making with pure drugs, 41-42

Solvent, 41
Spansules, 72
Specific action, 73
Spirits, 71
Spironolactone, 212
Sprays, 71
Steroids, 249
Stilboestrol. *See* Diethylstilbestrol
Stilphostrol. *See* Diethylstilbestrol
Stimulants, 234-35
    amphetamines, 235
    cerebrospinal stimulants, 235
    xanthines, 235
Stimulating expectorant, 193
Stock bottles, 36
Streptomycin, 140-41
Subcutaneous injection, 107-108
Sublingual tablet, 89
Subtrahend, 9
Sulfadiazine, 145
Sulfamethoxypyridazine, 144
Sulfathiazole, 55
Sulfisoxazole, 144
Sulfonamides, 144-45
Sulphur, 54
Suppositories, 72, 125-26
Suspensions, 70
Symbiosis, 139
Sympatholytic agents, 245
Sympathomimetic agents, 245
Synthetic antispasmodics, 200-201
Synthetic drugs, 54-55
Synthetic narcotic analgesics, 238
Syringes, 97-101
Syrups, 70

T
Tablets, 72
Tace. *See* Chlorotrianisene
Temperature conversion
    Celsius to fahrenheit, 23
    fahrenheit to Celsius, 22-23
Testosterone, 258
Testosterone propionate, 258
Tetracyclines, 141
Thiamine, 128
Thiazide compounds, 212
Thorium, 128
Thyroid gland, 219-21

Tincture of Belladonna, 205
Tinctures, 71
Toxoids, 168
Tranquilizers, 171
Triacetyloleandomycin, 142
Troches, 72

U
Uniform Narcotics Law, 66
United States Pharmacopoeia, 56
Urea, 211
Urinary antiseptics, 212-15
Urinary diuretics, 211
Urinary system disorders, medications for, 210-15
Urticaria, 154
U.S.P. *See* United States Pharmacopoeia
Uterine sedatives, 258
Uterine stimulants, 258

V
Vaccines, 168
Vaginitis, 125
Vasoconstrictors, 185
Vasodilators, 185
Verbal orders, 79
Vitamin A, 160
Vitamin B. *See* Thiamine
Vitamin B2. *See* Riboflavin
Vitamin B6. *See* Pyridoxin
Vitamin B12, 162
Vitamin C, 163
Vitamin D, 161
Vitamin E, 161
Vitamin K, 161
Vitamins, 159-63
    fat-soluble, 160-61
    uses of, 160
    water-soluble, 161-63

W
Wescodyne, 139
Whole numbers, 12

X
Xanthine diuretics, 211
Xanthines, 235

Y
Young's Rule, 45